MW00614614

The Art of Treatment Planning:
Dental and Medical Approaches
to the Face and Smile

Edited by
Rafi Romano, DMD, MSc

The Art of Treatment Planning: Dental and Medical Approaches to the Face and Smile

QUINTESSENCE PUBLISHING

London, Berlin, Chicago, Tokyo, Barcelona, Beijing, Istanbul, Milan, Moscow, New Delhi, Paris, Prague, São Paulo, Seoul and Warsaw

Dedication

To Michal, Emily, Lee-Ann, Illy, and Adam, my beloved family.

Rafi Romano

British Library Cataloguing in Publication Data
The art of treatment planning : dental and medical approaches to the face and smile
    1. Dentistry--Decision making. 2. Dentistry--Aesthetic aspects.
    I. Romano, Rafi
    617.6-dc22

    ISBN 978-1-85097-197-9

Copyright © 2010 Quintessence Publishing Co, Ltd
Quintessence Publishing Co, Ltd
Quintessence House
Grafton Road, New Malden, Surrey KT3 3AB
United Kingdom
www.quintpub.co.uk

Editor: Lisa C. Bywaters
Layout and Production: Ina Steinbrück
Printing and Binding: hoffmann druck; Nuremberg, Germany

Printed in Germany

Contents

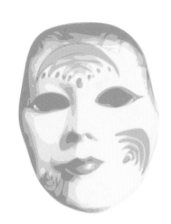

Section I:
Recent Innovations in Treatment Planning and Methodologies

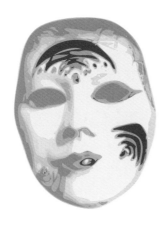

Section II:
Restoring Dental Function and Esthetics

Section III:
Innovative Concepts in
Orthodontic Therapy

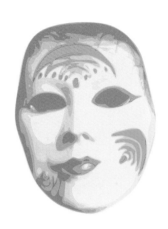

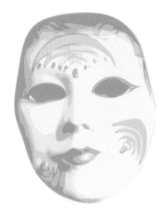

Section IV:
Achieving Facial Balance and Harmony

Section Editor: Michael Scheflan

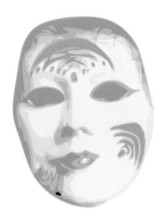

Section V:
Patient Communication and Motivation

Although innovations and new techniques emerge almost weekly, clinicians are often "trapped" in old protocols that they find safe and comfortable. Scant attention is paid to the serpentine path that led the clinician to choose one treatment option over another, and even less is given to the complex nature of beauty perception. My previous book, *The Art of the Smile* (Quintessence, 2004), addressed all aspects of smile analysis as approached by various disciplines. This book documents the rationale behind our treatment sequence while focusing our attention on the most innovative techniques and clinical procedures of our day.

Harmony, symmetry, proportion, soft and hard tissue health, and esthetics—these are among the goals of modern dentistry. Thirty years ago, when I started my dental education at the Hadassah School of Dental Medicine at Hebrew University, amalgam fillings were the most popular type of dental restorations, implants were a novelty, and light-cure technology had just been introduced. Those who believe that today's dental materials and procedures cannot possibly advance much further need only consider the ways in which computer technology and CAD/CAM capabilities have transformed other fields to know that the sky is still the limit.

This book examines the treatment process from multiple points of view in an effort to balance the very complex process of making a diagnosis, on the one hand, with the need for simplicity and coherence, on the other. Patients today demand individualized treatment plans that address not only their dental and/or esthetic problems but their self-image and personal expectations as well. I do not believe in the so-called cookbook approach adopted by many authors who provide "recipes" for any dental problem. "Make it simple!" was the essence of my instructions to the contributors, all of whom are world-renowned leaders in their various disciplines. My goal was to create a companion to *The Art of the Smile*: The two books can be read as a set or individually by the beginner and the advanced clinician alike, each seeking the tools necessary to achieve an optimal result.

We live in a world that continues to change at a galloping pace. As I write, a new American president is being sworn in—the first African American to hold that office. Although he has not reached the age of 50, the new president has succeeded in communicating his passion, enthusiasm, and beliefs in a whole new, nonconfrontational way. This is what we should strive for.

A spirit of teamwork pervades this book, which, like its predecessor, highlights the multidisciplinary nature of dentistry. Experts in

prosthodontics, periodontics, orthodontics, implantology, plastic surgery, patient management, and dental technology convey a similar passion and enthusiasm for their work and have done their best to transfer their feelings to the reader.

Acknowledgments

I was born to a dentist from the previous generation, who practiced in the days when the clinician had to know everything and rarely referred patients to specialists (who hardly existed). My father, Albert Romano, taught me to always see myself through the eyes of my patients, who rely on my advice and recommendations. We should respect our patients to the same degree that we respect our family and offer no treatment option we would not offer to our own relatives. I owe my career, my wisdom, and my personality to my father, and I hope I have fulfilled his expectations.

With their endless devotion, my own team did an outstanding job. I thank all of them, especially my personal assistant, Evelyn Rosenberg.

I would also like to thank Quintessence Publishing and especially the founder and owner, my friend, H. W. Haase, who supported and believed in me long before I became an established international speaker.

I would like to add a word of thanks to all the contributors, with special mention of André Saadoun for his particularly long and comprehensive chapter.

I would further like to thank Michael Scheflan for recruiting and choosing the contributors in the plastic surgery section of the book.

Last but certainly not least, I would like to thank my beloved wife, Michal, who makes it all possible by supporting me all of these years and taking care of our children in the most devoted and loving way possible. My gorgeous kids, Emily, Lee-Ann, Illy, and Adam, are my own reasons to smile. They give me the energy to keep going!

Recent Innovations in Treatment Planning and Methodologies

I

Rafi Romano
Liene Molly
Deborah Armellini
Devorah Schwartz-Arad

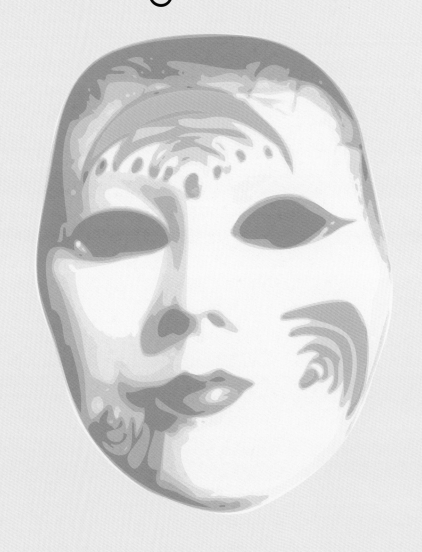

Dental and Paradental Disciplines Essential for Comprehensive Treatment Planning: A Literature Review

1

Rafi Romano, DMD, MSc

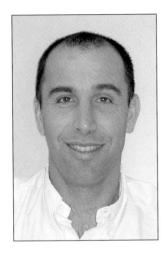

Rafi Romano, DMD, MSc

Rafi Romano is a specialist in orthodontics and dentofacial orthopedics. He maintains a private practice in Tel Aviv, Israel, limited to orthodontics with an emphasis on adult and esthetic orthodontics. He is also a clinical instructor in the Department of Orthodontics, Tel-Hashomer Hospital, IDF, Israel. Dr Romano is past president of the Israeli Orthodontic Society and past secretary-treasurer of the International Federation of Esthetic Dentistry. He is the former editor of the *Journal of the Israeli Orthodontic Society*, and the editor of 2 books: *Lingual Orthodontics*, (Decker, 1998) and *The Art of the Smile* (Quintessence, 2005).

Dr Romano is an active member of the European Academy of Aesthetic Dentistry, the American Association of Orthodontists, and the World Federation of Orthodontists. He lectures all over the world on esthetic orthodontics and adult multidisciplinary orthodontic treatment and delivers courses around the globe.

Email: rafi@drromano.com

Although most of any dental professional's career focuses on matters of esthetics and pain relief rather than general health issues, the current trends of each dental discipline (eg, prosthodontics, periodontics, orthodontics, endodontics, pedodontics, oral health) render clinicians more knowledgeable in their specific fields but almost completely ignorant of current practices in other fields.

Essential procedures for every case have evolved to include an interdisciplinary diagnosis and treatment plan, especially now that patients have more awareness of their general well-being, routine check-ups, and recourse to second and third opinions for every problem. Modern patients are defined by paradental problems such as breathing difficulties, temporomandibular disorders (TMDs), functional aberrations, and harmful habits, combined with psychological factors, that may affect how the underlying problem and proposed solution is perceived. These patients expect clinicians to solve not only the specific complaint with which they present at the dental clinic but also the multifactorial aspects that surround the problem.

Long-term maintenance and stability of a treatment has also become an important issue nowadays. Patients expect results that last a lifetime and an unlimited guarantee from the treating clinician. Although an unstable result usually stems from peripheral factors, not directly from imperfect dental care, patients tend to blame the clinician for not monitoring the problem and preventing it.

Proper dissemination of knowledge in the dental specialties is currently one of the biggest challenges to consistent improvement in care. The Internet is widely used by patients and clinicians, and information is easily accessed. Although conventions and meetings within the dental field aim to collect relevant and reliable information for clinicians who strive for continuing education, the amount of information is huge. Numerous innovations in techniques and dental materials constantly appear on a daily basis.

Fashion also plays an important role in treatment strategies, and beauty standards change occasionally. Tooth whitening, for example, is a relatively new trend that has affected the entire process of color selection for prosthetic restorations.

This chapter attempts to survey the innovations and updated trends in dental and paradental diagnosis. These trends should be taken into consideration when forming a comprehensive multidisciplinary treatment plan.

Face and Smile Analysis

Clinicians tend to rely too heavily on measurements and standards. For years orthodontists were required, in their postgraduate programs and

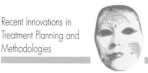

later board exams, to strive for an "ideal" dental and skeletal relationship. Recent studies show that no objective measure of the smile predicts whether that smile will be subjectively judged as attractive or unattractive.[1] Yet, an esthetic smile has become the main focus of many patients. In an effort to find the ultimate keys to a perfect smile, a French group tried to establish an analysis of 17 keys that guide the clinician to position the teeth in the face to build a harmonious, well-balanced, and attractive smile.[2] Unfortunately, this process remains a utopian concept since most patients are unlikely to fulfill every requirement for perfect alignment. Very rarely do the tooth anatomy, lip shape and thickness, mouth size, and ratios of all elements really match. Clinicians today understand the importance of the dynamic diagnosis versus the static one that was very common until a few years ago. Spontaneous smile can be completely different from the posed smile that is frequently used for the dental records. A posed smile displays a lower lipline and less tooth display and smile width. These features can affect the diagnostics of lipline height, smile arc, buccal corridors, and plane of occlusion. Videos are now recommended to record the true dynamic nature of a patient's spontaneous smile.[3]

More attention is given today to the effect of age on the smile. One study aimed to identify a consistent pattern in lip-line height during various functions. This was accomplished through analysis of lip-line heights and the effect of age in an adult male population. Subjects from three age groups (20 to 25 years, 35 to 40 years, and 50 to 55 years) were compared during spontaneous smiling, speech, and tooth display in the natural rest position. The study showed that upper lip length increased significantly (by almost 4 mm) in older subjects, an effect that must be considered by all dental specialists.[4] These results should be of particular interest to the orthodontist, who sometimes intrudes the upper central incisors, which will slowly disappear behind an aging patient's "falling" upper lip; the periodontist, who adds connective tissue graft to recessed gingiva; and the prosthodontist, who designs the length and shape of the teeth in this dynamic environment.

Implementation of all the above considerations into the treatment plan is likely to lead to miscorrelations between smile esthetics and the components of the objective grading system developed by the American Board of Orthodontics (ABO). Additional criteria should be incorporated into the assessment of overall orthodontic treatment outcomes, including variables that evaluate the smile.[5]

Although smile therapy is a relatively new specialty, society already has significant expectations for dental professionals' correct evaluation and treatment of the smile. Orthodontists and other specialists should be able to address this challenge and acquire the skills to identify various smile patterns, which will lead to better rehabilitation of all patients' smiles. Therefore, it is essential to understand that the smile is perceived

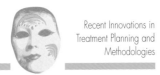

differently by different observers. One study asked groups, composed of orthodontic residents, operative dentistry residents, art students, or laypeople, to evaluate the attractiveness of a smile subjected to computerized variations. It was found that a smile that was medium-broad to broad, included a full incisor display with 2 mm of gingival exposure, and had a consonant smile arc was generally preferred in women. A broad smile with full incisor display and a flat smile arc was generally preferred in men. Variations in incisor angulations were judged as more acceptable than a midline deviation.[6] In other research, it was found that the threshold of orthodontists and prosthodontists to distinguish asymmetries of the maxillary central incisors' gingival margin was 0.5 mm, but laypeople were unable to distinguish asymmetry until the difference was 2.0 mm. Midline shifts were perceptible to orthodontists when equal to or greater than 1.0 mm, and to prosthodontists when equal to or greater than 3.0 mm; laypersons saw no alteration at these measurements. Perceptions of attractiveness in patients must be considered along with their esthetic expectations when planning treatment.[7]

The creation of a smile that is perfectly esthetic for a given individual is a challenge that requires precise treatment planning and cooperation between multiple specialties. Since esthetics is subjective and depends upon the perceptions of the patient and the clinician, it is a challenge to create specific guidelines or a systematic approach that leads to consistent results.[8]

What is the effect of each facial element (ie, lips, chin, and nose) on the attractiveness of the smile? The vertical dimension of the upper lip has been shown to have the greatest impact on smile esthetics. Any orthodontic treatment plan needs to consider the relationship of the maxillary incisors to the vertical thickness of the vermilion border of the upper lip if esthetic results are to be obtained.[9]

Many clinicians mention the "black triangles" in the corner of the mouth as responsible for the unattractiveness of the smile. Which hard and soft tissue factors are related to the amount of buccal corridor area (BCA) during a posed smile? The esthetic elements with the most influence on the amount of BCA are the lower anterior facial height (which defines the vertical pattern of the face), the amount of maxillary incisor exposure, and the sum of the tooth material. Minimal BCA will result in a more esthetic smile. No significant difference was seen in BCA between extraction and nonextraction groups, which traditionally had been named as the main variable that jeopardized the smile in this mode of treatment.[10]

The psychological factor, from observers' and patients' perspectives, probably plays the most important role in perception of smile esthetics. Recent research done in the Netherlands showed that tooth size and visibility and upper lip position were the most prevalent factors in how subjects rated the attractiveness of their own smile (social

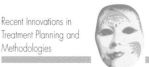

Recent Innovations in
Treatment Planning and
Methodologies

dimension). Color of teeth and gingival display were critical factors in satisfaction with smile appearance (individual dimension). Participants who showed full maxillary teeth and partial gingiva (2 to 4 mm) upon smile perceived their smile lines as most esthetic. Smiles with disproportionate gingival display were judged negatively and were correlated with personality traits of neuroticism and low self-esteem. Visibility and position of teeth correlated with dominant personality traits.[11]

Prosthodontics, orthodontics, periodontics, restorative dentistry, and plastic and reconstructive surgery are all specialties in which factors that influence smile esthetics should be analyzed. Clinicians also need to consider how morphology differs between ethnic groups. Smile norms for one population might be unsuitable for another group in regard to diagnosis and treatment planning.[12]

Paradental Elements that Influence Morphology and Function of the Face and Smile

Breathing

It is already common knowledge that transversal discrepancies of the maxilla and oral breathing have a strong correlation. Recent studies confirm that rapid maxillary expansion (RME) could also be an effective solution to upper respiratory and sleep-disordered breathing problems in growing children.[13] A recent Brazilian study revealed that measurements of upper airway space in patients with normal nasal breathing and Class II and III skeletal patterns are not affected by the type of malocclusion. The article emphasized that diagnosis and treatment planning require evaluation of upper airway space if esthetic and functional results are to be achieved.[14] Many clinicians overlook the integral relationship between breathing, swallowing, and speech with respect to disharmony, malfunction, and malocclusion of the maxillofacial components. Treatment of these aspects can and should be performed through a combination of orthodontics and surgery.[15]

Tongue

The tongue has active functions (during swallowing and speech) in addition to passive functions (in rest position). Tongue habits can create an anterior open bite or may occur alongside skeletal open bites as a factor that maintains or aggravates the condition. At times, tongue habits are a result of parafunctional habits such as thumb sucking. Unfortunately, tongue thrust habits are also responsible for relapses in many completed orthodontic treatments that were otherwise apparently successful.[16] Tongue thrust may contribute to poor occlusal intercuspation during

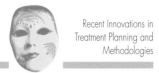

and after orthodontic treatment. On occasion, it appears that tongue thrust habits may actually develop as a result of the shifting spaces and tooth arrangements that occur during orthodontic therapy.[17]

The term *tongue thrust* is used rather than *tongue thrust swallow* because this is a habit generally associated less with the act of swallowing and more with the normal resting posture of the tongue. Because the tongue is held in a rest position the majority of time, it may be more destructive to the occlusion and maxillomandibular relationship compared to the force of the tongue during active behaviors like swallowing and speech.[18]

Temporomandibular disorders

Various factors such as excessive stress or malocclusion can decrease the adaptive capacity of the stomatognathic system and lead to the occurrence of TMD. Joint sounds frequently give the first indication of a TMD, although malocclusion is believed to be a predisposing factor.[19] Although some clinicians have claimed that devices can be used regularly in practice to diagnose and interpret dysfunction or pathologies of the temporomandibular joint, scientific evidence does not support this. Instruments that record jaw movements and interferences have not been proven to differentiate consistently between symptomatic or asymptomatic patients. Therefore, the diagnostic value of jaw-tracking or other electromyography devices and standard guidelines for methodology or interpretation of the data they generate cannot be established.[20]

Oral health–related quality of life (OHRQoL) measurement tools may be the most important diagnostic tool for useful interpretation of the psychological aspects of pain perception and its effects. With the information provided by these instruments, treatment plans can be adjusted accordingly for patients who suffer from various levels of TMD pain.[21]

Facial muscles

Recent technology that provides new solutions for the aging of the face has significantly altered practices for facial rejuvenation in cosmetic surgery. Of the minimally invasive techniques and materials now available for facial rejuvenation procedures, neuromuscular blocking agents (ie, botulinum toxin) and injectable fillers are the most commonly used.[22] Many patients are influenced by plastic surgeons and by their peers to undergo dramatic changes to their appearances through face-lift, nasal reconstruction, and orthognathic procedures. A recent study showed that patients' subjective evaluation of their esthetic outcomes after nasal reconstruction surgeries was significantly higher than the evaluation of an independent professional panel.[23] These findings should be remembered when a complete face and teeth diagnosis is made, and the clinician should always attempt to strive for the ultimate esthetic result.

Recent Innovations in
Treatment Planning and
Methodologies

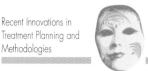

Psychology and patient management

Smiles are often judged by patients or laypeople as attractive or unattractive using subjective methods, and studies have shown that no objective measure of the smile can imitate this process in a way that consistently predicts a certain subjective perception.[1] Neither the Peer Assessment Rating (PAR) score nor patients' perceptions of the severity of their malocclusions have been demonstrated to have as much of an effect as a patient's overall self-concept on the perceived esthetic value of the dentofacial region.[24]   However, the psychological motivation behind patients' desire for treatment may present a serious ethical dilemma for the practitioner who offers esthetic interventions: Are these surgeries superficial interventions aimed primarily at material gain and profit, or are they procedures that truly benefit patients by solving the functional disharmonies behind the esthetic problem and, therefore, play an integral role in the health care system? Esthetic surgery with a goal to promote cosmetic procedures that play to patients' senses of vanity risks losing sight of what patients truly need from treatment and what the surgeon as a healer is able to provide. Therefore, clinicians must be careful that their services are not reduced to procedures with superficial value only, rather than representative of an advanced paradental specialty that serves a functional as well as a cosmetic purpose.[25]

What Is the Future of Esthetic Dentistry?

Current trends in esthetic dentistry encourage perfection, ultimate esthetics, and outstanding smiles—where all peripheral parameters align with the original dental treatment plan—yet these intentions may collide with the growing demand for minimally invasive techniques and individualized treatment plans that respect patients' preferences and expectations. The following chapters provide clinicians with tools to reach a balanced treatment plan that meets both extremes.

The future of esthetic dentistry will most likely bring more convenient and effective technologies that improve communication with patients and colleagues and simulation options that allow the clinician to offer and discuss a variety of alternative treatment plans.

References

1. Schabel BJ, Franchi L, Baccetti T, McNamara JA Jr. Subjective vs objective evaluations of smile esthetics. Am J Orthod Dentofacial Orthop 2009;135(4, suppl):72–79S.

2. Frindel F. The unattractive smile or 17 keys to the smile [in French]. Orthod Fr 2008;79(4):273–281.

3. Van Der Geld P, Oosterveld P, Berge SJ, Kuijpers-Jagtman AM. Tooth display and lip position during spontaneous and posed smiling in adults. Acta Odontol Scand 2008;66(4):207–213.

4. Van der Geld P, Oosterveld P, Kuijpers-Jagtman AM. Age-related changes of the dental aesthetic zone at rest and during spontaneous smiling and speech. Eur J Orthod 2008;30(4):366–373.

5. Schabel BJ, McNamara JA, Baccetti T, Franchi L, Jamieson SA. The relationship between posttreatment smile esthetics and the ABO Objective Grading System. Angle Orthod 2008;78(4):579–584.

6. Gul-e-Erum, Fida M. Changes in smile parameters as perceived by orthodontists, dentists, artists, and laypeople. World J Orthod 2008;9(2):132–140.

7. Pinho S, Ciriaco C, Faber J, Lenza MA. Impact of dental asymmetries on the perception of smile esthetics. Am J Orthod Dentofacial Orthop 2007;132(6):748–753.

8. Donitza A. Creating the perfect smile: Prosthetic considerations and procedures for optimal dentofacial esthetics. J Calif Dent Assoc 2008;36(5):335–340, 342.

9. McNamara L, McNamara JA Jr, Ackerman MB, Baccetti T. Hard- and soft-tissue contributions to the esthetics of the posed smile in growing patients seeking orthodontic treatment. Am J Orthod Dentofacial Orthop 2008;133(4):491–499.

10. Yang IH, Nahm DS, Baek SH. Which hard and soft tissue factors relate with the amount of buccal corridor space during smiling? Angle Orthod 2008;78(1):5–11.

11. Van der Geld P, Oosterveld P, Van Heck G, Kuijpers-Jagtman AM. Smile attractiveness. Self-perception and influence on personality. Angle Orthod 2007;77(5):759–765.

12. Levin L, Meshulam-Derazon S, Hauben DJ, Ad-El D. Self-reported smile satisfaction: Smile parameters and ethnic origin among Israeli male young adults. N Y State Dent J 2007;73(5):48–51.

13. Kiliç N, Oktay H. Effects of rapid maxillary expansion on nasal breathing and some naso-respiratory and breathing problems in growing children: A literature review. Int J Pediatr Otorhinolaryngol 2008;72(11):1595–1601.

14. Alves PV, Zhao L, O'Gara M, Patel PK, Bolognese AM. Three-dimensional cephalometric study of upper airway space in skeletal class II and III healthy patients. J Craniofac Surg 2008;19(6):1497–1507.

15. Loeb I, Boutremans E, Rey SM. Orthodontics, orthognathic surgery and their functional environment [in French]. Rev Med Brux 2008;29(4):273–276.

16. Stojanoviç L. Etiological aspects of anterior open bite [in Serbian]. Med Pregl 2007;60(3–4):151–155.

17. Chawla HS, Suri S, Utreja A. Is tongue thrust that develops during orthodontic treatment an unrecognized potential road block? J Indian Soc Pedod Prev Dent 2006;24(2):80–83.

18. Fraser C. Tongue thrust and its influence in orthodontics. Int J Orthod Milwaukee 2006;17(1):9–18.

19. Garcia AR, Zuim PR, Goiato MC, et al. Effect of occlusion on joint sounds in asymptomatic individuals. Acta Odontol Latinoam 2008;21(2):135–140.

20. Gonzalez YM, Greene CS, Mohl ND. Technological devices in the diagnosis of temporomandibular disorders. Oral Maxillofac Surg Clin North Am 2008;20(2):211–220.

21. Schierz O, John MT, Reissmann DR, Mehrstedt M, Szentpétery A. Comparison of perceived oral health in patients with temporomandibular disorders and dental anxiety using oral health-related quality of life profiles. Qual Life Res 2008;17(6):857–866.

22. Fedok FG. Advances in minimally invasive facial rejuvenation. Curr Opin Otolaryngol Head Neck Surg 2008;16(4):359–368.

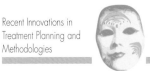

23. Moolenburgh SE, Mureau MA, Hofer SO. Aesthetic outcome after nasal reconstruction: Patient versus panel perception. J Plast Reconstr Aesthet Surg 2008;61(12):1459–1464.
24. Phillips C, Beal KN. Self-concept and the perception of facial appearance in children and adolescents seeking orthodontic treatment. Angle Orthod 2009;79(1):12–16.
25. Atiyeh BS, Rubeiz MT, Hayek SN. Aesthetic/cosmetic surgery and ethical challenges. Aesthetic Plast Surg 2008;32(6):829–839.

Treatment Planning and Transfer of Implants and Their Superstructures to the Clinical Field Through Guided Surgery

2

Liene Molly, DDS, MSc, PhD

Deborah Armellini, DDS, MSc

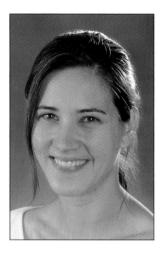

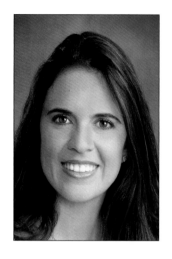

Liene Molly, DDS, MSc, PhD

Liene Molly graduated as a dentist from the Catholic University of Leuven, Belgium, in 2001. She performed a combined program in periodontology and doctoral training at the same university. Her PhD focused on immediate loading of dental implants. Together with her mentor, Prof D. van Steenberghe, she helped develop and improve the NobelGuide procedure, which was first called LITORIM. From 2006 to 2008 she was professor in the Department of Periodontology at the University of Maryland at Baltimore, where she was heavily involved in the undergraduate implant program and research projects in different fields. She is a reviewer for the *Journal of Oral Rehabilitation, Oral Surgery, Oral Medicine, Oral Pathology, Oral Radiology, and Endodontology,* and the *Journal of Periodontology.* She has published multiple peer-reviewed articles and book chapters and has lectured in countries all over the globe. Her main field of research is guided surgery.

Email: lienemolly@yahoo.com

Deborah Armellini, DDS, MSc

Deborah Armellini received her dental degree from the Universidad Central de Venezuela. After completing her training in prosthodontics at the University of Michigan, she embarked on a clinical fellowship in implant prosthodontics at the Hospital for Sick Children and the Bloorview MacMillan Children's Centre in Toronto. As an educator, she has taught at the University of Michigan, University of Toronto, and University of Maryland.

Dr Armellini is a diplomate of the American Board of Prosthodontics and a fellow of the Royal College of Dentists of Canada. Her main interests are dental implants, in particular, guided surgery. In addition, she is dedicated to providing complex oral rehabilitation and esthetic dentistry.

Some of Dr Armellini's research is related to shortened dental arches, success of treatment planning with guided surgery, and impact of implant dental treatments on patient's quality of life. She has published in peer-reviewed journals and lectured in national and international meetings.

Email: darmellini@umaryland.edu

General History of Guided Surgery

Guided surgery's roots trace back to 1908 at University College London, where Victor Horsley and Robert H. Clark developed the first guided surgery apparatus for animal experiments. Horsley and Clark referred to their procedure as *stereotactic surgery.*

From 1947 to 1949, two American neurosurgeons, Dr Ernest A. Spiegel and Dr Henry T. Wycis, and a Swedish neurosurgeon, Dr Lars Leksell, developed the first stereotactic device used for brain surgery in humans. By 1985, computers were being used for planning implants and developing methods to transfer that planning to the oral field. The optical or magnetic navigation system was created in France during the same era. Concurrently, at Catholic University in Leuven, Belgium, the Department of Periodontology and ESAT Radiology worked together on three-dimensional visualization and implant planning software, producing stereolithographic surgical guides to achieve accuracy in dental implant surgery.

The first guided surgery patients were treated using an open-flap technique and surgical guides based on stereolithographic copies of the three-dimensional planning models. After further modification of the technique, flapless surgery using stereolithographic surgical guides became possible.

Development of Guided Surgery in Dentistry

Implant placement has become a standard of care for dental treatment. The need for improved surgical techniques and the increase in prosthetic demands have led to the development of methods to obtain more accurate diagnoses. Several radiographic methods, used in combination with computer technology, have allowed for a new generation of implant placement procedures.[1] In addition, diagnostic software and navigation techniques have been developed. Periapical, bitewing, and panoramic radiographs are the most common radiographs used by clinicians but have limited use in advanced implant treatment planning because they are unable to give detailed information on anatomy, bone quality, and bone quantity. For more advanced treatments, the next step is computed tomography (CT). This medical imaging method uses digital geometry processing to generate a three-dimensional image of the interior of an object from a large series of two-dimensional radiographs taken around a single axis of rotation.[2,3] CT produces a volume of data that can be manipulated to demonstrate various structures based on their ability to block the x-ray beam. The data volume consists of a series of axial images that the computer can reformat to provide images in cross-sectional, panoramic, and three-dimensional views.

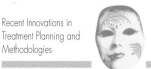

Recent Innovations in
Treatment Planning and
Methodologies

Contrary to other radiographic methods, CT does not require exposure of an image onto a radiographic film. Instead, files are viewed on a monitor using specific software. Because of the increased cost, the larger equipment, and the patient's higher exposure to radiation, this imaging modality is used mostly in more substantial reconstruction procedures.

To advance CT scan technology and provide greater application to the dental field, cone beam CT (CBCT) was developed. This imaging technology provides three-dimensional and cross-sectional views of the jaws and requires only a single rotation of the machine to scan the entire object. Scanning time takes 10 to 40 seconds depending on the quality of the image required. During the rotation, a high number of projections are rapidly captured on a large flat-panel receptor. Later, a reconstruction algorithm renders cross sections to build a three-dimensional image.[4]

CBCT has significant performance advantages over more traditional radiographic techniques (spiral and helical). Because the hardware also has advantages over traditional CT machines in terms of cost, size, weight, complexity, and radiation dose, CBCT has become the examination method of choice when making a risk–benefit assessment. It is possible to obtain more precise slices (0.2- to 0.4-mm thick) compared with traditional CT, where slices range from 0.5- to 1-mm thick. CBCT data can be imported, just as regular CT data can, into a software program to plan dental procedures. This technology is directly applicable to implant dentistry: When placing endosseous dental implants, a thorough preoperative plan, as can be obtained through CBCT data, is beneficial to reach optimal biomechanical and esthetic results.[5]

Several preoperative planning systems for oral implant surgery have been developed using CT as the source of three-dimensional images. Displaying a three-dimensional view in a software environment allows for easier implant planning by alerting the clinician to potential intraoperative complications[2,6] (eg, mandibular nerve damage, sinus perforations, fenestrations, or dehiscences). In addition, the software allows measurements of bone height, width, and density to be made. This permits detailed planning of the final implant position and orientation based on available images, which leads to a successful procedure. It is apparent that CBCT and related computer-driven techniques are the future of dentistry.

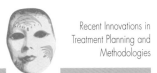

Recent Innovations in
Treatment Planning and
Methodologies

Treatment Planning for Fully and Partially Edentulous Patients

Model-based treatment planning

In model-guided surgery, information can be transferred from a clinical examination and/or assessment to the surgical field. Model-based treatment planning is a simple technique whereby the clinician predicts the position of the dental implant, as well as the selection of the prosthetic component, using clinical and radiographic measurements. The main advantage is that no further diagnostic aids are necessary to obtain a predictable plan.

This procedure requires an accurate model with large extensions in the buccal vestibule. A 0.20-mm sheet of a thermoplastic material is adapted to the model; this adapted form is then used to record the measurements from the bone-sounding procedure in the area of interest. At this point, the practitioner should know the amount of bone available. This information must be accurately transferred to the model onto which the surgical guide will be fabricated. A radiographic image is critical to plan the implant positioning in the model. The dummy implant should be placed in the desired position in the model, which relates to the position of the dental implant in the in vivo bone model. Creating this three-dimensional model allows the practitioner not only to plan the exact position of the implant but also to preplan the future prosthesis.

Indications

In general, model-guided surgery is appropriate in simple cases. Selected cases where no major grafting is necessary are ideal, as are the following:

- Cases where the anatomic characteristics or limitations are easily identified
- Cases with thin soft tissue where its management could complicate the esthetic outcome
- Cases where immediate implant placement into the extraction socket is indicated

Anatomic considerations

The main anatomic characteristics to consider when treatment planning dental implants are the maxillary sinuses for the maxilla and the inferior alveolar and mental nerves in the mandible. It is possible to determine the height, width, and length of bone present in the area of interest by outlining the underlying bone in a model. From this model, an ideal implant placement precluded by an ideal tooth positioning is possible. Consideration of various bone augmentation techniques,

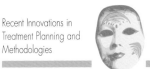

forces generated toward the implant restorations, and esthetic results are key factors in treatment planning.

Patient 1: Maxillary left second premolar

Patient 1 wished to have an immediate fixed solution to replace the maxillary left second premolar. Clinical examination revealed a slight buccal defect that had the potential to compromise the esthetic outcome of the restoration (Fig 2-1a). A polyvinyl siloxane impression was taken to capture the features of the buccal vestibule, and a type IV dental stone cast was fabricated. To make the necessary clinical measurements, a 0.20-mm thermoplastic sheet was used (Fig 2-1b). The bone-sounding measurements were transferred to the master cast to identify the quantity of bone available and to orient the implant in the best possible position. Periapical radiographs were then used as a reference to outline the roots of the adjacent teeth (Fig 2-1c). A regular platform (RP, 4.3-mm diameter) 13-mm-long implant was planned to achieve an esthetically oriented restoration for the tooth (Fig 2-1d). A surgical guide was then fabricated to transfer the treatment plan to the clinical field (Fig 2-1e). This planning allowed predictable placement of the immediate restoration without compromising the esthetics or biomechanics.

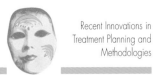

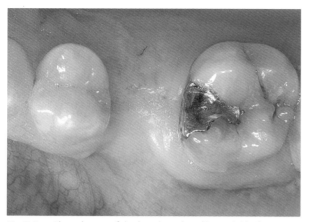

Fig 2-1a Clinical view of the length and width available for an implant restoration for Patient 1. A slight bone defect is present toward the buccal side of the ridge. With proper planning, this patient will not need bone grafting.

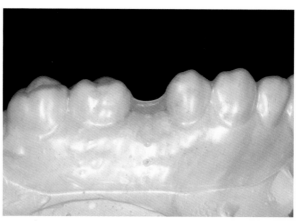

Fig 2-1b A 0.20-mm thermoplastic sheet is used to delineate and guide the bone-sounding procedure. Another set of marks should follow in the mesial and distal aspects of the center line.

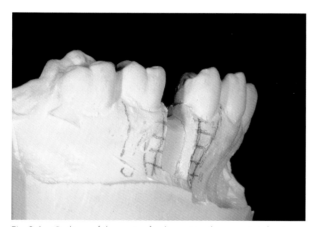

Fig 2-1c Outlines of the roots of adjacent teeth are painted onto the model.

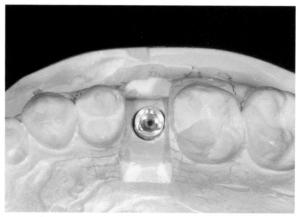

Fig 2-1d RP dummy implant (4.3-mm diameter, Replace Select [Nobel Biocare]) strategically placed in the stone cast to replace the maxillary left second premolar.

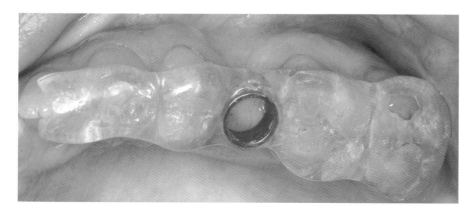

Fig 2-1e The surgical guide fabricated on the model must fit precisely in the oral field. An inspection window is used to verify the seating of the guide and can be viewed on the buccal aspect of the second molar.

Recent Innovations in
Treatment Planning and
Methodologies

Liene Molly, Deborah Armellini

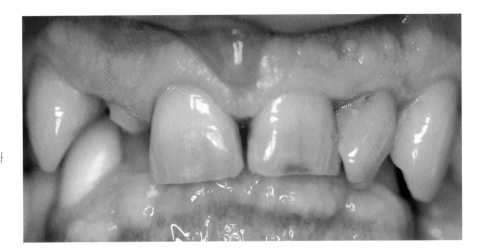

Fig 2-2a This anterior clinical photograph illustrates the status of the maxillary right lateral incisor. This tooth will be extracted, and an implant will be immediately placed using model-guided surgery.

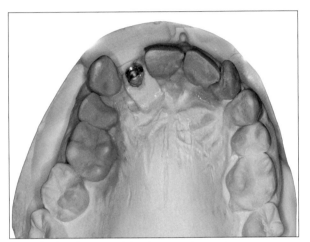

Fig 2-2b The placement of the dummy implant in the stone cast.

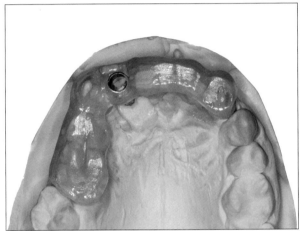

Fig 2-2c The fabrication of a model-based surgical guide to properly guide the implant placement to a position that is biomechanically advantageous and esthetically driven.

Patient 2: Maxillary right lateral incisor

Patient 2 presented to the clinic with a chief complaint of wanting the maxillary right lateral incisor replaced as quickly as possible. The treatment plan was to extract the tooth and immediately place a dental implant (Fig 2-2a). It is very difficult to successfully plan the position of the implant in the tooth socket as this may not be the most biomechanically or esthetically advantageous position. Therefore, in most cases, the implant is not to be placed in the same position as the root of the tooth. However, without proper guidance, it is very likely that the clinician will prepare the osteotomy following the root form. Model-guided surgery was selected to properly guide the placement of the implant. Clinical measurements (bone sounding) and periapical radiographs were taken, and the surgical guide was fabricated (Figs 2-2b and 2-2c).

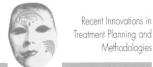

Computer-based treatment planning

Computer-guided surgery allows an image retrieved from the clinical presentation to be connected to the surgical field. The image is usually retrieved through a CT scan or two-dimensional radiographs (eg, intraoral radiographs or tomographs). These images can then be imported into a software program that allows for planning of oral implants. This computer-based treatment planning can incorporate prosthetic as well as anatomical, biomechanical, and mechanical needs, as long as the setup allows for a visualization of the superstructure that projects the correct occlusion and articulation. The necessary transfer to the surgical field can take place using optical or magnetic navigation, or may be achieved with scanning appliances.

Optical or magnetic navigation allows the practitioner to couple radiographs or models through a charge-coupled device (CCD) to video cameras and light-emitting diodes (LEDs) or magnetic charged devices attached to the area of interest. In one study, the accuracy of optical navigation was investigated by using two CCD video cameras to follow the three-dimensional coordinates of LED assemblies attached to the head, the mandible, and a handpiece for oral and maxillofacial surgery. Optical navigation systems were concluded to be a great asset in dental implant placement, orthognathic surgery, endoscopic surgery, and removal of foreign bodies.[7] The use of optical navigation implies the need for high-speed computers that can perform rapid recalculation of the three-dimensional environment. This recalculation is necessary to provide accurate images intraoperatively for situations when the patient moves, especially under local anesthesia. A combination of this optical navigation and surgical guides for implant surgeries would allow a flawless preoperative planning session, as well as intraoperative confirmation of planning accuracy. This protocol would become the ideal for every surgery and could also serve to verify the accuracy of scanning appliances without subjecting the patient to extraneous x-ray doses.

Computer-guided templates can be created using several techniques. Most of those available today are based on CT or CBCT images that are implemented into software. Several companies supply this kind of software (eg, implant3D [med3D], Osseoview [3D Diagnostix], coDiagnostiX/gonyX [IVS Solutions], VIP [BioHorizons], Implant Master [iDent], CADImplant [CADImplant], AccuDental [Medical Modeling], SimPlant [Materialise], NobelGuide [Nobel Biocare], and many others). This software sometimes allows for the visualization of the ideal superstructure. An esthetic treatment plan can thus be reached.

When static (scanning appliances) and dynamic (optical or magnetic navigation) computer-based methods of implant planning and surgery were compared, the static method appeared to be the recommended choice due to uncomplicated handling and low resource demands.[8]

Recent Innovations in
Treatment Planning and
Methodologies

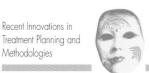

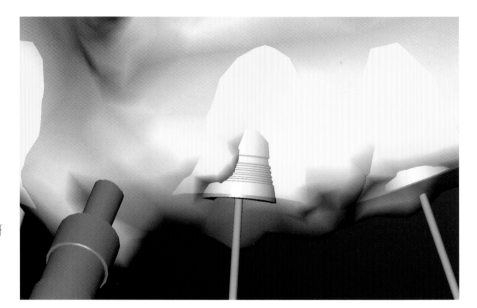

Fig 2-3 Dehiscences can easily be detected in three-dimensional computer software programs. An implant plan should be adjusted if dehiscences are detected, or a bone augmentation procedure should be planned before or during implant placement.

A reproduction of the ideal occlusion and, if immediate loading is applied, the articulation is extremely important for all software to include. Several techniques are currently used to achieve visualization of the ideal superstructure. In most cases, the ideal occlusion and articulation is mimicked via a guide, or *scanning appliance.* The scanning appliance must be visualized in correct relation to the bone, which is done by using differences in densities to help distinguish the appliance from other structures (eg, by coating the inside of the appliance with barium sulfate and imaging with software such as SimPlant), or by using a double CT-scan protocol where two images are superimposed by overlaying opaque structures (eg, gutta-percha markers using NobelGuide software). Most programs using three-dimensional images require conversion of DICOM (Digital Imaging and Communications in Medicine) files obtained from CT or CBCT scans.4

Since the various software solutions include similar features, the following procedures will be described using the NobelGuide program.

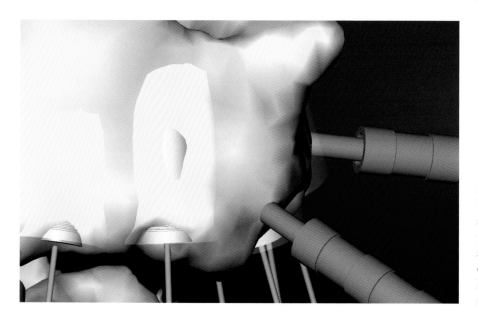

Fig 2-4 Fenestrations can easily be detected in three-dimensional software programs. A treatment plan should be adjusted if fenestrations are detected, or a bone augmentation procedure should be planned before or at implant placement.

Anatomic considerations

In the maxilla, the architecture of the alveolar arch and the outline of the maxillary sinus are the most important anatomic characteristics. In the area where an implant is to be placed, the height and width of bone, as well as the orientation of the arch versus the ideal tooth setup, will determine whether bone augmentation is indicated for ideal implant placement. The next steps are to *(1)* detect dehiscences (Fig 2-3) and/or fenestrations (Fig 2-4), *(2)* decide the most suitable augmentation techniques, and *(3)* provide possible treatment alternatives.

Patient 3: Full-mouth rehabilitation

The goal of Patient 3 was to have a fixed restoration in the mandible and the maxilla. In the mandible, the alveolar ridge presented clinically as a very thin ridge between both canines. The patient was told that a ridge augmentation would probably be necessary. Nevertheless, computer-guided surgery was planned to enable the most precise implant placement. After preparation of a scanning appliance, a double CT-scan protocol was followed (NobelGuide). The two images were converted, and computer-based treatment planning was deemed possible. The visuals also showed that, although the ridge was thin, it would be possible to plan three esthetically oriented RP (4.3-mm diameter) 13-mm implants (Fig 2-5). After reviewing the images, it became clear that with proper planning, the patient would not require bone grafting. In the posterior area, one more implant was planned on each side. Only one implant (5-mm diameter and 10-mm length) was chosen since the

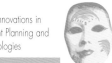

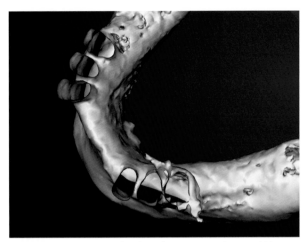

Fig 2-5a A very narrow alveolar ridge is seen in the mandible between the two canines, and an undercut is present in the buccal aspect. This condition often requires a bone graft.

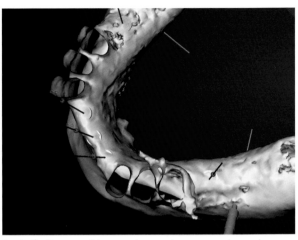

Fig 2-5b Planning of three implants in the narrow ridge in the anterior mandible. A bone-grafting procedure can often be avoided when computer-based treatment planning is administered.

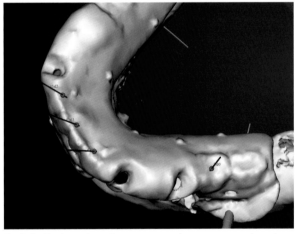

Fig 2-5c Verifying the esthetic outcome after accurate implant planning to allow for a screw-retained prosthesis.

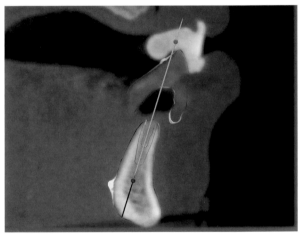

Fig 2-5d Cross-sectional view of one of the 4.3-mm-diameter implants in the anterior portion of the mandible, planned in the lateral incisor position.

opposing arch would also consist of 12 elements (Fig 2-6). In the maxillary arch, the clinical appearance of the alveolar ridge seemed satisfactory. The CT scan, however, shows limited bone in the posterior maxilla (Fig 2-7). Again, the clinical image differed from the radiologic image, which implied preoperative planning would most likely influence the method of treatment (discussed later).

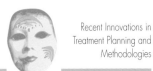

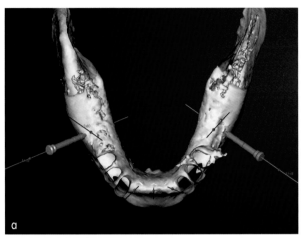
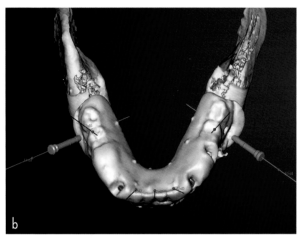

Figs 2-6a and 2-6b Complete planning of the mandible for Patient 3. (a) One implant is planned on each side in the posterior area, since the opposing jaw will include 12 elements. (b) The esthetic outcome of both anterior and posterior restorations can be verified. For all restorations, screw-retained superstructures are planned.

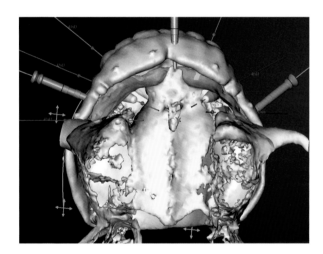

Fig 2-7 Direct view of the maxillary sinus in three dimensions shows the small amount of bone available in the posterior area of the maxilla in Patient 3. The available bone has a very low density, predicting low primary stability for implants.

Patient 4: Maxillary right first premolar

In Patient 4, the simulated positioning of the implant for the maxillary right first premolar revealed a fenestration in the buccal aspect (Fig 2-8). The angulation of the implant could be corrected according to the bony characteristics if angulated or customized abutments are chosen (Fig 2-9). If the angulation of the implant–abutment components is greater than 35 degrees in the planning, a bone graft should be considered.[9–12]

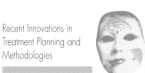

Liene Molly, Deborah Armellini

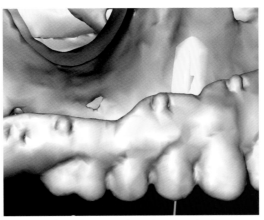

Fig 2-8 Implant planning in three-dimensional software in the location of the maxillary right first premolar shows a fenestration in the buccal aspect if planning is performed for a screw-retained restoration with straight abutments.

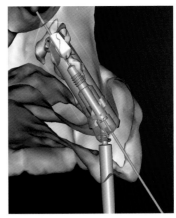

Fig 2-9 A similar view as described in Fig 2-8, but now the location of the implant has been adjusted and the planning has been modified for angulated abutments in the final restoration.

Whether the bone graft can be completed during or before implant placement depends on the extent of graft necessary. If the dehiscence is minor (eg, if only two implant threads are exposed in the treatment plan), guided bone regeneration with a resorbable membrane and bone-grafting material can be planned eventually.[13]

The infra-alveolar nerve in the mandible may be located in the upper one-third of the remaining alveolar arch, therefore possibly compromising the placement of long-enough implants in the posterior mandible. In partially edentulous patients, short implants with a surface that promotes osseointegration have proven to be successful.[14,15] Outcomes should be compared with those of implants placed in grafted bone. Additional investigation is still needed at this time to determine whether immediate loading is possible in partially edentulous cases where short implants are placed in the posterior areas.

In some areas, neighboring available bone can be used for placement of longer, angulated implants. In the maxilla, the choice of sinus elevation or angulated implants (ie, using the anterior jaw bone or the zygoma) sometimes needs to be considered. In the mandible, some bone augmentation procedures that would otherwise be necessary can be eliminated by using the retromolar area or by placing fewer implants in the interforaminal area, with the implant head angled to the posterior. Treatment planning these solutions, however, requires reliable software to enable precise transfers to the surgical area.

The architecture and available density of the bone determine the loading protocol. The current width of cortical bone, as well as the density of trabeculation in the bone marrow, should indicate overall bone density.

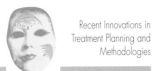

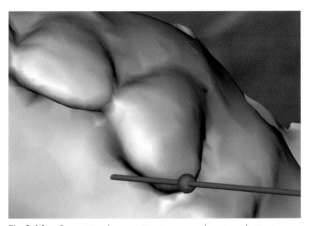

Fig 2-10a Correct implant positioning according to esthetic standards in the anterior maxilla. The angulation of the implant ensures that the screw opening for a screw-retained abutment is accessible in the cingulum of the incisors.

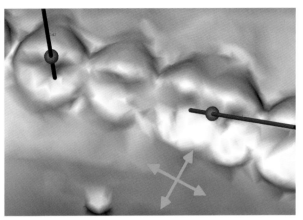

Fig 2-10b Correct implant positioning according to esthetic standards in the posterior maxilla. The angulation of the implants ensures that the screw openings for screw-retained abutments are accessible in the occlusal plane of premolars and molars.

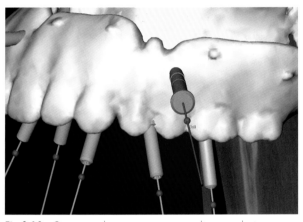

Fig 2-10c Correct implant positioning according to esthetic standards does not allow for implant access between two crowns, but within one element.

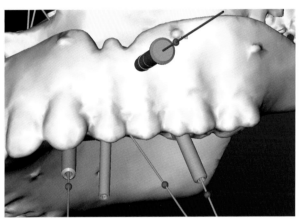

Fig 2-10d A 30-degree multiunit angulated abutment can be planned to adjust the angulation of the implant in relation to the crowns. This allows an esthetic outcome for the superstructure in the area of the premolars.

Esthetics

When planning implants, anatomic positioning is not the only important issue. In a society focused on esthetics, implant appearance cannot be overlooked. If screw-retained restorations are chosen, the screw opening should be positioned keeping ideal esthetics in mind. In anterior areas, the ideal position will be the cingulum of the restoration (Fig 2-10a); in posterior areas, the screw opening should be accessible in the occlusal plane of the restoration (Fig 2-10b). An abutment or implant should not be planned between two crowns (Fig 2-10c). The positioning of such an implant may thus require an angulated abutment (Fig 2-10d). If the implant or abutment angulation exceeds 35 degrees, cemented restorations could be chosen.

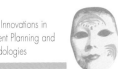

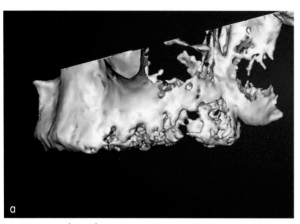

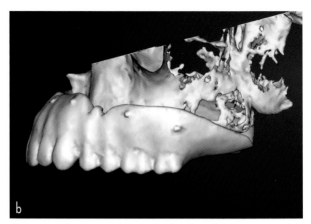

Figs 2-11a and 2-11b In Patient 3, a huge discrepancy exists between the bony architecture and the occlusal outline of the restoration. *(a)* The bony architecture of the maxilla can be detected. *(b)* The occlusal outline of the restoration on top of the bony architecture allows detection of any discrepancies.

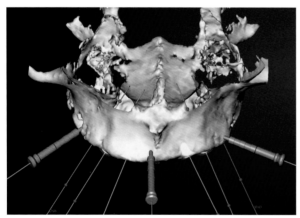

Fig 2-11c The apices of the implants are oriented opposite each other in the plan for Patient 3. The angulations are verified with the green lines.

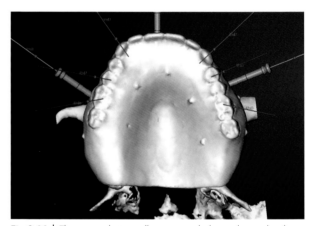

Fig 2-11d These angulations allow access holes in the occlusal plane of the restoration.

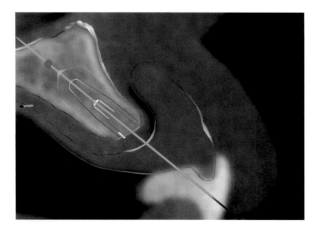

Fig 2-11e In the maxillary left canine region of Patient 3, the implant is submerged on the buccal aspect. In such planning, adjustment of hard tissues right after implant placement should be anticipated.

Recent Innovations in
Treatment Planning and
Methodologies

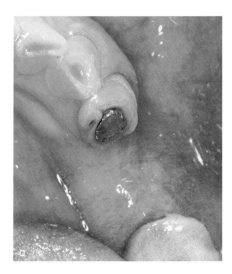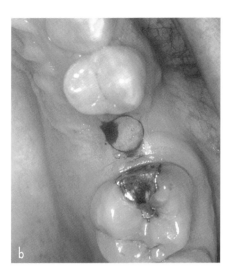

Fig 2-12a Preoperative soft tissue examination confirms that because of the amount of keratinized tissue available in this patient, flapless surgery will not be a problem.

Fig 2-12b A tissue punch through the surgical guide allows an exact outline of the implant/abutment position.

In Figs 2-11a and 2-11b, resorption of the alveolar arch has resulted in a huge discrepancy between the positioning of the bony arch and the tooth setup. Because of this discrepancy, it is necessary to plan implants angulated toward the occlusal plane. If fixed restorations are the goal, the apices of the implants will be tilted toward each other (Fig 2-11c). The planning process should be conducted with great care to use available bone effectively while preventing each implant surface from interfering with the osseointegration capacity (3 mm between the outer surfaces of two implant surfaces). The angulations among implants complicate the insertion of a fixed prosthesis. Avoidance of soft and hard tissue interference during the insertion path of the abutments or fixed superstructures is crucial; the potential for this type of interference should be inspected during planning (Figs 2-11d and 2-11e). Bone speculae around the shoulder of the implant should be removed during implant placement; however, a round bur or a bone mill could be useful. Thick soft tissue can be thinned or a gingivectomy or gingivoplasty in the angle of insertion could relieve the pressure on the tissue when the superstructure is inserted.

The clinician should also examine soft tissues preoperatively to determine whether they need to be augmented or manipulated. This will assist in evaluating the feasibility of flapless surgery (Fig 2-12). A minor flap treatment could prevent postoperative mucogingival problems around the abutment.

The abutment can be chosen based on the computer planning, in combination with a three-dimensional model created after planning through computer-aided design/computer-assisted manufacture (CAD/CAM) technology. The direct method requires a three-dimensional model created immediately from the three-dimensional images; the indirect method calls for a three-dimensional model made by

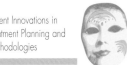

pouring a plaster cast from a CAD/CAM impression (eg, a CAD/CAM surgical guide). For single-tooth restorations, these computer-based treatment planning systems eventually will be able to design customized abutments during the planning phase. For multiple-tooth restorations, the base superstructure (eg, Procera zirconium or Procera titanium [Nobel Biocare] or CEREC [Sirona Dental Systems]) can also be customized in a software program. Whether this customization should be done preoperatively or when postoperative impressions are taken should be determined based on the accuracy of the transfer from the planning to the surgical field.

Biomechanics

Few programs check biomechanical aspects of a planning procedure.[16] More programs could implement this feature in the software to their benefit to understand whether all forces are distributed evenly over the planned implants.

The number of implants necessary to restore a full arch can be reduced to four in the mandible and even in the maxilla when insufficient bone structure is available to harbor more implants or if the patient cannot afford more implants.[17] For safety reasons, however, it is advisable to plan for a higher number of implants, especially in cases more prone to failure[18] (eg, patients who smoke, patients suffering from diabetes or other systemic diseases, or patients with functional habits such as bruxism).

Practical aspects

During the planning phase, the mechanical aspects of surgical guides and superstructures should be considered. Most surgical guides incorporate sleeves to guide the burs during the surgery. The insertion path of these access holes must not interfere with existing structures such as natural teeth (Fig 2-13). The sleeves must not collide and must also be stable enough in the guide to avoid fracture during surgery. A similar rationale accounts for the thickness of the surgical guide. If a surgical guide will be used, the mouth opening must be checked before surgery to prevent access problems. This especially applies to patients with a small mouth opening who need restorations in the posterior of the mandible.

The surgical guide also must be stable during surgery. In totally edentulous patients, the surgical guide can be connected to the bone with pins or may be attached to preexisting implants that allow connection of the surgical guide to the surgical area. In partially edentulous patients, a similar fixation method can be used, and secondary control through inspection windows in the guide within the dentate area could reveal a proper fit (Fig 2-14). It is important that the fixation methods planned in the software are transferred to the clinical field. The insertion path of those fixation methods must be clear; the mouth opening or soft

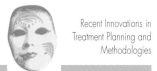

Recent Innovations in
Treatment Planning and
Methodologies

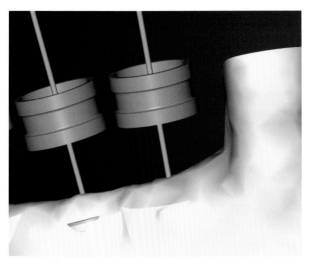

Fig 2-13 The access hole in the surgical guide allowing placement of the implant in the left lateral incisor in the mandible of Patient 3 must not interfere with the neighboring canine.

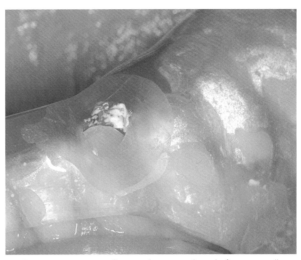

Fig 2-14 Inspection windows in the surgical guide for a partially edentulous patient reveal the fit of the guide. There must be no gap between the guide and the natural tooth.

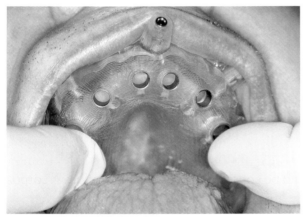

Fig 2-15 Soft tissue interference (eg, the lip or cheek tissue) can hinder the insertion path while seating the surgical guide. In this patient, the pins to anchor the surgical guide to the bone were oriented opposite the nose, and it was necessary to check whether the lip could be lifted enough to allow insertion of the anchor pins.

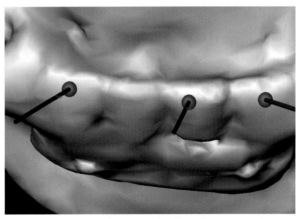

Fig 2-16 Abutment angulations can be planned preoperatively in a software environment. If the implant-cingulum or implant–occlusal plane angulation exceeds the possible abutment angulation, as shown here, a cement-retained restoration is necessary; in other situations, screw-retained restorations are possible (see Fig 2-10d).

tissue interference (cheek, lips, tongue, etc) can hinder the insertion paths and must thus be taken into account (Fig 2-15).

Planning abutment angulations in a software program can predict whether a screw-retained restoration will give an esthetic outcome or whether a cement-retained restoration is necessary (Fig 2-16). Computer-based treatment planning can also minimize free-ending pontics and predict with great precision the number and angulation of implants necessary to efficiently support the superstructure.

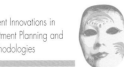

Case selection for guided surgery

Model-based versus computer-based treatment planning

The main difference between model-based and computer-based treatment planning is the use of radiographic information. The criteria used to select the best method of treatment planning are based on the clinical situation. During the initial consultation, a clinical impression of the site to be restored will be taken. That clinical impression should allow the clinician to do the following:

- Inspect the clinical width, length, and height of the alveolar arch
- Count the number of elements missing
- Estimate the thickness of the soft tissues (in dentate patients, the tissue type around existing teeth can predict the thickness in other areas)

The following anatomic features should also be checked:

- Angulation of the neighboring teeth
- Interocclusal width
- Position of the alveolar arch in relation to the neighboring teeth, to eliminate large discrepancies in the vertical (Fig 2-17a) and horizontal aspects (Fig 2-17b)
- Esthetic needs in a particular area

During the first consultation, a panoramic radiograph will be taken. An apical radiograph of the edentulous zone will most likely be available to provide deeper insight into the anatomic situation. If this combination of information—clinical and radiographic—clarifies there is enough bone available to predictably place an implant with sufficient primary stability, then model-guided surgery can be planned. If questions remain concerning anatomic outlines, then more information should be obtained through CT and CBCT. The patient will thus be exposed to a higher radiation dose only when necessary. If those radiographs are processed, they should be used to their full extent, and computer-based treatment planning should be performed.

Immediate placement versus delayed placement

The placement of an implant immediately after tooth extraction is called *immediate placement.* This can be compared to the standard protocol, which prescribes a period to allow for initial healing (6 to 8 weeks post-extraction) before an implant should be placed in an extraction socket. The major benefit of immediate placement is the shorter time frame in which the patient can be treated; some authors also claim immediate placement prevents collapse of the socket walls. However, disadvantages to immediate placement could include nonintegration of the implant due

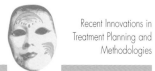

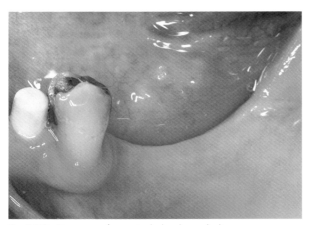

Fig 2-17a Detection of a vertical alveolar arch discrepancy means that bone onlay grafting will be required.

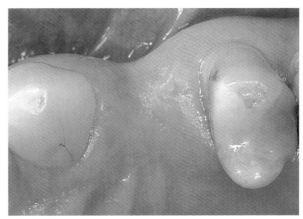

Fig 2-17b Detection of a horizontal alveolar arch discrepancy means that bone grafting will be required before or at implant placement.

to remaining residual infection of the tooth that was extracted or bone resorption after implant placement, both of which create less favorable esthetic outcomes.[19] Because no clear research perspectives have been established, no implants should be placed immediately after extraction of teeth with extensive periapical or periodontal lesions. Thorough curettage, as well as socket preservation techniques, should preserve the alveolar arch contours to the maximum extent possible. In extraction sockets that show no signs of inflammation, however, immediate placement can help to preserve the alveolar arch contour even better by using the osseoconductive implant as a filler material. Guided surgery can clearly facilitate the immediate placement of implants in extraction sockets and even allows for predicting primary stability. Model-based treatment planning or computer-based treatment planning can be used for these implants. The tip of each implant will mostly be planned in one of the walls or even outside the extraction socket to increase primary stability and improve the esthetic outcome of the restoration (Fig 2-18).

Immediate loading versus delayed loading

In early experiences with dental implants, an extended submerged healing phase was necessary to obtain successful osseointegration.[20] High levels of predictability in more recent implant therapy have initiated a reevaluation of several aspects of the traditional Brånemark implant protocol, which called for a 6-month healing phase.[21–24] The newer protocols directly challenge the healing process by introducing loading during wound healing.[25] Due to the variety of terminology among protocols, a consensus of several definitions was established.

Immediate loading was defined as the condition where a restoration is placed in occlusion with the opposing dentition within 48 hours after implant placement. *Early loading* was defined as a restoration in contact

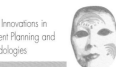

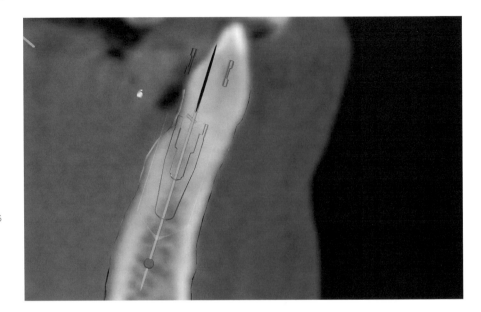

Fig 2-18 The tip of the implant is planned outside the extraction socket to augment the primary stability of the implant and to allow the access hole to exit in the cingulum of the restoration.

with the opposing dentition placed at least 48 hours, but not later than 3 months, after implant placement.[26] On the other hand, *delayed loading* was defined as attachment of the prosthesis via a second procedure that takes place between 2 months and 3 to 6 months (the conventional healing period) after implant placement. Clinical parameters for the success of early or immediate loading have also been established. Loading could be even further delayed to allow an extended healing period in a compromised host or unfavorable site conditions.[25]

Immediate loading of dental implants shortens treatment time and makes it possible to provide the patient with instant satisfactory results. However, additional research is still needed regarding long-term hard and soft tissue healing before a final definition can be determined for immediate loading. The decision of immediate loading will be made using several factors:

- Presence of parafunctional habits
- Presence of infection
- Quality of bone
- Primary stability of the implant
- Type of implant surface to enhance osseointegration
- Systemic conditions of the patient
- Biomechanics in the present oral cavity

Flap versus flapless

The appropriateness of flapless surgery depends on the software used in planning and the anatomic situation. The accuracy of the different computer-based treatment planning systems is not always equivalent, but the obtained result mostly lies within 10 degrees and 2 mm from the original plan.[2,27,28] Taking these accuracy limits and the anatomy into consideration, the clinician can determine whether a flap procedure is necessary to evaluate the bone contour and eventually decide whether bone augmentation is indicated. Information gained via radiographic images or a model created from clinical measurements during treatment planning plays a key role in helping the clinician evaluate the quality and quantity of the soft tissue, along with the hard tissue, and how this will impact the final esthetic outcome.

The main rationale for flap surgery is to keep the incision line away from the implants, thereby possibly preventing infection. By raising a flap, however, postoperative recession of the soft tissue and resorption of bone becomes a possibility. Advantages of a flapless approach include minimal surgical trauma due to the small size of the incision, as well as less postoperative pain, swelling, and discomfort. Therefore, soft tissue healing is far more predictable.[29]

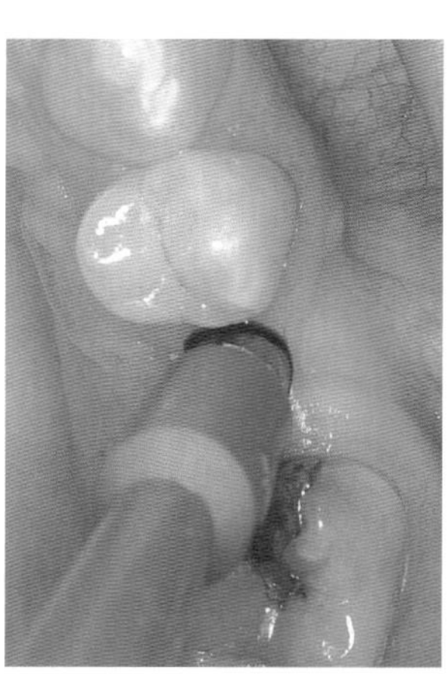

Fig 2-19 In Patient 1, the punch outlines the implant head position. Sufficient soft tissue surrounds the outline, so a punch-out soft tissue removal technique along with flapless surgery can follow.

Transfer of the Planning to the Clinical Field

Surgical intervention

A surgical guide should be fabricated to allow the exact planned position of the implants to be properly transferred to the clinical field. As previously mentioned, optical or magnetic navigation could be used, but this technique will not be discussed in this chapter.

Model-based

During model-based treatment planning, a stone model incorporating the planned implant is fabricated. That model also shows the thickness and position of the soft tissues. An accurate surgical guide of clear acrylic resin with inspection windows was made on top of the model in Fig 2-1e. The restoration is also planned based on this model. To transfer the implant planning to the surgical field, the surgical guide is placed on top of the remaining teeth. Appropriate fit of the surgical guide allows it to click over the remaining teeth without any supporting fixation, and inspection windows provide a built-in safety check. A punch outlines the position of the implant head. If sufficient soft tissue surrounds that outline, a punch-out soft tissue removal technique along with flapless surgery can follow (Fig 2-19).

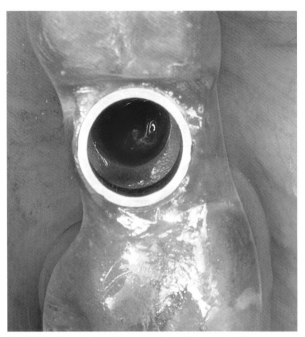

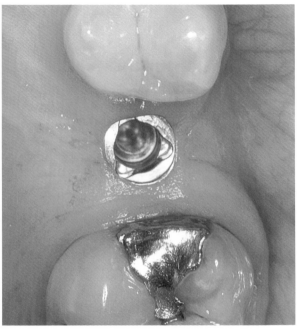

Fig 2-20a The punch outline, seen through the guide, shows no mucogingival contraindications to flapless surgery.

Fig 2-20b The nicely guided placed implant seen after attaching the surgical guide to the neighboring teeth and preparing the osteotomy through the guide.

Patient 1

In Patient 1, the punch outline showed no mucogingival contraindication to flapless surgery, and after clicking the surgical guide onto the neighboring teeth, the implant osteotomy could be prepared. An RP (4.3-mm diameter) 13-mm-long implant was placed with good primary stability and could immediately be loaded (Fig 2-20).

Patient 2

In Patient 2, the surgical guide was fabricated to allow implant placement immediately after extraction. When the patient came in for surgery, a small flap was raised, and the tooth was carefully extracted, avoiding any fracture of the buccal plate. It was possible to maintain most of the surrounding bone, which enabled the clinician to proceed as planned and obtain primary implant stability (Fig 2-21a). The surgical guide could be properly seated over the neighboring teeth using the built-in inspection windows (Figs 2-21b and 2-21c). An RP (4.3-mm diameter) implant was inserted in the prepared guided osteotomy with perfect primary stability (Fig 2-21d). The insertion torque during implant placement was recorded with the OsseoCare device (Nobel Biocare). Allograft material was placed as filler material to decrease the loss in vertical dimension between the implant and the neighboring canine. A resorbable membrane and some sutures were applied to allow primary osseointegration preceding implant loading (Fig 2-21e).

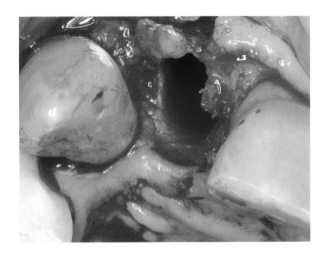

Fig 2-21a A small flap is raised to allow for a conservative extraction procedure. Most of the surrounding bone can be maintained, which enables primary implant stability.

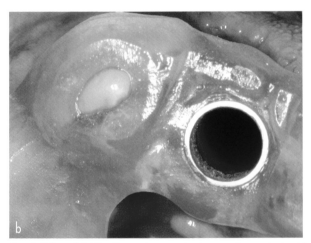

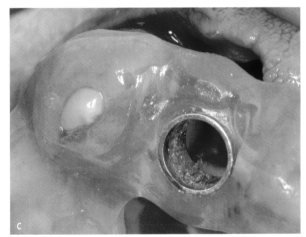

Figs 2-21b and 2-21c These photographs illustrate the surgical guide placed in the oral field. The inspection windows confirm the position that matches the seating on the model.

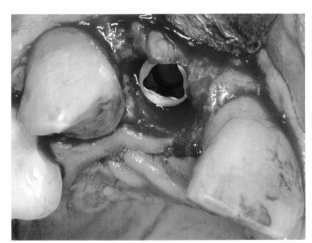

Fig 2-21d The dental implant, an RP 4.3-mm-diameter Replace Select, is placed into the prepared guided osteotomy. The implant achieved a perfect primary stability.

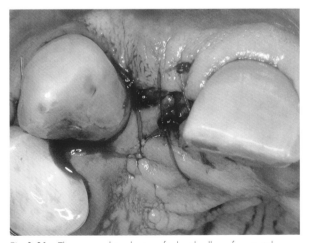

Fig 2-21e The covered implant grafted with allograft material (LifeNet) and a resorbable Ossix membrane (ColBar).

Recent Innovations in
Treatment Planning and
Methodologies

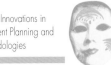

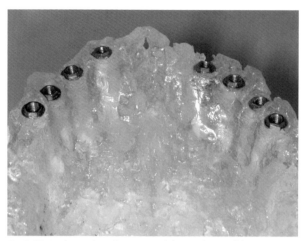

Fig 2-22 Implants placed in a stereolithographic model.

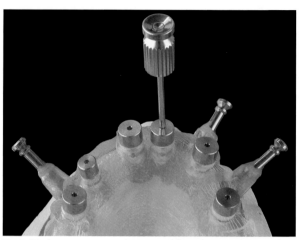

Fig 2-23 A master cast can be created from the stereolithographic surgical guide.

Computer-based

Once a computer-based treatment plan has been made, most software programs will use CAD/CAM to manufacture a surgical guide. This can be done through creation of the model or direct fabrication of the surgical guide, depending on the setup of the software program. Most companies use stereolithography to manufacture either the model with exact positioning of the implants, which allows fabrication of a surgical guide (Fig 2-22), or the surgical guide, which allows reproduction of a model (Fig 2-23).

Because more information is available in computer-based treatment planning compared with model-based treatment planning, the surgical guide can be anchored in the bone. In partially edentulous patients, the inspection windows on the guide allow the clinician to check for proper fit (Fig 2-24). In totally edentulous patients, the relation to the antagonist jaw can be used as an indicator for proper surgical guide fixation (Fig 2-25). After the surgical guide is attached, a punch can outline the soft tissues, similar to the model-guided surgery. Again, flap or flapless surgery can be performed, and the osteotomies can be prepared through guided surgery (Fig 2-26). The implants can be placed immediately after osteotomy preparation, and if indicated, the restorative phase can take place immediately after implant insertion (Fig 2-27).

Restorative phase

Model-based

Various restorative options can be planned before model-guided placement of the implant. The final decision depends mostly on the primary stability that is determined at implant placement.

Recent Innovations in
Treatment Planning and
Methodologies

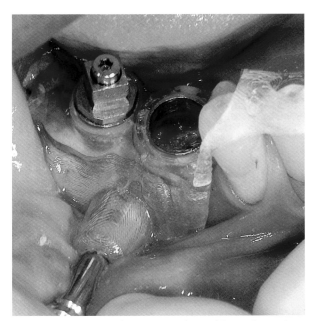

Fig 2-24 Inspection window in a partial stereolithographic guide to verify accurate seating.

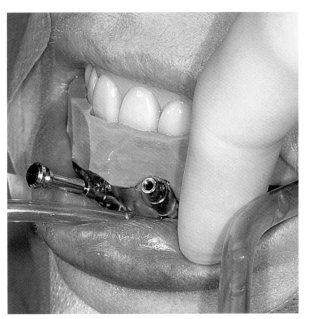

Fig 2-25 The surgical guide for an edentulous mandible should be seated in correct relation to the maxilla through the use of a surgical index.

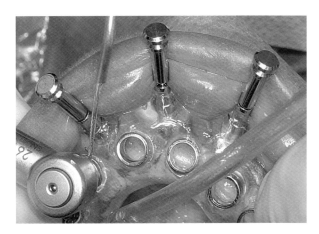

Fig 2-26 Preparation of an implant osteotomy through the use of a computer-based surgical guide.

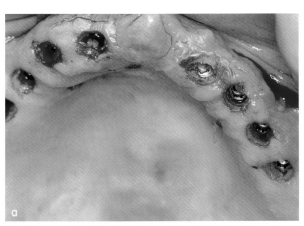

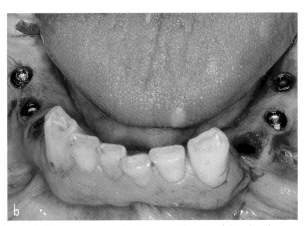

Figs 2-27a and 2-27b Clinical view of implants placed immediately after guided surgery using a flapless procedure in a fully edentulous jaw (a) and in a partially edentulous jaw (b).

Recent Innovations in
Treatment Planning and
Methodologies

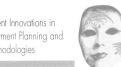

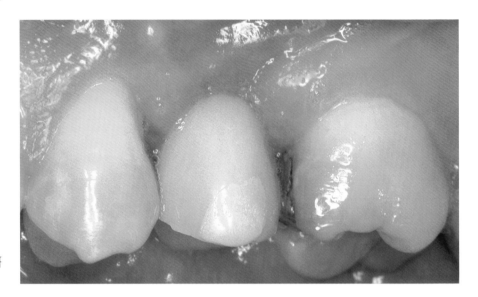

Fig 2-28 Immediate placement of a provisional acrylic resin crown.

Immediate loading

The main advantage of model-guided surgery is that the abutment choice and the restoration can be made on the model preoperatively. The selection of the abutment depends on the selected prosthesis design and the number of implants to be restored; splinting should be taken into consideration in cases with multiple adjacent implants. Immediately after the implant is inserted, a temporary abutment with the preplanned acrylic resin provisional crown can be placed.

After a 2-month healing process, prefabricated customized abutments can be used to restore the implant in a more definitive manner. In some cases, the prefabricated customized abutment can be delivered at the time of surgery. After primary osseointegration involving a healing time of 2 to 6 months, the definitive crown can be cemented, bypassing the impression and/or abutment try-in appointment. For example, Patient 1 underwent treatment planning for the immediate replacement of the maxillary left second premolar. In this particular case, the decision was made to place an immediate cement-retained crown. For that purpose, a provisional abutment (Nobel Biocare) was screwed into place. A prefabricated acrylic resin provisional crown (made on the planning model) was then cemented on the abutment (Fig 2-28).

Delayed loading

In cases where the implant is restored after a healing period of 2 to 3 months, the definitive restoration can be fabricated in the immediate postoperative period. Since the placement of the implant in the planning model is analogous to the real placement in the oral cavity, it is appropriate to create the abutment and crown on the planning model.

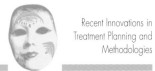

This technique requires accurately mounted casts, and the clinician must ensure no major changes or modifications in the oral cavity have taken place postoperatively.

Computer-based
Immediate loading

The possibility of placing the restoration immediately after surgical placement of dental implants is a unique opportunity that can only be done with proper planning. Three-dimensional software specifically designed for this procedure not only allows predictable placement of the implants at the planned position but also aids in creation of the superstructure even in cases that are anatomically and restoratively difficult. The Procera software is recommended for this purpose. The provisional superstructure, using expandable or multiunit abutments, is placed immediately after the implants are inserted. Titanium provisional multiunit copings (Nobel Biocare) or a cast titanium framework layered with acrylic resin can be used within an acrylic resin–reinforced prosthesis as a provisional superstructure. After 6 to 12 months, the final prostheses can be fabricated.

Delayed loading

Computer-guided surgery offers the advantage of establishing a logical continuity between diagnosis, prosthetic planning, and surgical phases. The surgical guide dictates the position of the dental implant. This guide can be used to fabricate the master model, which allows the creation of the provisional and eventually the definitive prostheses. Occasionally, it is necessary to verify the master model. A jig can confirm that the relationship of all implants in the master model is identical to their relationship in the oral cavity. The superstructure can then be fabricated with the various laboratory techniques available to the clinician. Restoration materials (usually acrylic resin or porcelain) are also chosen by the practitioner.

Conclusion

Proper patient selection, combined with model-based or computer-based treatment planning, allows for predictable delivery of high-quality results in guided surgery. When careful planning leads to properly executed guided surgery, flapless procedures in selected cases and even immediate loading become possible.

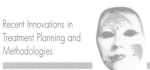

Acknowledgments

We would like to acknowledge our dear colleague Dr Orlando Alvarez from Chili for allowing us to borrow some of his beautiful pictures and Dr Jessica Adams for her efforts during the treatment of the clinical cases as a dedicated fourth-year dental student at UMB and as a head start in periodontics.

References

1. Wanschitz F, Birkfellner W, Watzinger F, et al. Evaluation of accuracy of computer-aided intraoperative positioning of endosseous oral implants in the edentulous mandible. Clin Oral Implants Res 2002;13:59–64.
2. Jacobs R, Adriansens A, Verstreken K, Suetens P, van Steenberghe D. Predictability of a three-dimensional planning system for oral implant surgery. Dentomaxillofac Radiol 1999;28(2):105–111.
3. Gher ME, Richardson AC. The accuracy of dental radiographic techniques used for evaluation of implant fixture placement. Int J Periodontics Restorative Dent 1995;15(3):268–283.
4. Jabero M, Sarment DP. Advanced surgical guidance technology: A review. Implant Dent 2006;15:135–142.
5. Verstreken K, Van Cleynenbreugel J, Martens K, Marchal G, van Steenberghe D, Suetens P. An image-guided planning system for endosseous oral implants. IEEE Trans Med Imaging 1998;17(5):842–852.
6. Fortin T, Bosson JL, Coudert JL, Isidori M. Reliability of preoperative planning of an image-guided system for oral implant placement based on three-dimensional images: An in vivo study. Int J Oral Maxillofac Implants 2003;18:886–893.
7. Tsuji M, Noguchi N, Shigematsu M, et al. A new navigation system based on cephalograms and dental casts for oral and maxillofacial surgery. Int J Oral Maxillofac Surg 2006;35:828–836.
8. Mischkowski RA, Zinser MJ, Neugebauer J, Kübler AC, Zöller JE. Comparison of static and dynamic computer-assisted guidance methods in implantology. Int J Comput Dent 2006;9:23–35.
9. Clelland NL, Gilat A. The effect of abutment angulation on stress transfer for an implant. J Prosthodont 1992;1(1):24–28.
10. Clelland NL, Gilat A, McGlumphy EA, Brantley WA. A photoelastic and strain gauge analysis of angled abutments for an implant system. Int J Oral Maxillofac Implants 1993;8(5):541–548.
11. Clelland NL, Lee JK, Bimbenet OC, Brantley WA. A three-dimensional finite element stress analysis of angled abutments for an implant placed in the anterior maxilla. J Prosthodont 1995;4(2):95–100.
12. Erneklint C, Odman P, Ortengren U, Karlsson S. An in vitro load evaluation of a conical implant system with 2 abutment designs and 3 different retaining-screw alloys. Int J Oral Maxillofac Implants 2006;21:733–737.
13. Buser D, Dula K, Hirt HP, Schenk RK. Lateral ridge augmentation using autografts and barrier membranes: A clinical study with 40 partially edentulous patients. J Oral Maxillofac Surg 1996;54:420–432.
14. Renouard F, Nisand D. Short implants in the severely resorbed maxilla: A 2-year retrospective clinical study. Clin Implant Dent Relat Res 2005;7 (1 suppl):104S–110S.
15. Renouard F, Nisand D. Impact of implant length and diameter on survival rates. Clin Oral Implants Res 2006;17(suppl 2):35–51.
16. Olsen S, Ferguson SJ, Sigrist C, et al. A novel computational method for real-time preoperative assessment of primary dental implant stability. Clin Oral Implants Res 2005;16:53–59.

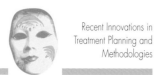

Recent Innovations in Treatment Planning and Methodologies

17. Maló P, Rangert B, Nobre M. "All-on-Four" immediate-function concept with Brånemark System implants for completely edentulous mandibles: A retrospective clinical study. Clin Implant Dent Relat Res 2003;5(suppl 1):2–9.

18. van Steenberghe D, Quirynen M, Molly L, Jacobs R. Impact of systemic diseases and medication on osseointegration. Periodontol 2000 2003;33:163–171.

19. Esposito MA, Koukoulopoulou A, Coulthard P, Worthington HV. Interventions for replacing missing teeth: Dental implants in fresh extraction sockets (immediate, immediate-delayed and delayed implants). Cochrane Database Syst Rev 2006;4:CD005968.

20. Brånemark PI, Hansson BO, Adell R, et al. Osseointegrated implants in the treatment of the edentulous jaw. Experience from a 10-year period. Scand J Plast Reconstr Surg Suppl 1977;16:1–132.

21. Adell R, Lekholm U, Rockler B, Brånemark PI. A 15-year study of osseointegrated implants in the treatment of the edentulous jaw. Int J Oral Surg 1981;10(6):387–416.

22. Brånemark PI, Adell R, Albrektsson T, Lekholm U, Lundkvist S, Rockler B. Osseointegrated titanium fixtures in the treatment of edentulousness. Biomaterials 1983;4(1):25–28.

23. Albrektsson T, Brånemark PI, Hansson HA, Lindström J. Osseointegrated titanium implants. Requirements for ensuring a long-lasting, direct bone-to-implant anchorage in man. Acta Orthop Scand 1981;52(2):155–170.

24. Szmukler-Moncler S, Piattelli A, Favero GA, Dubruille JH. Considerations preliminary to the application of early and immediate loading protocols in dental implantology. Clin Oral Implants Res 2000;11:12–25.

25. Cochran DL, Morton D, Weber HP. Consensus statements and recommended clinical procedures regarding loading protocols for endosseous dental implants. Int J Oral Maxillofac Implants 2004;19(suppl):109–113.

26. Attard NJ, Zarb GA. Immediate and early implant loading protocols: A literature review of clinical studies. J Prosthet Dent 2005;94:242–258.

27. Van Steenberghe D, Malevez C, Van Cleynenbreugel J, et al. Accuracy of drilling guides for transfer from three-dimensional CT-based planning to placement of zygoma implants in human cadavers. Clin Oral Implants Res 2003;14:131–136.

28. Di Giacomo GA, Cury PR, de Araujo NS, Sendyk WR, Sendyk CL. Clinical application of stereolithographic surgical guides for implant placement: Preliminary results. J Periodontol 2005;76:503–507.

29. Campelo LD, Camara JR. Flapless implant surgery: A 10-year clinical retrospective analysis. Int J Oral Maxillofac Implants 2002;17:271–276.

Immediate Loading of Implants Placed into Fresh Extraction Sockets

Devorah Schwartz-Arad,
DMD, PhD

Recent Innovations in
Treatment Planning and
Methodologies

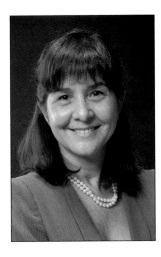

Devorah Schwartz-Arad, DMD, PhD

Devorah Schwartz-Arad received her DMD and PhD degrees from the Hebrew University, Jerusalem, Israel. She is a specialist in oral and maxillofacial surgery and was a senior lecturer in the Department of Oral and Maxillofacial Surgery at the School of Dental Medicine, Tel Aviv University, until 2008.

Dr Schwartz-Arad is a member of the Specialty Examination Board for Oral and Maxillofacial Surgery (Ministry of Health, Israel) and was the president of the Israeli Association of Oral Implantology. Dr Schwartz-Arad has published numerous scientific articles and abstracts and presented more than 100 papers at scientific meetings in Israel, Europe, and the United States. She has been awarded several academic and professional awards, including membership in the Israel Academy of Sciences and the Israel Cancer Association.

Dr Schwartz-Arad is the owner and senior surgeon of a day-surgery center that specializes in bone grafting, dental implantology, and orthognathic surgery.

E-mail: dubi@dsa.co.il

The first evidence of successful immediate total teeth replacement with endosseous alloplastic implants in a living person seems to date from about AD 600. The mandible, possibly from a Mayan woman, was found by Dr and Mrs Wilson Popenoe in Honduras in 1931 and has three pieces of shell serving as replacements for the natural incisors. A recent radiograph revealed "osseointegration" of the shells.

Rationale for Immediate Placement

Immediate implant placement into fresh extraction sites is considered a predictable and acceptable procedure and has been gaining popularity over the past decade.[1–7] The rationale behind immediate placement is based in part on observations that it might contribute to bone preservation.[8,9] Early extraction and immediate placement could lead to a favorable crown-implant ratio, better esthetics, and a favorable interarch relationship.[1,9] Diagnosis and treatment planning are key factors in achieving successful outcomes after placement and restoration of implants inserted immediately after tooth extraction.[10,11]

Gap filling

Following tooth extraction, a socket often presents dimensions that may be considerably greater than the diameter of a conventional implant. Botticelli et al concluded that a marginal defect wider than 1 mm may heal with new bone and a high degree of osseointegration with an implant surface.[12] Their study reported that a marginal defect lateral to the implant gradually filled in with newly formed bone. This de novo bone formation originated within the walls of the surgically prepared defect. Bone-to-implant contact was first established in the apical portion of the gap. This new bone tissue was in the coronal direction continuous with a dense, nonmineralized, "implant-attached" soft tissue that, over time, also became mineralized to increase the height of the zone of bone-to-implant contact. These results suggest that healing of a wide marginal defect around an implant is characterized by appositional bone growth from the lateral and apical bone walls of the defect.[13] Provided the gap size of any remaining defect is 2 mm or smaller, no additional regeneration procedures should be necessary.[14]

Human immediate postextraction implants were also found to have a high percentage of bone-to-implant contact.[15] Furthermore, immediate loading did not appear to impair osseointegration of an immediate postextraction implant compared with an unloaded postextraction implant.[16]

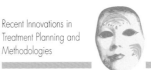

Recent Innovations in
Treatment Planning and
Methodologies

Primary closure

Primary closure of the extraction socket in immediate placement may be difficult depending on the size of the opening left by the extracted tooth. The absolute need for bone augmentation and primary flap closure for implants placed into fresh extraction sites has never been proven. Immediate implant placement into the site of a single extracted tooth can be successful even without primary closure.[17,18] This is most important in the anterior maxilla, the so-called esthetic zone.

Immediate Loading

Time of loading has been rigidly controlled in clinical investigations so that implants can heal under unloaded conditions. The reason for this lies in the significant association between successful osseointegration and the absence of loading. In the past, immediate loading of dental implants resulted in fibrous encapsulation.[14]

Immediate loading can be considered in some clinical cases. Once the parameters for success were defined, immediately loaded implants have proven to be at least as successful as implants placed under a standard loading protocol. Controlling micromotion is the key difference between the success and failure of osseointegration of immediately loaded implants. Micromotion can be reduced through broad anteroposterior distribution of the immediately loaded implants combined with cross-arch stabilization of the edentulous arches with a rigid prosthesis. Stability of the individual implant also is important. To increase implant stability, anchorage of the cortical bone, especially in the maxilla, may be necessary.

An implant-supported restoration offers a predictable treatment option for tooth replacement.[16,19–21] The high success rate of dental implants has led to an improvement in quality of life for many patients. Clinicians have recognized that the difficulty of providing anterior tooth replacements lies in preserving the hard and soft tissue components that surround natural teeth. Immediately loading implants into fresh extraction sockets benefits patients by decreasing healing time, reducing resorption of the alveolar bone, and achieving optimal esthetic results.[22]

Immediate Placement with Immediate Loading or Provisionalization

The objective of immediate provisionalization or loading of dental implants is to combine tissue preservation with the bone preservation

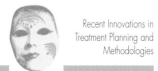

that follows immediate placement. Immediate provisionalization results in fewer surgical interventions and a simpler solution for the patient.

A recent study by the author found that, after a mean follow-up of 15.6 months, provisionalization of implants that were immediately placed proved to be a predictable procedure with a high implant survival rate (97.6%).[23]

Histologic observations from different animal and human studies have shown that immediately loaded implants can have a direct bone-to-implant interface without any fibrous tissue formation.[16,24] It has not been established how much bone is preserved when implants are placed immediately into fresh extraction sockets, and further research is warranted to clarify the bone remodeling process.[25,26] Success in immediate placement and loading of implants is based on several clinical parameters. Therefore, this treatment concept can be applied in everyday clinical practice to properly selected cases that have good primary stability and sites with a fully preserved extraction socket with no bone dehiscence. Immediate provisionalization should be proposed only if an appropriate initial insertion torque has been applied to the implant.[27]

A growing number of clinical publications report implant placement in extraction sockets combined with immediate function.[16,23,28–34] The concept of immediate placement and immediate loading or provisionalization warrants discussion of the following four treatment options:

- Single-tooth replacement: extraction of a single tooth followed by immediate implant placement and immediate provisionalization
- Replacement of multiple adjacent teeth: extraction of a few adjacent teeth in a partially edentulous arch, followed by immediate placement of implants with immediate provisionalization
- Total arch replacement: extraction of a few hopeless teeth resulting in a completely edentulous arch, followed by placement of implants that coincide with extraction sockets; then immediate provisionalization and loading
- Total mouth replacement (two arches): extraction of a few, hopeless teeth resulting in a completely edentulous patient, followed by placement of implants that coincide with extraction sockets in both arches; then immediate provisionalization and loading

Single-tooth replacement

As patients become more aware of treatment alternatives, replacement of a single tooth by means of single-implant restoration is an increasingly popular treatment option, especially among young patients[35,36] (Fig 3-1). The single-implant restoration has been reported to achieve a high level of surgical and prosthetic success.[37–40] Among the advantages of the imme-

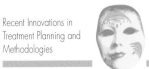

diate-loading protocol are *(1)* a significant reduction in the number of surgical procedures required and *(2)* elimination of the need for a provisional prosthesis between the surgical and prosthetic phases of treatment. This procedure has demonstrated a predictable clinical success and the possible preservation of the existing osseous and gingival morphology.[41] Results of recent studies showed that immediate restoration of implants placed immediately in fresh extraction sites can provide a safe treatment option, with success rates of 94% to 98%.[23,33]

Atraumatic tooth extraction is essential for successful immediate implant placement and the maintenance of the buccal plate (see Fig 3-1c). Two of the most important factors and main prerequisites for immediate loading are sufficient initial implant stability and insertion torque of about 40 N/cm. When a single-tooth implant is immediately loaded, the implant-abutment connection should also be stable; primary stability is fundamental.

The single-tooth replacement does not represent immediate functional loading since clinicians normally prevent any occlusal function of the provisional restoration. Therefore, these types of restorations are classified as immediate provisionalizations only.

One of the strongest advantages of this treatment protocol is immediate placement of the restoration, which eliminates the need for a provisional removable prosthesis and leads to satisfactory esthetic results. Moreover, a stage-two surgery is unnecessary, and excellent soft tissue healing occurs predictably, with a stable mucogingival junction in relation to the adjacent teeth and with the preservation of the interproximal papillae. These clinical outcomes reduce the necessity of further surgical procedures to improve the gingival architecture.

Fig 3-1a In this case, the maxillary right canine is scheduled for extraction due to root fracture. Single-tooth replacement through immediate provisionalization is chosen as the treatment method.

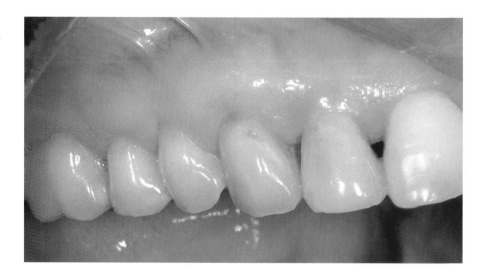

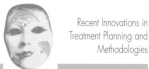

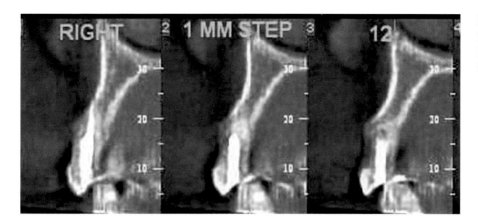

Fig 3-1b A preoperative computed tomography scan reveals a thin buccal plate in the area of this canine.

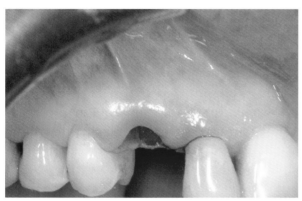

Fig 3-1c The canine is atraumatically extracted without damage to the buccal plate and the adjacent papillae.

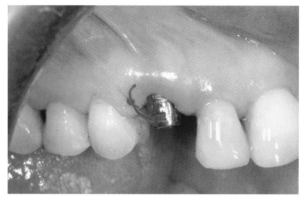

Fig 3-1d An implant is immediately placed into the fresh extraction socket without raising a flap.

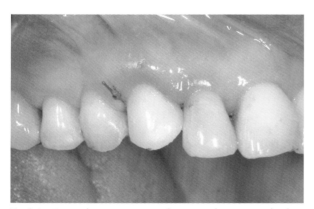

Fig 3-1e An acrylic resin provisional crown without any occlusal contacts is fabricated and placed.

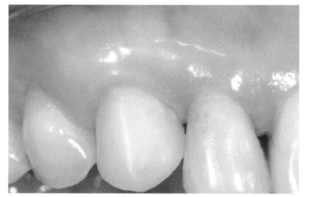

Fig 3-1f Six months later, a healthy soft tissue around the provisional crown is evident.

Recent Innovations in
Treatment Planning and
Methodologies

Replacement of multiple adjacent teeth

Replacement of multiple adjacent teeth with fixed implant restorations in the anterior maxilla is poorly documented. Because the mechanism of tissue behavior in the context of the esthetic outcome is still not fully understood, the esthetic results are not always predictable.[42–45] The distance of the bone crest from the restoration's contact point is related to the presence of the interimplant papillae.[7,46] This may imply that preservation of this bone crest is imperative for interimplant papilla regeneration.[7,11,17,18]

The effect of immediate implants on the shape and quality of noncompromised bone (eg, in the maxillary premolar and anterior mandibular regions) is less important, but it becomes a major contributor to success when bone shape and quality are compromised (eg, anterior maxillary region and posterior regions of both arches). The preservation of alveolar ridge dimensions immediately after tooth extraction has been documented.[47,48]

Immediate loading of multiple adjacent implants in a partially edentulous arch seems to result in success rates even higher than those for single-tooth replacements[23] (Fig 3-2). This might be caused by the distribution of forces among the adjacent implants and the absence of rotational forces that act on a single implant.

As with single-tooth implants, the clinician is advised to eliminate any function of the provisional restoration for the first 3 to 6 months, which is the waiting period prior to final restoration.

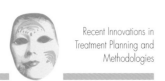

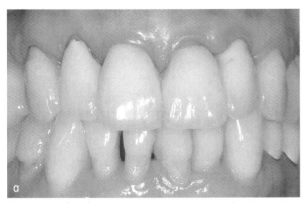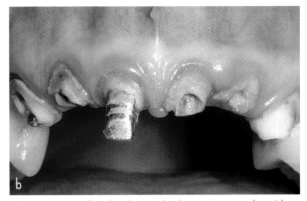

Figs 3-2a and 3-2b Immediate provisionalization of multiple adjacent implants in a partially edentulous arch. The patient was referred for extractions and immediate implant placement in the sites of all six anterior maxillary teeth.

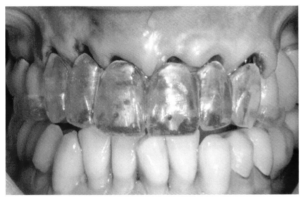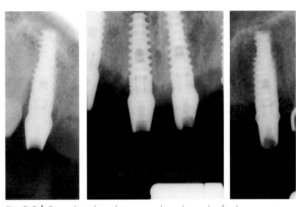

Fig 3-2c Teeth are extracted atraumatically, and a surgical guide is used for implant placement.

Fig 3-2d Four dental implants are placed into the fresh extraction sockets of the two central incisors and canines.

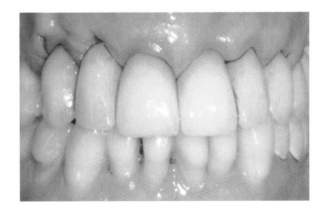

Fig 3-2e A prefabricated provisional fixed partial denture is inserted, taking care to avoid occlusal loading.

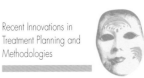

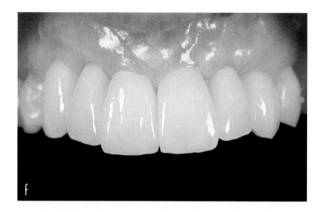

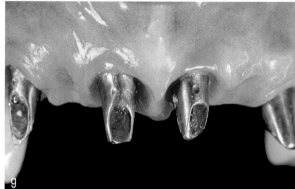

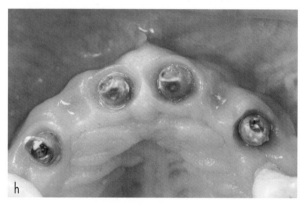

Figs 3-2f to 3-2h Six months later, healing of the soft tissue is remarkable with preservation of the interimplant papillae.

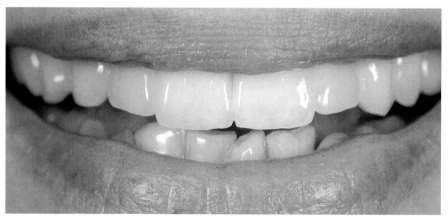

Fig 3-2i After an additional 6 months, the definitive restoration is delivered.

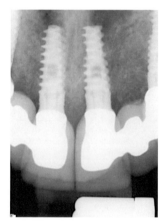

Fig 3-2j A radiograph taken 3 years post-rehabilitation reveals bone height preservation. (Restoration by Dr Nitzan Bichacho, Tel-Aviv, Israel.)

Full arch or full mouth replacement

Fixed implant-supported reconstructions in fully edentulous patients are a well-established treatment method if the implants are allowed to heal unloaded for 3 to 6 months. Long-term data show that this kind of reconstruction can be successful for many years.[3–5,49,50] Unfortunately, patients undergoing such therapy are required to wear a provisional restoration for several months since a certain healing time is traditionally recommended after tooth extraction and implant placement before the implants can be loaded.

Several studies have shown that implants placed immediately after tooth extraction can be as successful as implants placed into healed sites.[23,28,51,52] The success rate for immediately placed implants is estimated to be higher than 95%.

Immediate implant placement for fixed full-arch restorations can be a viable treatment option for patients with severe periodontal disease[3] (Fig 3-3). In patients being considered for total arch reconstruction, strategic extractions may be appropriate[53]; questionable teeth can be preserved as temporary abutments to support a provisional restoration (see Figs 3-3c, 3-3d, and 3-3f to 3-3h). Loading should be adjusted to those supporting teeth.

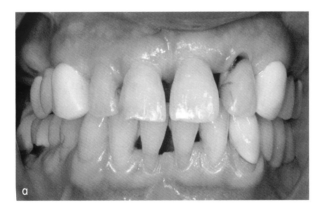

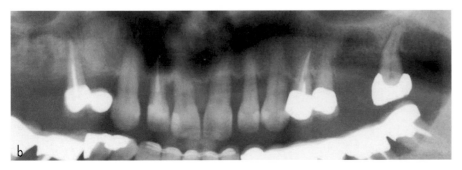

Figs 3-3a and 3-3b Full-arch rehabilitation through immediate provisionalization is a treatment option for patients with periodontal disease. In this patient, all maxillary teeth are scheduled for extraction and immediate replacement using dental implants.

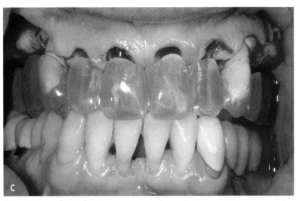
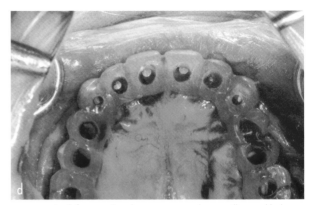

Figs 3-3c and 3-3d Extraction is performed, leaving the two maxillary canines and a left second molar to preserve the maxillomandibular relationship during the provisionalization and to support the provisional restoration. A surgical flap is not raised in the anterior region. Implants are placed using a surgical guide.

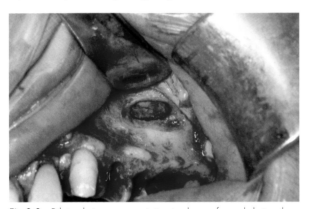
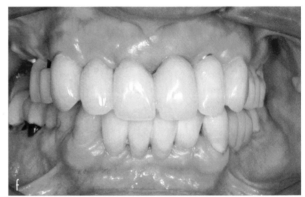

Fig 3-3e Bilateral sinus augmentation is also performed during the same surgery.

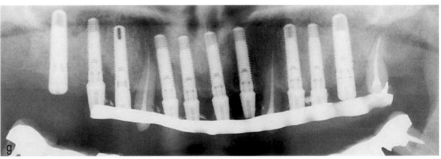

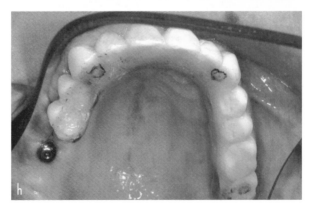

Figs 3-3f to 3-3h A provisional restoration is placed immediately postoperatively. Occlusal loads are balanced so that the remaining teeth provide most of the support.

Recent Innovations in Treatment Planning and Methodologies

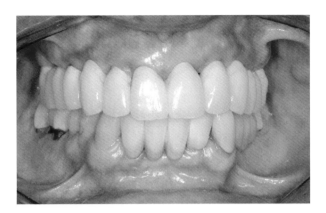

Fig 3-3i Nine months later, after canine and molar extraction, the final restoration is delivered.

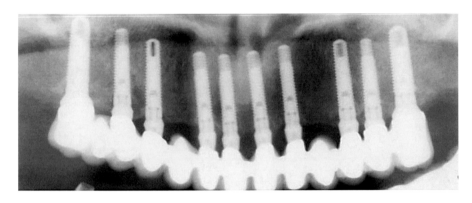

Fig 3-3j Panoramic view of the maxilla 3 years after rehabilitation. (Restoration by Dr Dani Maor, Tel-Aviv, Israel.)

Contrary to a single implant or a few immediate provisionalizations, true functional loading can occur only in edentulous cases (when all residual teeth are extracted) with implant-supported rehabilitation (Fig 3-4).

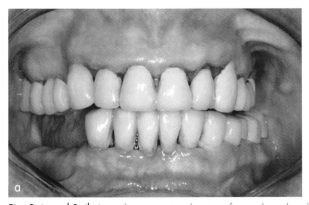

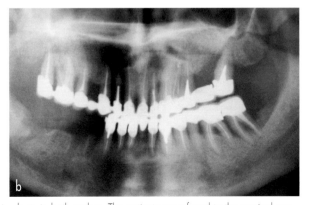

Figs 3-4a and 3-4b Immediate provisionalization of immediate dental implants in both arches. The patient was referred to the surgical center for extraction of all her teeth and immediate rehabilitation.

Recent Innovations in
Treatment Planning and
Methodologies

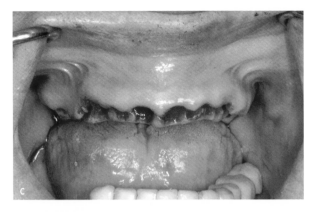

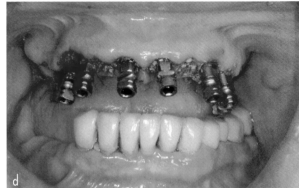

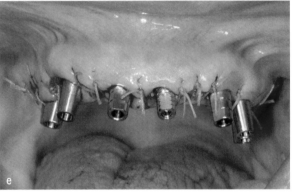

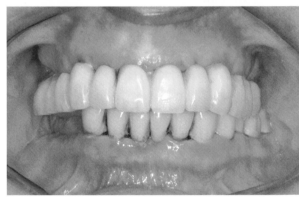

Figs 3-4c to 3-4e To preserve the vertical dimension of the face, the procedure is divided into two stages, performed one after the other in the same surgical session. In the first stage, all maxillary teeth are carefully extracted, and implants are placed in the maxilla.

Fig 3-4f Following maxillary implant placement, a provisional fixed partial denture is adopted with the guidance of the remaining mandibular teeth.

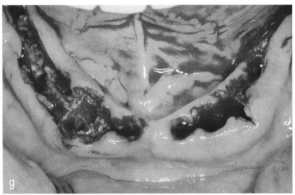

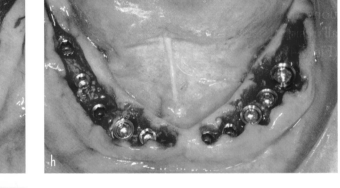

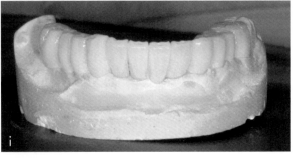

Figs 3-4g to 3-4i In the second stage, all mandibular teeth are extracted, implants are placed, and a provisional mandibular fixed partial denture is seated with the guidance of the maxillary restoration. (Restoration by Dr Abraham Schnieder, Tel-Aviv, Israel.)

Recent Innovations in
Treatment Planning and
Methodologies

Tips for Success

Several important parameters should be taken into consideration to achieve successful implant placement with immediate loading:

- Primary stability is crucial (at least 40 N/cm is recommended). An implant with stability less than 30 N/cm should not be loaded.
- Flapless surgery is preferable, especially in the esthetic zone. When planning a flapless procedure, measure the soft tissue thickness with a probe. Add this tissue thickness to the drilling depth for correct site preparation.
- Gap filling is optional but recommended in the esthetic zone.
- Membrane is not necessary.
- Implant placement should be slightly palatal for better esthetics, especially in the anterior maxilla (with augmentation at the buccal area).
- Rigid fixation is to be used when more than one implant is involved.
- The provisional crown or fixed partial denture should not be in occlusal contact except in cases of total arch provisionalization when all residual teeth are extracted. In these cases, the occlusal contacts should include all implants at the palatal/lingual area; contact in the incisal tips should be avoided to prevent off-axis forces on the implants.
- Cross-arch stabilization is essential in full arch cases.
- Strategic extraction should be considered when it allows placement of longer implants, which leads to better prognosis and prosthetic positioning, especially in the esthetic zone.

Acknowledgment

The author would like to thank Dr Liran Levin for his profound help and support in the preparation of this chapter.

References

1. Schwartz-Arad D, Chaushu G. The ways and wherefores of immediate placement of implants into fresh extraction sites: A literature review. J Periodontol 1997;68:915–923.
2. Schwartz-Arad D, Chaushu G. Placement of implants into fresh extraction sites: 4 to 7 years retrospective evaluation of 95 immediate implants. J Periodontol 1997;68:1110–1116.
3. Schwartz-Arad D, Chaushu G. Full-arch restoration of the jaw with fixed ceramometal prosthesis: Immediate implant placement. Int J Oral Maxillofac Implants 1998;13:819–825.
4. Chaushu G, Schwartz-Arad D. Full-arch restoration of the jaw with fixed ceramometal prosthesis: Late implant placement. J Periodontol 1999;70:90–94.

Recent Innovations in
Treatment Planning and
Methodologies

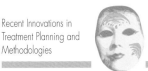

5. Schwartz-Arad D, Gulayev N, Chaushu G. Immediate versus non-immediate implantation for full arch fixed reconstruction following extraction of all residual teeth: A retrospective comparative study. J Periodontol 2000;71:923–928.

6. Schwartz-Arad D, Yaniv Y, Levin L, Kaffe I. A radiographic evaluation of cervical bone loss associated with immediate and delayed implants placed for fixed restorations in edentulous jaws. J Periodontol 2004;75:652–657.

7. Kupershmidt I, Levin L, Schwartz-Arad D. Inter-implant bone height changes in anterior maxillary immediate and non-immediate adjacent dental implants. J Periodontol 2007;78(6):991–996.

8. Denissen HW, Kalk W, Veldhuis HA, van Waas MAJ. Anatomic consideration for preventive implantation. Int J Oral Maxillofac Implants 1993;8:191–196.

9. Orenstein IH, Synan WJ, Truhlar RS, Morris HF, Ochi S. Bone quality in patients receiving endosseous dental implants. DICRG Interim Report No. 1. Implant Dent 1994;3:90–96.

10. Becker W. Immediate implant placement: Treatment planning and surgical steps for successful outcomes. Br Dent J 2006;26;201(4):199–205.

11. Becker W, Sennerby L, Bedrossian E, Becker BE, Lucchini JP. Implant stability measurements for implants placed at the time of extraction: A cohort, prospective clinical trial. J Periodontol 2005;76(3):391–397.

12. Botticelli D, Berglundh T, Buser D, Lindhe J. The jumping distance revisited: An experimental study in the dog. Clin Oral Implants Res 2003;14(1):35–42.

13. Botticelli D, Berglundh T, Buser D, Lindhe J. Appositional bone formation in marginal defects at implants. Clin Oral Implants Res 2003;14(1):1–9.

14. Jung UW, Kim CS, Choi SH, Cho KS, Inoue T, Kim CK. Healing of surgically created circumferential gap around non-submerged-type implants in dogs: A histomorphometric study. Clin Oral Implants Res 2007;18:171–178.

15. Cornelini R, Scarano A, Covani U, Petrone G, Piattelli A. Immediate one-stage postextraction implant: A human clinical and histologic case report. Int J Oral Maxillofac Implants 2000;15(3):432–437.

16. Guida L, Iezzi G, Annunziata M, et al. Immediate placement and loading of dental implants: A human histologic case report. J Periodontol 2008;79:575–581.

17. Becker W, Goldstein M, Becker BE, Sennerby L. Minimally invasive flapless implant surgery: A prospective multicenter study. Clin Implant Dent Relat Res 2005;7(1 suppl):21S–27S.

18. Schwartz-Arad D, Chaushu G. Immediate implant placement: A procedure without incisions. J Periodontol 1998;69(7):743–750.

19. Esposito M, Grusovin MG, Coulthard P, Thomsen P, Worthington HV. A 5-year follow-up comparative analysis of the efficacy of various osseointegrated dental implant systems: A systematic review of randomized controlled clinical trials. Int J Oral Maxillofac Implants 2005;20:557–568.

20. Schwartz-Arad D, Herzberg R, Levin L. Evaluation of long-term implant success. J Periodontol 2005;76(10):1623–1628.

21. Schwartz-Arad D, Laviv A, Levin L. Failure causes, timing, and cluster behavior: An 8-year study of dental implants. Implant Dent 2008;17(2):200–207.

22. Garber DA, Salama MA, Salama H. Immediate total tooth replacement. Compend Contin Educ Dent 2001;22:210–216,218.

23. Schwartz-Arad D, Laviv A, Levin L. Survival of immediately provisionalized dental implants placed immediately into fresh extraction sockets. J Periodontol 2007;78(2):219–223.

24. Romanos GE, Testori T, Degidi M, Piattelli A. Histologic and histomorphometric findings from retrieved, immediately occlusally loaded implants in humans. J Periodontol 2005;76:1823–1832.

25. Covani U, Bortolaia C, Barone A, Sbordone L. Bucco-lingual crestal bone changes after immediate and delayed implant placement. J Periodontol 2004;75:1605–1612.

26. Schropp L, Kostopoulos L, Wenzel A. Bone healing following immediate versus delayed placement of titanium implants into extraction sockets: A prospective clinical study. Int J Oral Maxillofac Implants 2003;18:189–199.

Recent Innovations in
Treatment Planning and
Methodologies

27. Ottoni JM, Oliveira ZF, Mansini R, Cabral AM. Correlation between placement torque and survival of single-tooth implants. Int J Oral Maxillofac Implants 2005;20:769–776.

28. Grunder U. Immediate functional loading of immediate implants in edentulous arches: Two-year results. Int J Periodontics Restorative Dent 2001;21(6):545–551.

29. Aires I, Berger J. Immediate placement in extraction sites followed by immediate loading: A pilot study and case presentation. Implant Dent 2002;11(1):87–94.

30. Cooper LF, Rahman A, Moriarty J, Chaffee N, Sacco D. Immediate mandibular rehabilitation with endosseous implants: Simultaneous extraction, implant placement, and loading. Int J Oral Maxillofac Implants 2002;17(4):517–525.

31. Crespi R, Capparè P, Gherlone E, Romanos GE. Immediate occlusal loading of implants placed in fresh sockets after tooth extraction. Int J Oral Maxillofac Implants 2007;22(6):955–962.

32. Degidi M, Piattelli A, Carinci F. Immediate loaded dental implants: Comparison between fixtures inserted in postextractive and healed bone sites. J Craniofac Surg 2007;18(4):965–971.

33. Barone A, Rispoli L, Vozza I, Quaranta A, Covani U. Immediate restoration of single implants placed immediately after tooth extraction. J Periodontol 2006;77(11):1914–1920.

34. Ferrara A, Galli C, Mauro G, Macaluso GM. Immediate provisional restoration of postextraction implants for maxillary single-tooth replacement. Int J Periodontics Restorative Dent 2006;26(4):371–377.

35. Naert I, Koutsikakis G, Duyck J, Quirynen M, Jacobs R, van Steenberghe D. Biologic outcome of single-implant restorations as tooth replacements: A long-term follow-up study. Clin Implant Dent Relat Res 2000;2(4):209–218.

36. Romeo E, Lops D, Margutti E, Ghisolfi M, Chiapasco M, Vogel G. Long-term survival and success of oral implants in the treatment of full and partial arches: A 7-year prospective study with the ITI dental implant system. Int J Oral Maxillofac Implants 2004;19:247–259.

37. Gotfredsen K. A 5-year prospective study of single-tooth replacements supported by the Astra Tech implant: A pilot study. Clin Implant Dent Relat Res 2004;6(1):1–8.

38. Levin L, Sadet P, Grossmann Y. A retrospective evaluation of 1,387 single-tooth implants: A 6-year follow-up. J Periodontol 2006;77(12):2080–2083.

39. Levin L, Laviv A, Schwartz-Arad D. Long-term success of implants replacing a single molar. J Periodontol 2006;77(9):1528–1532.

40. Levin L, Pathael S, Dolev E, Schwartz-Arad D. Aesthetic versus surgical success of single dental implants: 1- to 9-year follow-up. Pract Proced Aesthet Dent 2005;17(8):533–538.

41. Kan JY, Rungcharassaeng K, Lozada J. Immediate placement and provisionalization of maxillary anterior single implants: 1-year prospective study. Int J Oral Maxillofac Implants 2003;18:31–39.

42. Belser UC, Schmid B, Higginbottom F, Buser D. Outcome analysis of implant restorations located in the anterior maxilla: A review of the recent literature. Int J Oral Maxillofac Implants 2004;19(suppl):30–42.

43. Buser D, Martin W, Belser UC. Optimizing esthetics for implant restorations in the anterior maxilla: Anatomic and surgical considerations. Int J Oral Maxillofac Implants 2004;19(suppl):43–61.

44. Higginbottom F, Belser U, Jones JD, Keith SE. Prosthetic management of implants in the esthetic zone. Int J Oral Maxillofac Implants 2004;19(suppl):62–72.

45. Belser UC, Buser D, Higginbottom F. Consensus statements and recommended clinical procedures regarding esthetics in implant dentistry. Int J Oral Maxillofac Implants 2004;19(suppl):73–74.

46. Tarnow DP, Elian N, Fletcher P, et al. Vertical distance from the crest of bone to the height of the interproximal papilla between adjacent implants. J Periodontol 2003;74:1785–1788.

47. Orenstien IH, Synan WJ, Truhlar RS, Morris HF, Ochi S. Bone quality in patients receiving endosseous dental implants. DICRG Interim Report No. 1. Implant Dent 1994;3:90–94.

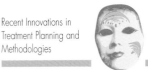

Recent Innovations in
Treatment Planning and
Methodologies

48. Haas R, Donath K, Födinger M, Watzek G. Bovine hydroxyapatite for maxillary sinus grafting: Comparative histomorphometric findings in sheep. Clin Oral Implants Res 1998;9:107–116.

49. Brånemark PI, Hansson BO, Adell R, et al. Osseointegrated implants in the treatment of the edentulous jaw. Experience from a 10-year period. Scand J Plast Reconstr Surg Suppl 1977;16:1–132.

50. Adell R, Eriksson B, Lekholm U, Brånemark PI, Jemt T. Long-term follow-up study of osseointegrated implants in the treatment of totally edentulous jaws. Int J Oral Maxillofac Implants 1990;5:347–359.

51. Rosenquist B, Grenthe B. Immediate placement of implants into extraction sockets: Implant survival. Int J Oral Maxillofac Implants 1996;11:205–209.

52. Grunder U, Polizzi G, Goené R, et al. A 3-year prospective multicenter follow-up report on the immediate and delayed-immediate placement of implants. Int J Oral Maxillofac Implants 1999;14:210–216.

53. Kao RT. Strategic extraction: A paradigm shift that is changing our profession. J Periodontol 2008;79(6):971–977.

Recent Innovations in
Treatment Planning and
Methodologies

Restoring Dental Function and Esthetics

II

Bernard Touati
André P. Saadoun
Tidu Mankoo
Wyman Chan
Sergio Rubinstein
Cobi J. Landsberg
Galip Gürel

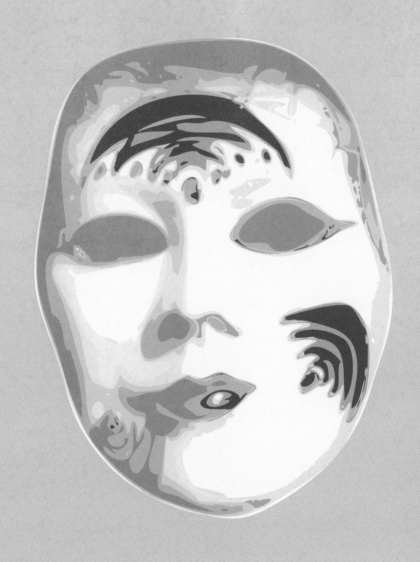

Treatment Planning for Esthetic Anterior Single-Tooth Implants

4

Bernard Touati, DDS, MS

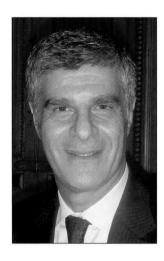

Bernard Touati, DDS, MS

Bernard Touati is a doctor of dental surgery and dental sciences (DDS-MS) and visiting professor at the Hebrew University Hadassah, School of Dental Medicine in Jerusalem. From 1976 to 1985 he was assistant professor in prosthodontics (University of Paris 5). Dr Touati is the past president of the European Academy of Esthetic Dentistry and the founder and past president of the French Society of Esthetic Dentistry. He is also a member of the American Academy of Restorative Dentistry and the American Academy of Esthetic Dentistry. He is the co-academic director of the Global Institute for Dental Education and the editor-in-chief of *Practical Procedures and Aesthetic Dentistry* (USA). Dr Touati is an international lecturer and author of numerous publications all over the world, including the bestselling textbook *Esthetic Dentistry and Ceramic Restorations* (Martin Dunitz, London). He is coeditor of the book *The Art of the Smile* (Quintessence, USA) and main author of the book *Esthetic Integration of Digital Ceramic Restorations* (Montage Media, USA). He has been awarded the Legion of Honor in France.

Email: esthdent@club-internet.fr
       contact@34montaigne.fr

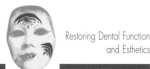

Restoring Dental Function
and Esthetics

Implant dentistry is quite different from restorative dentistry performed on natural teeth in that implant restorations are transmucosal and engage the three-dimensional biologic space. Unlike normal mucosa, which attaches to root surfaces through collagen bundles deeply inserted in the cementum (ie, Sharpey fibers), peri-implant mucosa is only adherent to titanium or zirconium oxide implant surfaces. Therefore, the mechanical resistance of connective tissue adhesion is low, and peri-implant mucosa easily recedes when bone support is deficient. In restorative dentistry, every effort is made to be noninvasive; in implant dentistry, however, the very nature of the specialty requires that the vast majority of procedures be invasive. This chapter provides an overview of some treatment planning principles the clinician should consider for successful esthetic integration of the anterior single-tooth implant with the natural dentition.

Evaluation of Soft Tissue Esthetic Integration

In current clinical practice, the phenomenon of osseointegration is considered a predictable biologic event that is expected of the various materials and designs of available implants. Although hard tissue integration is now a matter of routine, esthetic integration of a dental implant with the surrounding soft tissues remains a challenge for both novice and experienced clinicians to achieve on a predictable basis. The pink esthetic score (PES) is a method designed to provide an objective appraisal of the esthetic appearance of soft tissue around single-tooth implants. With this method, the clinician visually evaluates the following seven anatomic variables in the peri-implant areas and then in the surrounding mucosa of adjacent or contralateral natural teeth[1]:

1. Mesial papilla
2. Distal papilla
3. Soft tissue level
4. Soft tissue contour
5. Soft tissue texture
6. Soft tissue color
7. Alveolar process deficiency

A numeric score (0, 1, or 2) is applied to each variable based on the clinician's visual assessment. The final PES reflects the total of these scores, up to a maximum value of 14. Although the final value may vary from one clinician to another, the PES for a single-tooth implant generally has been found to be a lower value when compared to the PES of a reference natural tooth. The preoperative PES of the implant site can be used as the reference value that can help the clinician determine the potential for successful immediate implant placement and loading or the need for additional procedures to improve soft tissue esthetics for the final restoration.[2]

Prevention of Tissue Recession

In the esthetic zone, implants are primarily indicated *(1)* after tooth loss from trauma or infection or *(2)* in healed sites under a preexisting fixed partial denture or provisional restoration. Because of the circumstances that necessitate implant placement, the surrounding hard and soft tissues are frequently already deficient and unable to mimic the architecture and color of the unaffected gingiva and interdental papillae. The challenge of placing implant-supported restorations that blend in with the natural dentition requires the clinician to establish a perfect treatment plan with a biologic emphasis. To effectively preserve the esthetics, the treatment plan should use whatever appropriate tools and technology are available to maximize the connective tissue volume and avoid tissue recession. Therefore, the clinician's primary objective during the initial consultation is to determine which materials and procedures are necessary to provide a long-term, stable solution to hard or soft tissue deficiencies.

Tissue grafting or regeneration

The gingival biotype is an essential factor in soft tissue management of implants and should be considered at the planning stage. Thin and medium biotypes require special care because they frequently display unesthetic soft tissue recession, sometimes even with perforation. For this reason, the clinician must obtain informed consent from the patient and plan for grafts of biomaterials, autogenous bone, and/or connective tissue before or during implant placement. Grafts serve to thicken hard or soft tissues and thereby provide stability and esthetics to the surrounding implant mucosa. Experience has shown that it is mandatory to graft connective tissue in extraction sites with a thin gingival biotype to avoid medium-term and long-term soft tissue recession.[3] A pouch grafting procedure is preferred to a flap procedure, which results in greater restriction of the blood supply.[3]

Only a few clinical situations allow for conservative treatment that preserves rather than regenerates tissue. One example is an extraction site with a thick gingival biotype and a socket that does not show any loss in crestal bone height and width or any soft tissue recession. As discussed above, when this clinical situation exists in a patient with a thin biotype, preservation alone is not sufficient to provide long-term soft tissue stability, and grafting procedures are required.

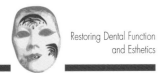

Restoring Dental Function
and Esthetics

Choice of materials

A proper treatment plan for anterior single-tooth implant cases requires the clinician to choose and perform the surgical procedures that allow the peri-implant tissue to be stable and indistinguishable from the adjacent tissue in the long term, even if these procedures are more invasive. In addition, the treatment plan should consider how the following factors will work with the chosen procedure to affect the final outcome optimally:

- Implant type
- Abutment design
- Abutment material
- Schedule for loading the definitive abutment (ie, early loading or delayed loading)
- Provisional restoration submergence profile

The current prosthetic trend is to load definitive abutments as soon as possible, preferably during implant placement, and leave them undisturbed so as not to disrupt the mucosal barrier with multiple implant-abutment disconnections. It is therefore recommended to precisely plan, whenever possible, the final placement of the implant(s) via a model-guided or computer-guided technique. A titanium or, even better, zirconia abutment can be fabricated using computer-aided design/ computer-assisted manufacture (CAD/CAM), inserted at time of surgery, and prescanned. A concave abutment placed transmucosally, such as the Nobel Curvy Abutment (Nobel Biocare), or a platform switching technique thickens the connective tissue and provides better mechanical resistance and stability. This planning requires precision in the diagnostic phase, anticipation of the factors involved in three-dimensional placement of the implant, and the laboratory prefabrication of abutments and provisional restorations.[3]

The proper anatomic placement of the implant should allow the formation of a biologic space that will not affect the esthetic outcome; the PES of the final restoration site should be good or excellent. This generally calls for placement of zirconia abutments (at least in thin and medium gingival biotypes) and all-ceramic restorations, or one-piece screw-retained zirconia-based ceramic restorations, as seen in the following clinical example.

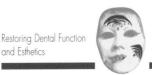

Clinical Case

The clinical example shown in Fig 4-1 demonstrates the successful placement of an implant in the maxillary left central incisor position in a woman in her 60s. Treatment planning included evaluation of hard and soft tissues and the regeneration necessary for long-term stability. After the initial extraction site was allowed to heal with a resin-bonded fixed partial denture for 4 months, a provisional restoration was placed that would allow for soft tissue adaptation over a period of 10 weeks. These procedures, combined with the definitive restoration that was chosen, achieved esthetic soft tissue integration and stability.

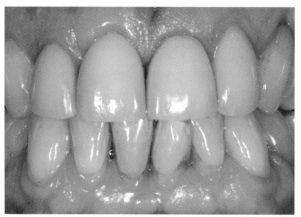

Fig 4-1a Initial clinical presentation of a woman in her 60s; the maxillary left central incisor needs to be extracted.

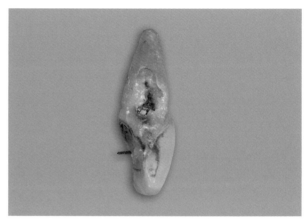

Fig 4-1b After the tooth is extracted, external root resorption can be seen.

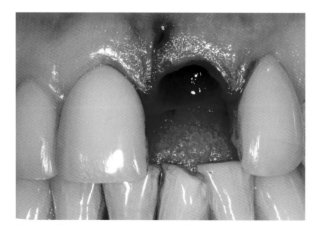

Fig 4-1c The extraction socket displays the buccal bone plate and fistula.

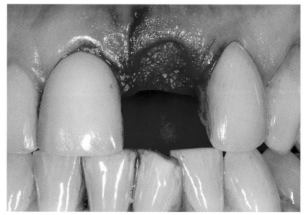

Fig 4-1d Guided bone regeneration using Tarnow's ice cream cone technique for the socket. The ice cream cone technique is aimed at regenerating bone in an extraction socket by placing a membrane along the bone walls (the cone) and filling it with a bone substitute (the ice cream).

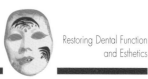

Restoring Dental Function and Esthetics

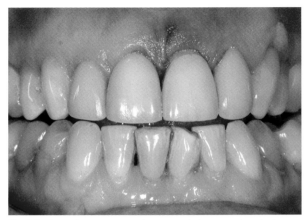

Fig 4-1e Immediate provisionalization with the natural tooth during the regeneration phase.

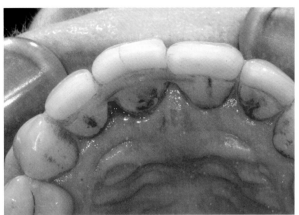

Fig 4-1f Palatal view of the resin-bonded fixed partial denture.

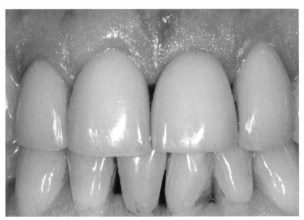

Fig 4-1g Clinical view of the healing site 7 days postoperatively.

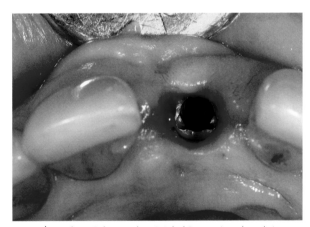

Fig 4-1h Replace Select implant (Nobel Biocare) is placed 4 months after site development.

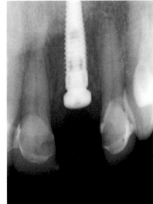

Fig 4-1i Radiograph of the Nobel Curvy provisional abutment with concave transmucosal aspect connected to the implant.

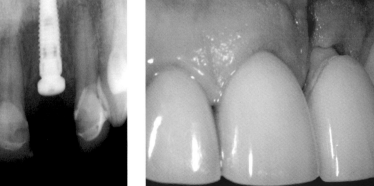

Fig 4-1j Provisional crown is undercontoured cervically to promote soft tissue vertical growth.

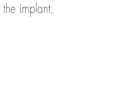

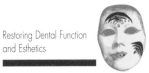

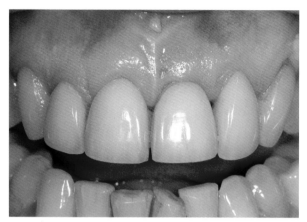

Fig 4-1k Soft tissue healing and thickening 10 weeks after provisionalization.

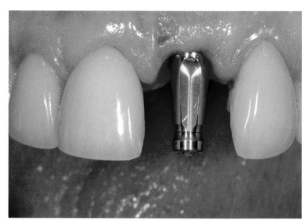

Fig 4-1l Definitive impression coping is placed.

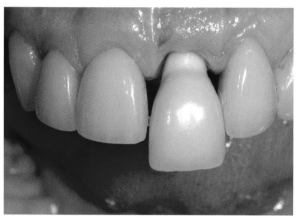

Fig 4-1m The definitive restoration, a Procera (Nobel Biocare) one-piece zirconia-based screw-retained crown with undercontoured transmucosal aspect, is loaded onto the coping.

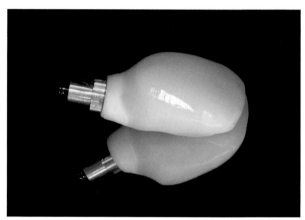

Fig 4-1n Note the submucosal buccal concavity of this monobloc crown.

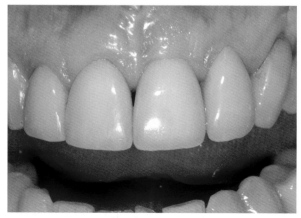

Fig 4-1o Postoperative clinical appearance of soft tissue integration warrants a good PES in relation to the preoperative site.

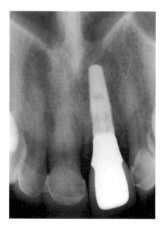

Fig 4-1p Postoperative radiograph of the definitive restoration shows good stability.

Restoring Dental Function and Esthetics

Conclusion

There is no magic recipe for "perfect" treatment that meets the challenge of preserving soft tissue esthetics after an invasive procedure, and several surgical and material options may be clinically successful in different hands. A successful plan that will ultimately allow soft tissue integration should undercontour the transmucosal aspect of the definitive restoration and provide immediate esthetic tissue support after immediate implant placement. Modern implant dentistry must provide patients with long-term stability and optimal esthetics through use of responsible treatment plans that minimize tissue trauma, protect the blood supply, limit the manipulation of prosthetic components, and incorporate biocompatible materials such as titanium and zirconia.

References

1. Fürhauser R, Florescu D, Benesch T, Haas R, Mailath J, Watzek G. Evaluation of soft tissue around single-tooth implant crowns: The pink esthetic score. Clin Oral Implants Res 2005;16(6):639–644.
2. Fürhauser R, Haas R, Mailath-Pokorny J, Watzek G. Prospective Evaluation of Soft Tissue Around Immediate Implant Restorations [Proceedings of the 16th Annual Scientific Congress of the EAO, 25–27 Oct 2007, Barcelona]. Munich: European Association for Osseointegration, 2007.
3. Touati B, Etienne JM, Van Dooren E. Esthetic Integration of Digital Ceramic Restorations. New Jersey: Montage Media, 2008.

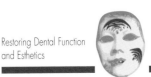

Multifactorial Parameters in Peri-Implant Soft Tissue Management

5

André P. Saadoun,
DDS, MS

Restoring Dental Function
and Esthetics

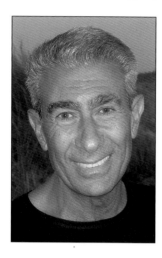

André P. Saadoun, DDS, MS

André Saadoun received his degree in dental surgery from the Faculty of Paris and completed his post-graduate certificate in periodontology at the University of Pennsylvania and his postgraduate certificate in implantology at the University of California in Los Angeles. Dr Saadoun is a faculty member of the Global Institute of Dental Education (Los Angeles) and the Dental XP Program of Education (Atlanta).

He previously served as an associate professor in the Department of Periodontics at the University of Southern California. He is also visiting professor at the Hadassah Jerusalem University.

Dr Saadoun is a diplomate of the American Academy of Periodontology, a diplomate of the International Congress of Oral Implantology, Member of Honor of the American Dental Implant Association, and president of the Rencontres Méditerranéennes de Dentisterie. He received the French Medal of Chevalier de l'Ordre National du Merite.

An internationally renowned lecturer in periodontology and implantology, Dr Saadoun has written more than 150 articles and several book chapters. He is associate editor of the Implant Site Development. He is also on the editorial board of scientific journals including *Practical Procedures and Aesthetic Dentistry, Implant Dentistry, Dental Implantology Update, Journal of Periodontology,* and *European Journal of Esthetic Dentistry.*

Dr Saadoun maintains a private practice in Paris limited to esthetic periodontics and implant surgery.

Email: andre.p.saadoun@wanadoo.fr

Restoring Dental Function
and Esthetics

Implant protocols for the replacement of missing anterior teeth or compromised edentulous ridges have evolved considerably over the years to a less invasive approach. The primary goals of implant treatment have shifted from merely functional replacement of one natural tooth to an esthetically driven, functional replacement of the entire tooth system.[1] At the same time, patient demand for esthetic smile enhancement continues to increase.[2]

Osseointegration is easily obtained if the basic surgical implant principles are respected. Esthetic predictability in the anterior zone is a different issue, however, and a greater challenge due to the variety of anatomical and biologic considerations and patient expectations. The predictability of implant success is related not only to the characteristics of the implant system used but also to the training and experience of the surgical team and their attention to detail during the surgical and prosthetic stages.[3] Esthetic success can be achieved through the development of a systematic treatment approach and proper understanding of the parameters that affect the outcome at the tooth-implant interface.[4] For soft tissue contours to be considered esthetic, they must include (1) a harmoniously scalloped gingival line; (2) a lack of abrupt vertical differences in clinical crown lengths between adjacent teeth; (3) a convex buccal mucosa with sufficient thickness; and (4) distinct papillae.[5] Natural-looking esthetics for single-tooth implants depends on several factors, including the patient's smile line (high/medium/low), gingival margin position, and bone foundation (Fig 5-1). Other influences on esthetics include preoperative and postoperative considerations such as implant design and position, soft and hard tissue profile, and final prosthetic support (Box 5-1). If, upon evaluation of the surgical site, all criteria are met, the primary goal of therapy should be to preserve the favorable hard and soft tissue architecture.[9]

Contemporary implant therapy is based on biologically driven concepts; if the physiologic relationship between different components of tissues is not biologically correct, optimal esthetics cannot be achieved[10,11] (Fig 5-2).

Box 5-1 Keys to success in esthetic implant restoration[6–8]
- Detailed preoperative diagnosis of the smile and surgical site
- Precise and atraumatic surgical technique
- Pre- or perioperative bone preservation/augmentation
- Continuous management of peri-implant soft tissue
- Accurate three-dimensional implant position/angulation
- Acceptable implant stability quotient (ISQ) at insertion and exposure
- Integration mechanism with delayed or immediate placement
- Optimal emergence profile influenced by the abutment/provisional crown
- Regulation of occlusal forces
- Material biocompatibility of the restoration

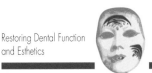

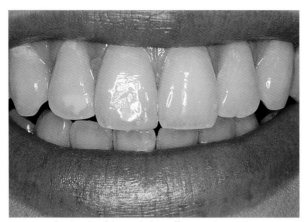

Fig 5-1a The height of the smile line affects implant esthetics.

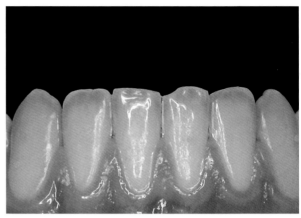

Fig 5-1b The harmony, color, inflammation level, and quality/quantity of gingiva should be evaluated.

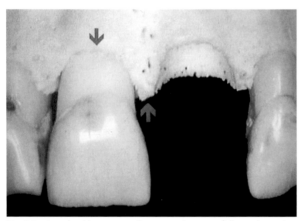

Fig 5-1c In a healthy patient, the gingival margin follows the underlying occlusal/cementoenamel junction (CEJ) contour.

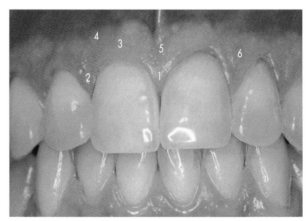

Fig 5-1d Normal tooth shape, position, relationship with bone, gingiva, and proximal contact points are also important factors. Numbers designate the pink esthetic scores (PES).

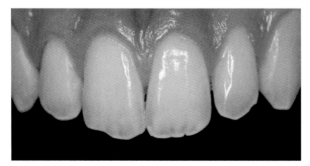

Fig 5-1e Interdental papillae depend on the interproximal bone height and the interproximal teeth contact point.

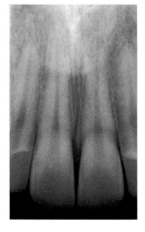

Fig 5-1f The relationship between the contact point and the peak of bone can be observed on a periapical radiograph.

Restoring Dental Function
and Esthetics

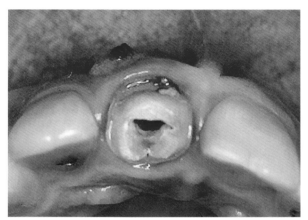

Fig 5-2a Right maxillary central incisor fractured in an accident.

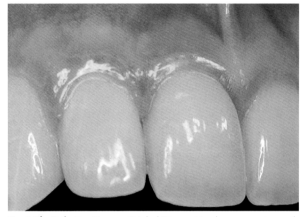

Fig 5-2b Definitive Procera (Nobel Biocare) implant restoration with esthetic stable gingival proximal contour.

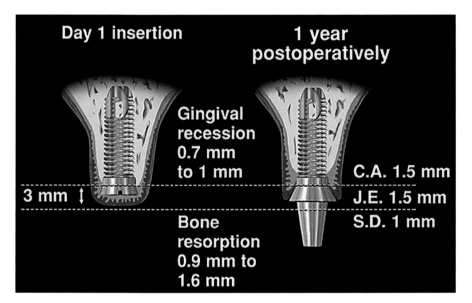

Fig 5-3 The majority of submerged implants lose approximately 0.9 to 1.6 mm of crestal bone after implant abutment connection and in the first year of function. (CA, connective attachment; JE, junctional epithelium; SD, standard deviation.)

Regardless of the procedures or materials used, hard and soft tissue recession will occur (Fig 5-3). The cervical and interproximal crest of bone is traditionally expected to resorb to the first thread of the implant, which flattens the bony crest in addition to the gingival architecture as the papillae follow the bone.[12,13] This resorption is one of the most common parameters evaluated in osseointegrated implant studies and allows the dynamic aspect of peri-implant bone and its reaction to the implant surface to be quantified. One year postoperatively, the bone is usually stable and shows negligible subsequent changes.[14]

Facial soft tissue recession generally occurs in the first year after implant loading.[15] Despite significant differences in experiment design, several studies have concluded that gingival recession is unavoidable, and

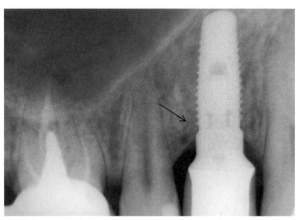

Fig 5-4a Arrow shows interproximal bone loss to the first implant thread. (Restoration by Dr B. Touati, Paris France.)

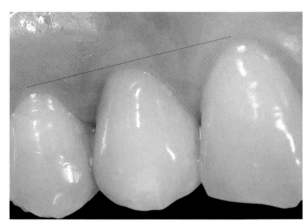

Fig 5-4b Clinical photograph of the same restoration with limited gingival recession. (Restoration by Dr B. Touati, Paris, France.)

most occurs within 6 months postoperatively.[15–17] A majority of sites experience 0.5 to 1.5 mm of recession within 1 month of implant placement or abutment connection. One clinical study reported 1.3 mm of recession from 1 month to 1 year, then an additional loss of 0.4 mm from 1 to 3 years.[18] Another study found an average of 1.6 mm of recession in the mandible and 0.9 mm in the maxilla.[19] Small and Tarnow[16] demonstrated that 50% of soft tissue recession occurs after only 6 weeks (0.6 mm) and reaches a stable level at 9 months. Thick keratinized tissue and areas with large amounts of attached gingiva show less recession. No significant difference has been determined between the two-stage and single-stage surgeries, nor between one- and two-piece implants.

Gingival recession could be related to the gingival biotype, occlusal trauma, pathology, or incorrect position of the implant (Fig 5-4). It could also be induced by the acuity of the facial contours of the abutment-restoration complex or attributed to the resorption of the thin zone of buccal cortical bone. Without a full understanding of the involved biologic parameters, such as maintenance or augmentation of the biologic width, the nature of bone defects and edentulous spaces, interdental papilla, the pink esthetic score (PES), and other related implant factors, no clinician will be able to achieve predictable and stable esthetic success with implant restoration[10] (Fig 5-5). The full preoperative analysis of the patient's biologic profile guides the clinician's diagnosis and treatment plan and is essential to success in esthetic implantology.

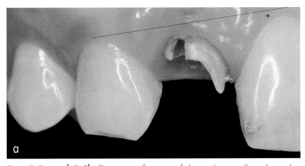
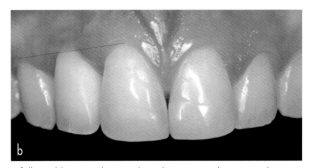

Figs 5-5a and 5-5b Traumatic facture of the right maxillary lateral incisor, followed by immediate implant placement and provisionalization.

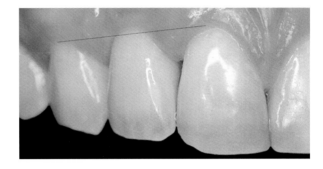

Fig 5-5c Definitive ceramic restoration shows significant gingival recession. (Restoration by Dr B. Touati, Paris, France.)

Implant Considerations

Implant concept evolution

The current trends in esthetic implantology have evolved dramatically in recent years to represent a paradigm shift. Contemporary treatment plans take into consideration issues such as the following features of implant design[20,21]:

- Grooves extending to the top of the collar
- Minimal tissue invasion
- Capacity for immediate placement and loading
- Narrow transgingival components
- Concave transmucosal profile in the abutment design
- Abutment or provisional restoration that provides immediate gingival support
- Biocompatible abutment/restoration
- Reduced load, inducing less bone remodeling

Twenty years ago, the key to management of successful implant therapy followed the concept of "the implant comes to the bone." Open flap procedures were routinely performed to allow visualization of important anatomical structures. One-piece or two-piece implants were used in two-stage surgery that involved submerged placement in stage-one surgery and exposure of the implant in stage-two surgery, necessitating a delayed loading procedure. Time from stage-one to stage-two surgery was 3 months in the mandible and 6 months in the maxilla. Pain, edema, and functional discomfort were common, and the rate of success was 85% to 90%. The overall procedure was complex, and results were not predictable.

Today, the theme of implant therapy is "the bone comes to the implant." In contemporary procedures, flap elevation is limited or eliminated in 50% to 75% of all cases. The majority of patients undergo single-stage surgery, resulting in fewer overall procedures and a reduction in pain and trauma. Now that immediate loading is an option in selected cases, the total treatment time is shorter, although this still involves some risk. Patient comfort, satisfaction, and acceptance of treatment have been significantly improved by modern techniques, and the rate of success is now considered to be greater than 95%. With simplified protocols, the predictability of implant placement and loading is better than ever.

Implant design and components

Morphologic changes have been made in implant design and surface components over the years to increase implant stability during placement.

Implant design

Two types of implant design are currently available. Parallel-walled implants (Fig 5-6a) display a two-piece external abutment connection and a two-piece internal abutment connection, while tapered implants (Fig 5-6b) include a two-piece internal abutment connection and are available with an integrated abutment.

An implant with a slightly tapered design and a double-thread configuration compresses the low-density bone along the entire length of the implant during insertion, preventing bone necrosis while progressively increasing implant stability.[22] This implant design also offers an increased bone-to-implant contact surface. The tapered design, in terms of the consequences of the forces on the peri-implant bone, results in improved osteogenesis versus the parallel-walled implants. Tapered implants also facilitate better primary stability in unfavorable bone types because of the lateral bone compression during insertion.

Anatomically shaped implants, which are adapted to the type of bone density, have improved clinical results and decreased failure rates to 2.3%.[23]

With favorable success rates and stable bone levels, in addition to satisfactory esthetic and soft tissue outcomes, the NobelDirect one-piece implant (Nobel Biocare) is a viable clinical concept that supports the hypothesis that it is possible for one-piece implants to achieve results similar to those of two-piece implants, but with a simpler and more patient-pleasing clinical protocol.[24,25]

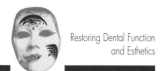

Restoring Dental Function and Esthetics

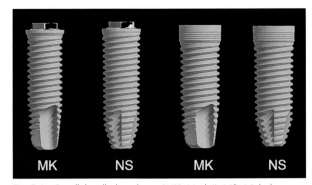

Fig 5-6a Parallel-walled implants. (MK, Mark II; NS, Nobel Speedy.)

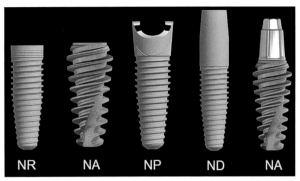

Fig 5-6b Tapered implants. (NR, Nobel Replace; NA, Nobel Active; NP, Nobel Perfect; ND, Nobel Direct.)

The soft tissue color around titanium implants may be affected by the surface characteristics of the implant and abutment.[26] It is possible to improve gingival esthetics by coloring the implant neck, most effectively with light pink, to mask the underlying titanium implant. This may be a feasible approach to establish improved peri-implant soft tissue esthetics.[27]

Innovative implant surfaces, designs, and customized abutments have contributed significantly to the support of crestal soft tissues by helping to engineer the supporting bone and contour the soft tissues. Identification of the form and quantity of the underlying alveolar bone and the surrounding soft tissue biotype, along with meticulous implant placement, improves esthetic predictability.[28] Yet despite these efforts, optimal implant esthetics in the esthetic zone still remains a challenge to the restorative dentist.[29]

Body

Implants with a microthread design emphasize the bone-to-implant contact in the neck area, in comparison with implants without microthreads. These microgrooves allow better healing when the implants are loaded because they increase the available surface area of the implant by up to 15%, improving acceleration of osseointegration by 30% to 50%[30] (Fig 5-7). This is accomplished through the osteoconductive effect of the fibrin clot retention on the implant surface, which reduces healing time regardless of bone type. During the initial osteogenesis and bone remodeling on a TiUnite (Nobel Biocare) implant surface, the bone cells will colonize the microthreads before filling the threads.[31] As a result, more patients with lower bone density are now indicated for implant therapy, and success rates have significantly increased.

Surface

The processing of the implant surface may influence the interaction between the bone and the implant.[32] More bone at the bone-implant

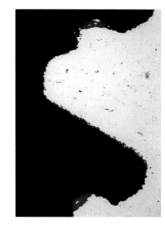

Fig 5-7a The grooves inside the threads of the implant accelerate the osseointegration process (Courtesy of Dr B. Schüpbach and Dr R. Glauser, Zurich, Switzerland.)

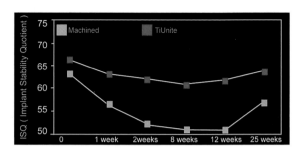

Fig 5-7b Stability of the rough-surface implant versus machined-surface implant over a period of 25 weeks. (Courtesy of Dr R. Glauser, Zurich, Switzerland.)

interface and higher removal torque have been observed with rough-surface implants compared with machined-surface implants.[33] In unfavorable situations, such as poor bone density, a rough-surface implant may provide better results than a smooth-surface implant.

The TiUnite surface of some implants displays the following biomechanical advantages over implants with machined surfaces[34,35]:

- Reduced healing period of 3 to 4 weeks versus 6 to 8 weeks (see Fig 5-7b)
- Higher treatment predictability and failure risk reduction
- New options in advanced clinical indications

Collar

Crestal bone will remodel around the machined junction of an implant. Therefore, subcrestal placement of machined-surface implant collars will result in additional bone loss. The inability of the bone to maintain contact with the machined collar appears to be a factor in the marginal bone loss that occurs in healed sites.[36,37]

No statistically significant difference in bone loss around polished collars has been detected between machined-surface implants (Osseotite [Biomet 3i] and rough-surface implants (TiUnite), or among the various regions of the oral cavity.[38] A rough surface and microthreads at the implant neck increase the bone-implant interface, which not only reduces crestal bone loss[39] but also improves early biomechanical adaptation against loading in comparison with the machined neck design.[40] It is suggested, however, that the progression of peri-implantitis induced by ligature, if left untreated, is more pronounced at implants with a moderately rough surface than at implants with a polished surface.[41]

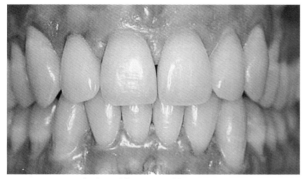

Fig 5-8a Type I: thick and flat gingival biotype.

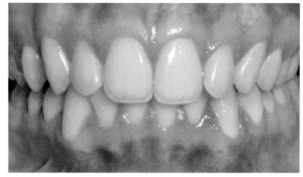

Fig 5-8b Type II: thin and scalloped gingival biotype.

Table 5-1 Classification of biotypes[43]

Class I	Thick biotype	Single tooth	Intact hard and soft tissue
Class II	Thin biotype	Single tooth	Intact hard and soft tissue
Class III	Thick/thin	Multiple teeth	Intact hard and soft tissue
Class IV	Thick/thin	Multiple teeth	Compromised hard or soft tissue

Gingival Biotype

Two gingival biotypes have been described.[42] A thick, flat biotype is referred to as *type I biotype* (Fig 5-8a). This biotype is characterized by *(1)* minimal distance between the gingival margin and the peak of the papilla; *(2)* a flatter, thicker underlying osseous form; *(3)* denser, more fibrous tissue; and *(4)* a larger amount of keratinized attached gingiva. A thin, scalloped biotype is referred to as *type II biotype* (Fig 5-8b). This biotype displays *(1)* a distinct difference in location of the gingival margin versus the peak of the papilla; *(2)* a scalloped osseous form often combined with dehiscences or fenestrations; *(3)* delicate, friable soft tissue; and *(4)* very little keratinized attached gingiva. These types have been further divided into classes (Table 5-1).

Gingival thickness is related to gingival height and thickness of the buccal plate. The thicker the buccal plate, the less bone resorption. The thicker the gingiva, the less gingival recession.[44] A study on peri-implant circumferential biologic space reformation found that thick gingival biotypes experienced internal cortical bone resorption and minimal external resorption.[45] However, no gingival recession and, therefore, no soft tissue deformity occurred (Fig 5-9a). Thin biotypes also experienced

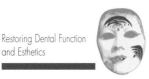

Restoring Dental Function
and Esthetics

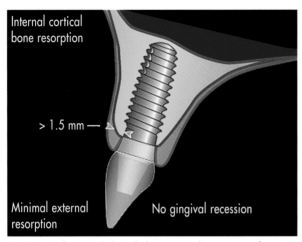

Internal cortical bone resorption

> 1.5 mm —

Minimal external resorption   No gingival recession

Fig 5-9a Biologic and clinical phenomena characteristic of type I biotype.

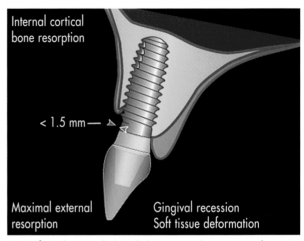

Internal cortical bone resorption

< 1.5 mm —

Maximal external resorption   Gingival recession Soft tissue deformation

Fig 5-9b Biologic and clinical phenomena characteristic of type II biotype.

internal cortical bone resorption, but displayed significant external resorption, gingival recession, and soft tissue deformities (Fig 5-9b). Consequently, any marginal bone remodeling around teeth likely results in no gingival changes in type I biotypes (Figs 5-10a and 5-10b) but induces gingival recession in type II biotypes (Figs 5-10c and 5-10d).

In their study on peri-implant mucosal dimensions on anterior single-tooth implants, Kan et al[46] found that dimensions around a stage-two implant are slightly greater than the dimensions of the mucosa surrounding natural teeth. Thus, the 3- to 6-month postoperative healing period is important for the esthetic zone to achieve maturity and stability of the peri-implant mucosa prior to the final impression-taking procedure and ceramic restoration.

Counterboring during implant site preparation is not recommended, especially with thin and medium biotypes, as it reduces the crestal bone thickness and often affects the biologic space.

If an implant system with a narrow neck is inserted palatally with a soft tissue graft and/or a xenograft added on the buccal side, with an undercontour labial to a transmucosal component, a thin biotype could be artificially modified to a thick biotype and could minimize the gingival recession.[47]

Prior to extraction, the osseous crest around both central incisors, assuming the absence of periodontal disease, roughly follows the scalloped nature of the cementoenamel junctions (CEJs), resulting in an average scallop depth of 3 mm; the average interproximal bone height is 3 mm coronal to the facial crest of bone. Because the soft tissue typically follows the bone, the osseous scallop results in a gingival scallop of 3 mm. When teeth are present, the gingiva on the facial aspect of the tooth is positioned so that, on average, the free gingival margin is 3 mm coronal to the crest of bone. However, the interdental papillae are

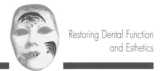

Restoring Dental Function and Esthetics

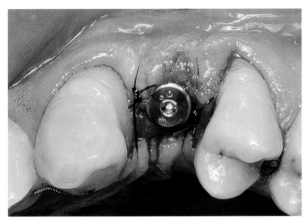

Fig 5-10a Nonsubmerged implant placement in patient with a type I biotype.

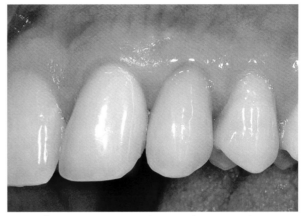

Fig 5-10b Implant restoration with no significant gingival recession. (Restoration by Dr B. Touati, Paris, France.)

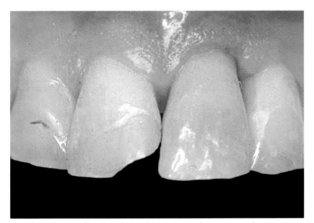

Fig 5-10c Immediate implant placement with provisionalization in a patient with a type II biotype.

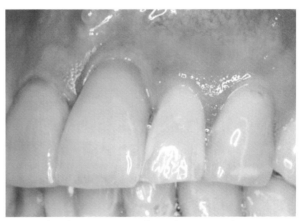

Fig 5-10d Implant restoration with significant gingival recession after 1 year. (Restoration by Dr P. Zyman, Paris, France.)

generally 4.5 to 5.0 mm coronal to the interproximal crest of bone, 1.5 mm on average more coronal to the crest of bone than the facial tissue. This additional 1.5 mm, along with the 3 mm average osseous scallop, results in the tip of the papillae being an average of 4.5 to 5.0 mm coronal to the facial free gingival margin.[48]

It is necessary to understand what happens to the osseous scallop and papilla height above bone after tooth removal and immediate implant placement.[49]

Management of gingiva at implant sites

A minimally invasive approach and proper three-dimensional (3D) implant placement are common requirements for soft tissue management regardless of gingival biotype. While type I biotypes need tissue

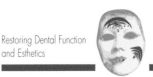

preservation only, type II biotypes may call for augmentation (see Table 5-1). Proper choice of biocompatible abutments and restorations also affects the soft tissue outcomes and allows more esthetic predictability.

Class I and Class II

A negative submergence profile is necessary (flat transmucosal prosthetic component in Class I, undercontour in Class II) for gingival stability in these cases. The clinician should determine whether adequate vertical tissue is available in Class II patients; if not, approaches such as orthodontic extrusion, bone grafting with membrane, or connective tissue grafting should be considered to increase tissue thickness.

Class III and Class IV

The more teeth extracted in the esthetic zone, the more the hard and soft tissues are compromised. This increases the difficulty of the case and often requires site reconstruction (guided bone regeneration or connective tissue grafting), strategic placement and quantity of implants, or further pontic site development.

Biologic width

Numerous articles have described the existence of the soft tissue barrier, often called *biologic width,* and its impact on the long-term functional and esthetic success of treatment.[50,51] Biologic width separates the internal and external environments, whether it surrounds a natural tooth or implants (Fig 5-11). The epithelium and the connective tissues contribute to the establishment of the tissue interface, which may prevent infiltration of oral bacteria and their byproducts. The formation of biologic width depends on gingival tissue thickness before implant placement, and crestal bone loss may occur during this process in cases with thin gingival tissue.[52]

Natural teeth

The biologic width is a 3D anatomical and histologic structure always supracrestal around natural teeth.[53] The biologic width surrounding the natural tooth consists of 1 mm of hemidesmosomes (junctional epithelium) and 1 mm of connective tissue attachment (Sharpey fibers), which comprises bundles of collagen fibers that insert in the root cementum in a direction perpendicular to the tooth. These collagen fibers cannot be stretched or compressed without violating the biologic width.

The biologic width is rich in cells, fibroblasts, and blood vessels, and follows the scalloped contour of the CEJ. It helps to contour the cervical bone crest, and upon probing, the tip of the periodontal probe will stop at the apical part of the junctional epithelium.

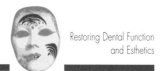

Restoring Dental Function and Esthetics

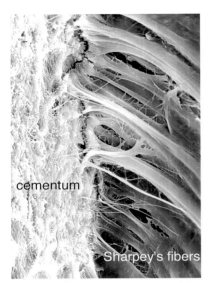

Fig 5-11a Electron microscope view of the biologic width around the natural tooth showing the Sharpey fibers. (Courtesy of Dr P. Schüpbach, Zurich, Switzerland.)

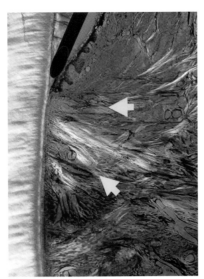

Fig 5-11b Electron microscope view of the biologic width around the natural tooth showing the perpendicular direction of the Sharpey fibers (arrows). (Courtesy of Dr P. Schüpbach, Zurich, Switzerland.)

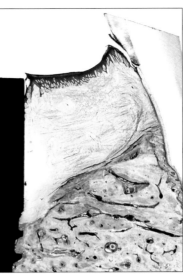

Fig 5-12 Biologic width around an implant on the left side with circumferential fibers and a tooth on the right side with perpendicular fibers. (Courtesy of Dr P. Schüpbach, Zurich, Switzerland.)

Titanium implants

The biologic width always occurs subcrestally around the implant[35,54–57] (Fig 5-12). The biologic width around implants includes the junctional epithelium at a depth of 2.40 mm in machined implants and 1.09 mm in rough-surface implants. Connective tissue is generally 1.50 mm in machined implants and 1.31 mm in rough-surface implants. No significant difference has been found between one- and two-piece implants, or those placed with single-stage or two-stage surgery. The biologic width follows the circular flat implant platform and contours the implant abutment junction. Upon probing, the tip of the periodontal probe will stop at the coronal part of the bone crest.

Dense collagen longitudinal fibers and circular bundles are seen around the implant surface, but unlike in natural teeth, they form in a parallel direction as they do not have any cementum into which they can insert.[54,58] These fiber bundles are rich in collagen but poor in cells, fibroblasts, and blood vessels. This results in mucosal scar tissue adhesion, weak anchorage, and poor mechanical resistance. The fibers can be stretched or compressed without violating the biologic width.

The connective tissue attachment around implants shows functional orientation (longitudinal cut) and circumferential orientation (perpendicular cut). Because no true anchorage of supra-alveolar connective tissue can occur on the implant, a brittle adhesion substitutes. As the connective tissue interface is considered of paramount importance to support the epithelium and block its apical migration, this lack of

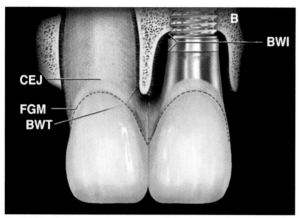

Fig 5-13a Schematic representation of the biologic width around an implant and adjacent tooth. B, bone; BWI, implant biologic width; CEJ, cementoenamel junction; FGM free gingival margin; BWT, tooth biologic width. (Courtesy of Dr N. Elian and Dr D. Tarnow, New York, NY.)

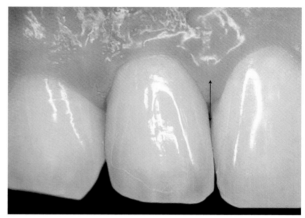

Fig 5-13b Clinical interdental papilla regeneration (arrow) adjacent to the implant restoration. (Courtesy of Dr B. Touati, Paris, France.)

mechanical resistance can potentially endanger the prognosis of dental implants. Tearing can occur at the connective tissue–implant interface as a consequence of mastication or a lack of soft tissue stability, which can then induce an apical migration of the junctional epithelium, bone resorption and pocket formation, or gingival recession.[21] Bacterial invasion is more destructive around implants than around natural teeth because of the limited peri-implant vascularization.

Rough-surface implants (eg, TiUnite) have exhibited less epithelial downgrowth, a smaller connective tissue seal, and less bone remodeling than machined-surface implants.[59]

Biologic Width Relationships

Tooth-implant relationship

When an implant is correctly placed adjacent to a tooth with a healthy periodontium, the interproximal bone is maintained at its original level because the biologic width at the tooth site remains undisturbed (Fig 5-13). Less than 5 mm between the implant-tooth contact point and the crest of interproximal bone results in a papilla similar to that between two teeth with a healthy periodontium.

Implant-implant relationship

The challenge of multiple implant placement occurs when adjacent teeth are already missing or need to be removed (Fig 5-14). Consider the loss of two maxillary central incisors and the response of the papillae origi-

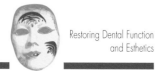

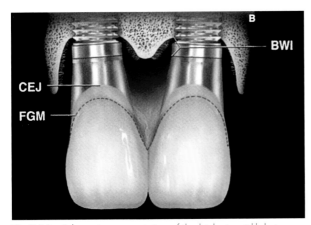

Fig 5-14a Schematic representation of the biologic width between two adjacent implants. B, bone; BWI, implant biologic width; CEJ, cementoenamel junction; FGM, free gingival margin. (Courtesy of Dr N. Elian and Dr D. Tarnow, New York, NY.)

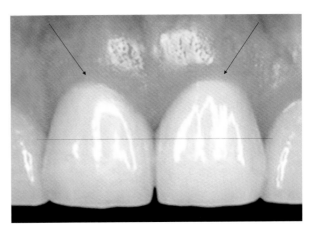

Fig 5-14b Clinical view of central incisors inter-implant papilla regeneration apical to the proximal papilla adjacent to the natural teeth (arrows indicate implant restorations).

nally between these teeth and the adjacent remaining lateral incisors. The interproximal bone on the lateral incisors determines the papilla height between the central and lateral incisors. The facial bone level and tissue thickness at each central incisor site will determine the final facial gingival margin. In addition, just as in the single-tooth situation, if the final facial gingival margin is less than ideal, it is much easier to augment height and thickness on both central incisors with a soft tissue procedure than it is to improve the papilla height. The real challenge in implant placement at the central incisor location is to evaluate what happens to the papillae afterwards.[60,61] Maintenance of the interproximal crest of bone is critical to preservation of the height of the papilla between adjacent implants. To do this, 3 mm of space must be retained between the platforms of the adjacent implants.[62] It is also necessary to understand that, as stated earlier, papilla height is 4.5 to 5.0 mm above bone between a tooth and an adjacent implant.

It appears that when adjacent implants are placed, the papilla height above the bone reduces from 4.5 mm to between 3.0 and 3.5 mm.[62] With the conventional two-piece implant, approximately 1.0 to 1.5 mm of peri-implant bone loss generally occurs up to the first thread in the first year following implant exposure and restoration. With a one-piece implant, there is no gap between implant and abutment at the bone proximity, and bone resorption is limited to approximately 0.7 mm in the first year. Even if the interproximal crest of bone is maintained, the inter-implant papilla will end up 1.0 to 1.5 mm apical to its original level, simply from the change in soft tissue levels. If this 1.0- to 1.5-mm difference is added to any reduction in interproximal crestal bone height, it is easy to comprehend why the maintenance of inter-implant papilla height is different.[48]

Only 2.3 to 4.0 mm of soft tissue height (average 3.4 mm) can be expected to form over the inter-implant crest of the bone. To compensate for the missing papilla, the contact point between two implant restorations should be moved apically, or the interproximal bone height increased. This modification is mandatory because of insufficient interproximal tissue.[60]

The implant is placed so that the platform is level with the facial crest of bone. However, since the bone is scalloped, the interproximal platform of the implant may be as much as 3 mm apical to the interproximal crest of bone. It is recommended to leave the implant collar above the bone crest to minimize bone resorption after abutment connection and implant restoration.

Biologic space regeneration

The mechanisms of protection in the peri-implant bone/mucosa correspond to those in the gingiva surrounding a tooth. In esthetic zone sockets, thin buccal bone exhibits a tendency to resorb until its thickness is stabilized. If the implant is placed at the same buccopalatal position as the natural tooth, it will often have insufficient buccal bone thickness (0.5 to 1.0 mm). Between the regeneration of the biologic space (height and width) and upon loading, however, the cervical bone will experience resorption around the neck of the implant to reestablish the biologic space.

If the vestibular bone wall is less than 2 mm, it will resorb apically in patients with a thin biotype. The result is gingival recession, buccal bone concavities, deformed ridge contour, compromised tissue color, and poor esthetics. If the buccal bone wall is thicker than 2 mm, an infrabony defect will develop around the implant collar.

In the presence of keratinized mucosa, collagen fibers tend to be perpendicular to the implant surface, which may result in better anchorage of the implant. Implants that are placed within mobile, non-keratinized lining mucosa, however, have collagen fibers oriented mostly parallel to the implant surface. Functionally oriented fibers may impede the downgrowth of the junctional epithelium and result in an osteoclastic remodeling of the alveolar bone crest. Without cementum to anchor the collagen fibrils, the mechanism for implant-fiber anchorage is clearly different from that in the natural dentition. The mechanical interlocking of the collagen fibers in the pores of the oxidized implants may improve anchorage.

The surface texture of implants may substantially affect the orientation of connective tissue collagen fibers at the implant surface. Perpendicularly oriented collagen fibers are found, in particular, when the surface contains microscopic irregularities (eg, acid-etched surfaces or porosities in plasma-sprayed titanium surfaces).[57]

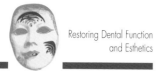

This biologic process should be explained to the patient prior to the implant treatment. Patients with a type I biotype should be informed of the risk of longer implant restoration due to the probability of gingival recession and the need for surgical augmentation of hard or soft tissues or a restoration on the adjacent tooth.[63]

Forced eruption

Implant placement, especially in a type I biotype, is sometimes impossible because of the complexities of bone and soft tissue augmentation necessary to increase tissue thickness, height, stability, and esthetic predictability. The clinician could relocate the hard and soft tissues orthodontically by forced eruption (1 mm per month). This procedure is performed until the tooth is extracted and the thin soft tissue has gained vertical thickness nonsurgically, at which time immediate placement and provisionalization can be done[64] (Fig 5-15).

Forced eruption relocates the bone housing and keratinized gingiva coronally within certain limits.[65] Advantages of this nonsurgical approach include prevention of bone resorption after extraction and enhancement of poor soft tissue levels (gingival recession, missing papillae with inadequate interproximal bone).

The orthodontic extrusion technique requires (1) an active movement period of 8 weeks to increase hard and soft tissue by 4 to 5 mm and (2) a stabilization time of 4 to 6 months to maintain the new hard and soft tissue levels.[43] Overcorrection is necessary to compensate for the approximately 1 mm of peri-implant bone loss (up to the first thread) and the soft tissue recession that occurs within the first year of implant loading. The definitive restoration with a negative emergence profile is placed 3 months after the stabilization period. Loading time does not seem to significantly affect the degree of osseointegrated bone-to-implant contact or the composition of newly formed peri-implant bone.

Extraction timing and implant placement

Treatment or extraction of a tooth in the esthetic zone is often a complex test of the clinical team's knowledge and ability to reach the ultimate goal of an esthetic and functional restoration that will last for years to come. All of this must be done with the patient's emotional and financial status taken into account.[66]

Restoration and maintenance of the health, function, and esthetics of soft tissue around single-tooth implants depend mainly on integrity of the attachment apparatus of the adjacent teeth. The collagen fibers normally function as the supportive network required to maintain function and form in hard and soft tissue around natural teeth. Extraction destroys these adjacent collagen fibers.[67]

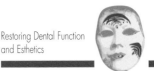

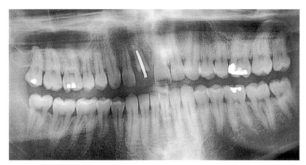

Fig 5-15a Pretreatment panoramic radiograph showing a fractured right maxillary central incisor with a long post core.

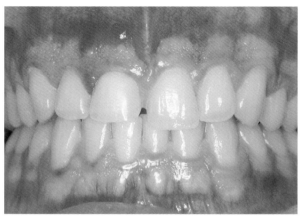

Fig 5-15b Clinical photograph of the restored tooth treated with a post and core.

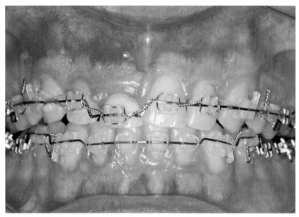

Fig 5-15c Forced eruption is begun using buccal brackets. Note the coronal position of the gingival margin on the right central incisor.

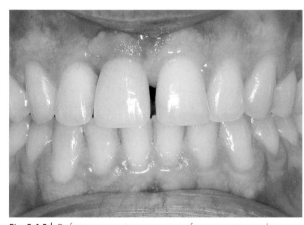

Fig 5-15d Definitive ceramic restoration after extraction and immediate implant placement. Note the perfect gingival harmony between the two central incisors.

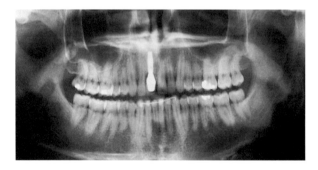

Fig 5-15e Final panoramic radiograph showing the implant and the ceramic restoration. (Orthodontics by Dr E. Serfaty, Paris, France.)

The inability of connective tissue fibers to insert into implant surfaces dictates the inferiority of the "implant zone of connective tissue contact" compared with the natural dental connective tissue attachment and its ability to resist infection and support and maintain the configuration, texture, and color of the periodontal and gingival tissues.

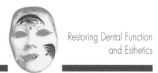

Restoring Dental Function and Esthetics

The loss of a single anterior tooth can be difficult for almost any patient, but replacing it with an implant or a fixed partial denture results in a predictable esthetic outcome unless significant hard and soft tissue were also lost. The loss of multiple anterior teeth, especially if they were adjacent, is a much larger esthetic challenge that often requires the combination of implants and ovate pontics to achieve an acceptable esthetic result. Accounting for this difference are the biology of the periodontium and the response of the bone and soft tissues when one tooth versus multiple teeth are lost.[48]

Biologic healing process considerations

The risk of adverse esthetic outcomes for implants placed into extraction sockets must be carefully evaluated by the clinician. Vertical soft tissue is a contour-correlated behavior with marginal bone modeling, which is a significant issue in the esthetic zone. Most bone remodeling occurs within 3 to 6 months of tooth extraction.[68,69]

Implant placement timing should be based on the morphologic, dimensional, and histologic changes that result from several biologic processes (intra-alveolar and extra-alveolar) that always follow tooth extraction.[70] These include a combination of horizontal and vertical bone growth into the socket and alveolar ridge resorption. Those alterations are more pronounced during the first 3 months postextraction. Long-term absence of teeth leads to a ridge collapse within 3 to 12 months and can also reduce the ridge height so that implant placement becomes a challenge.

Postextraction (Fig 5-16a), the greatest amount of bone loss occurs in the horizontal dimension and is more pronounced on the buccal side. Vertical resorption is also a significant risk factor in the buccal plate. Postextraction resorption can be prevented using immediate implant placement, early delayed placement,[71,72] or a socket preservation procedure.[73,74] The thinner the buccal plate, the greater the reduction of the buccopalatal/buccolingual ridge dimension. The result is a buccal concavity and a loss of height that has clinical ramifications.[75]

After bone resorption, the diminished arch form also reduces the mesiodistal distance of the interproximal bony spaces, affects the health and quality of the interdental papillae, and jeopardizes the definitive esthetic outcome.

When teeth are extracted in the esthetic zone, grafting of the ridge may be a prerequisite to maximize the esthetic outcome. Careful postextraction circumferential examination of the alveolus is essential. If the socket walls are thick and intact, ridge preservation should not be necessary since the surrounding bone walls may be able to withstand postoperative resorption. If a dehiscence, a fenestration, or a thin bone wall is observed, ridge preservation/augmentation should be performed to

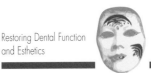

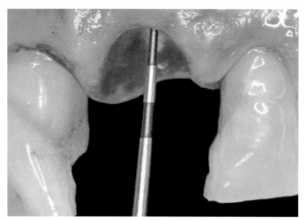

Fig 5-16a Buccal cortical bone sounding should always be done after an extraction.

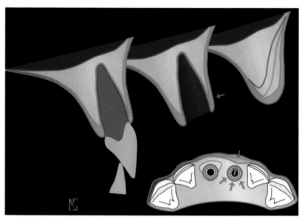

Fig 5-16b Following tooth extraction, osseous and gingival tissue contours are negatively impacted by bone resorption.

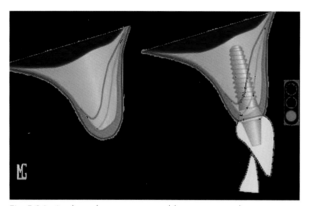

Fig 5-16c Implant placement is possible in an optimal position (green light).

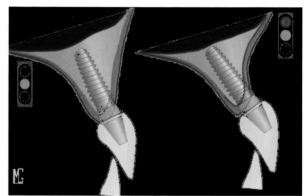

Fig 5-16d Implant placement may be possible with some resorption (yellow light) or may not be possible if bone volume is insufficient (red light).

minimize changes in the ridge dimensions. If the socket is left to heal without grafts and no ridge preservation is performed, the following scenarios can be clinically encountered (Figs 5-16b to 5-16d):

- Implant placement may be possible in an ideal position, but a bone dehiscence may occur at implant placement because of insufficient bone volume, thus requiring a regenerative procedure.
- Implant placement may be possible, but in a nonideal position, and the functional and esthetic restoration may be compromised.
- Implant placement may not be possible because of a lack of sufficient bone volume, thus requiring a ridge augmentation procedure prior to implant placement.[43]

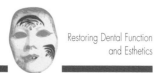

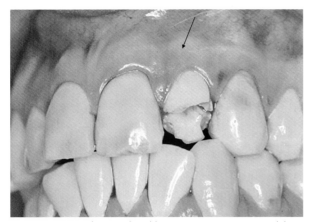

Fig 5-17a Optimal gingival and bone contour *(arrow)* around the fractured left lateral incisor.

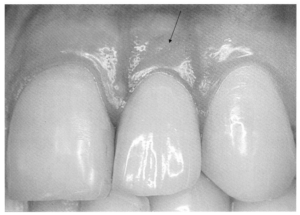

Fig 5-17b Immediate implant placement and provisionalization did not prevent buccal bone resorption and related gingival deformity/recession *(arrow)*.

The postextraction resorption of the thin buccal bone around prominent maxillary roots results in a deformed localized edentulous ridge, which can be a challenge for optimal implant placement. Inclusion of osteoconductive Bio-Oss grafting material (Geistlich) at the time of the extraction is beneficial to the patient, as its use has been reported to result in a loss of less than 20% of the buccal plate in 80% of cases.[76] Immediate implant placement may not limit the postextraction resorption process. The peri-implant bone resorption is more important when the cortical alveolar sockets are thin and close to the implant collar (Fig 5-17).

Final implant selection should take into consideration the mesiodistal space and the confines of the tooth socket and should avoid the coronal portion at the labial plate in order to prevent its perforation, bone resorption, and soft tissue recession. The implant is placed into sound bone along the palatal wall of the extraction site, 1 to 2 mm away from the buccal wall of the socket.[77] This will avoid trauma to the buccal plate and allow the gap to be filled with an allograft material. Therefore, for an optimal buccopalatal position, the first drilling must be more palatal, and the emergence profile is on the cingulum.

The need for bone grafting depends on the thickness of the labial plate rather than the size of the gap. Although a thick labial plate is generally resistant to resorption and grafting is unnecessary, allograft bone grafting is frequently used to prevent collapse and minimize resorption of the buccal labial plate, regardless of the gap size.[6] Maintaining a gap of less than 1.5 mm between the implant and the labial plate may facilitate secondary bone fill with an autogenous blood clot and establish a thicker, more stable bone, thus increasing resistance to bone resorption.[78,79] Evaluations of the bone-implant interface after gap induction of various dimensions have indicated that gaps greater than

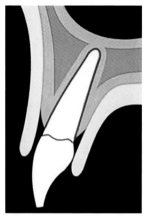 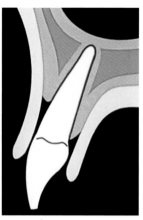 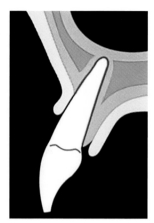

Fig 5-18a Classification of extraction sockets. In a type I defect, facial soft tissue and bone are present at a normal level.

Fig 5-18b In a type II defect, soft tissue is present, but buccal bone is reduced or partially missing. (Modified from Elian et al.[60] Reprinted with permission.)

Fig 5-18c A type III defect has missing buccal soft and hard tissue.

2 mm do not spontaneously fill with bone when bone grafting and guided tissue regeneration are not performed.[80,81]

Care is taken not to involve the buccal alveolar plate and to leave a space of at least 2 mm between the implant shoulder and buccal wall for all implant placements. This gap is filled with an autogenous bone graft and xenograft mixed with platelet-rich plasma (PRP) after immediate implant placement.

Careful preparation of the osteotomy and the palatal socket wall in the esthetic zone should be undertaken to place the implant with maintenance of a horizontal defect depth of 2 mm. Oversized implants that fill the socket or reduce this depth to less than 2 mm should be avoided.

The extent of the horizontal resorption may be limited to 25% of the original buccal dimension with the use of anorganic bone grafts and/or barrier membranes. The relationship between remodeling in the buccal crestal bone region and soft tissue esthetic outcomes is unknown.[82]

Classification of extraction sockets

Different extraction classifications have been described, but the simplest practical one is based on the pre-extraction defect morphology of the site.[74]

In a type I defect, the facial soft tissue and buccal plate of bone of the tooth are at normal levels in relation to the CEJ and remain intact postextraction (Fig 5-18a). Type I sockets are the easiest and most predictable sockets to treat if the soft tissue biotype is thick and flat, in contrast to a thin, highly scalloped biotype.[46]

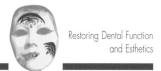

Restoring Dental Function and Esthetics

Type II defects, in which soft tissue is present but buccal bone is reduced, are the most difficult to diagnose. These lead to a less-than-ideal esthetic result, particularly when immediate implant placement is performed (Fig 5-18b). The socket repair technique uses a resorbable membrane on the internal wall of the alveolar buccal cortical bone that covers a slow-resorbing allograft material condensed in the alveolar socket.[74]

Type III defects have markedly reduced facial soft tissue and buccal bone (Fig 5-18c). These sockets are very difficult to treat and require soft tissue augmentation with additional connective tissue or bone–connective tissue grafts in a staged approach to rebuild lost tissue.[71]

Implant placement timing

Hard tissue management could be performed before the start of and during stage-one surgery; and soft tissue management could be performed either before or during stage-one or stage-two surgery.[83] However, the sooner the soft tissue surgical procedures are performed, the better the final gingival level should be achieved.

Site development prior to implant placement

The simplified socket repair technique procedure is as follows[74]:

1. The hopeless tooth is extracted.
2. A collagen membrane is contoured into a modified V shape.
3. The membrane is placed into the socket lining on the internal side of the buccal bone.
4. Allograft material is delivered into the socket.
5. The membrane is sutured to the palatal tissue with absorbable sutures.
6. The buccal tissue is prevented from migrating into the healing socket.
7. A bonded provisional crown with an ovate pontic is placed.
8. The implant is placed 6 months postextraction.
9. After implant exposure, a healing abutment or implant abutment is placed with the provisional crown.
10. Final restoration with natural esthetics is placed after gingival maturation.

Complex site development (Fig 5-19) is necessary when the patient presents with a combination of high lip line and gummy smile, thin biotype with multiple teeth displaying class I or II gingival recession, and/or soft tissue defect with horizontal/vertical resorption of the edentulous ridge.

In this procedure, AlloDerm membrane (BioHorizons) is inserted below the buccal flap on the labial plate to prevent labial cortical bone resorption or to cover the existing gingival recession with an advanced coronal flap.

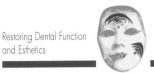

Fig 5-19a Right lateral view of missing maxillary left central incisor in a patient with a high lip line, gummy smile, and multiple areas of gingival recession.

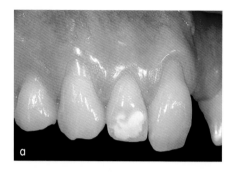
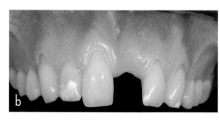

Fig 5-19b Anterior view showing the gingival disharmony between the crest and adjacent teeth.

Fig 5-19c Left lateral view of deformed ridge covered with thin gingiva.

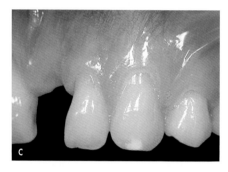
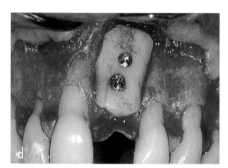

Fig 5-19d Retromolar bone graft screwed and fixed to the ridge defect with two screws.

Fig 5-19e AlloDerm membrane (BioHorizons) sutured over the bone graft and used to cover multiple exposed roots.

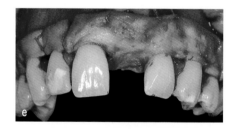
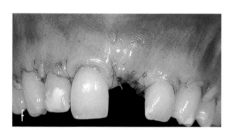

Fig 5-19f Advanced coronal flap sutured over the bone graft and AlloDerm membrane.

Fig 5-19g Anterior view of convex edentulous crest with full coverage of the multiple recessions 6 months later.

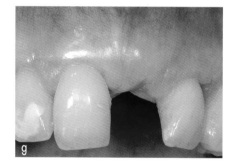
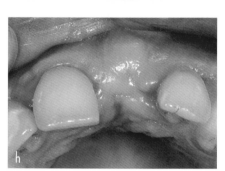

Fig 5-19h Occlusal view of developed site ready for implant placement. (Surgery by Dr M. Silberg, Robinson Township, PA.)

If a bone defect is encountered, implant placement may not be possible, and bone grafting with a fixed membrane will be necessary before an implant can be placed.[84] A major disadvantage of this staged approach is the duration of treatment with the following sequences for site development prior to implant placement:

- 3 to 9 months postextraction for bone block, guided bone regeneration, or connective tissue graft
- Implant placement 6 months later

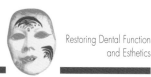

- Provisionalization/definitive restoration
- Soft tissue esthetics stability

Autogenous graft procedures or barrier membranes alone do not appear to improve crestal ridge preservation around implants.[85] Local bone grafting seems to create sufficient bone volume for implant placement after 6 months, but individual variations in resorption pattern and other complications make the grafting procedure unpredictable for long-term prognosis.[86] Therefore, significant resorption of the autogenous graft may be present, which reduces the impact of grafting on the esthetic outcome.[87] A Bio-Oss allograft with Bio-Gide membrane (Geistlich) prevents and limits resorption of an autogenous onlay graft.[88]

Submerged two-stage

The submerged two-stage approach (Fig 5-20) consists of the following steps[72]:

1. Delayed implant placement 2 to 3 months postextraction; late implant placement 4 to 6 months postextraction
2. Hard/soft tissue architecture reconstruction accomplished in conjunction with implant placement as necessary
3. Submerged implant placed with bone/connective tissue graft
4. Implant exposure 6 to 9 months later
5. Abutment connected to the implant and placement of the provisional crown
6. Definitive restoration placed 3 to 6 months later
7. Interproximal support re-established

Nonsubmerged single-stage

This approach considers the 3D position of the implant and allows the placement of a one-piece implant or a two-piece implant with a healing abutment with the following procedure (Fig 5-21):

1. Flapless extraction
2. Hard/soft tissue architecture preservation
3. Interproximal support preservation
4. 3D implant placement
5. Abutment connected to the implant and placement of the provisional crown
6. Definitive restoration placed 6 months later

Immediate implant placement

The implant housing should have adequate bone height on the interproximal surfaces of the teeth to support the formation of papillae. The

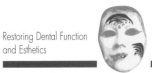

Fig 5-20a Mobile maxillary right central incisor.

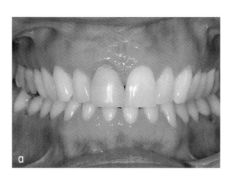
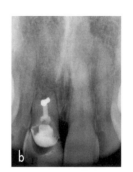

Fig 5-20b Periapical radiograph showing apical root resorption of the right central incisor.

Fig 5-20c The central incisor is extracted employing a minimally traumatic technique.

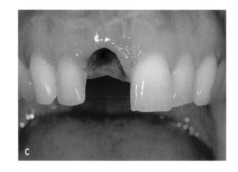
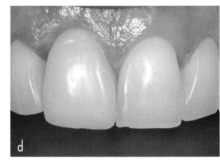

Fig 5-20d Bonded bridge with convex pontic to replace the extracted tooth.

Fig 5-20e Envelope flap showing surgical bone dehiscence.

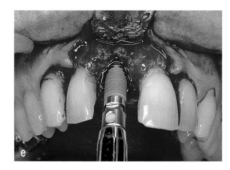
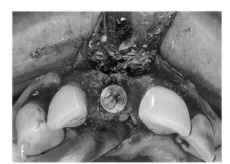

Fig 5-20f Implant in place with the thin facial bone.

Fig 5-20g Bone graft is placed in the socket and over the buccal plate.

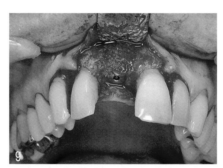

Fig 5-20h Flap closure. (Surgery by Dr M. Salama, Atlanta, GA.)

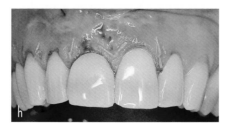
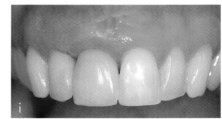

Fig 5-20i Definitive implant-supported ceramic restoration. (Restoration by Dr H. Salama, Atlanta, GA.)

Restoring Dental Function and Esthetics

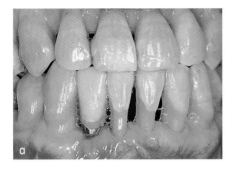

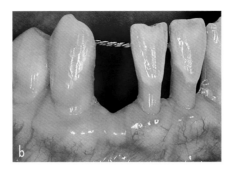

Fig 5-21a Loose mandibular right lateral incisor with a metal-ceramic restoration.

Fig 5-21b Ridge aspect after 8 weeks of healing following extraction of the tooth.

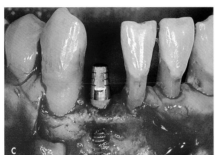

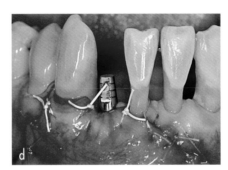

Fig 5-21c Flap elevation and placement of one-piece implant.

Fig 5-21d Bone graft and resorbable membrane are placed over the fenestration defect before closure of the flap.

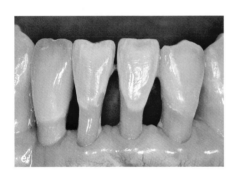

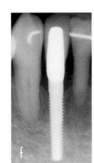

Fig 5-21e Definitive implant-supported ceramic restoration.

Fig 5-21f Postoperative radiograph of the implant restoration. (Surgery by Dr S. Leziy, Vancouver, BC. Restoration by Dr B. Miller, Vancouver, BC.)

buccopalatal bone should permit implant placement in a position and orientation that approaches that of the adjacent tooth with respect to the mesiodistal interproximal bone.[89]

A gap is generally left between the facial/coronal portion of the implant and the extraction socket to minimize contact trauma to the labial bone during osteotomy and placement of the correct implant design. A gap of less than 2 mm between the collar and the alveolar border seems to limit bone resorption because this gap fills with new bone during the healing process.[90] If the gap is more than 2 mm, an allograft is necessary.[91]

Therefore, in immediate implant placement after extraction, the clinician should ensure that the implant is placed slightly to the palatal aspect in order to avoid trauma to the buccal plate and allow an allograft to fill in the gap (Fig 5-22). An optimal buccopalatal position requires that the first drilling be more palatal, and the emergence is on the cingulum.

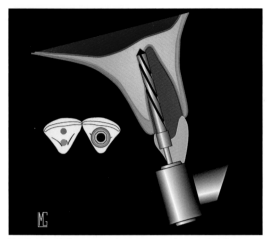

Fig 5-22a Following tooth extraction, the initial drilling should be done on the palatal wall of the socket.

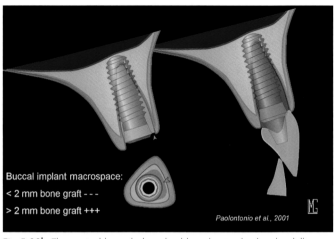

Buccal implant macrospace:
< 2 mm bone graft - - -
> 2 mm bone graft +++

Paolontonio et al., 2001

Fig 5-22b The cortical buccal plate should not be involved in the drilling nor touched by the implant.

Immediate implant placement after extraction in the esthetic zone presents several challenges[49,92–94]:

- Esthetic, because of the visibility of the restoration
- Functional, because of its impact on anterior guidance
- Phonetic, because of the tongue support on the palatal surface
- Psychologic, because of the patient's postoperative comfort
- Timing, because implant placement must be planned along with the extraction

Flapless surgery in extraction sites (Fig 5-23) and healed sites (Fig 5-24) with nonfunctional provisionalization has many advantages[95–97]:

- Critical preservation of the facial bone/maintenance of socket vascular supply
- Maintenance of the architectural form of the restorative gingival interface
- Preservation or improvement of esthetics
- Optimization of implant length using the primary native bone beyond the apex
- Primary stability and healing with full osseointegration
- Immediate placement of transmucosal abutment
- Immediate insertion of provisional restoration
- Patient's psychologic acceptance because of increased comfort and esthetics
- Placement of the definitive restoration 3 to 6 months later for single implant
- Placement of the definitive restoration 8 to 12 weeks later for multiple implants

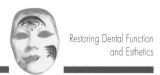

Restoring Dental Function
and Esthetics

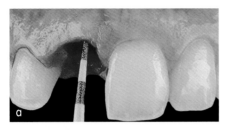
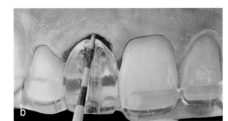

Fig 5-23a In extraction sites, the buccal cortical plate is evaluated immediately postextraction.

Fig 5-23b A surgical guide identifies the precise 3D position of the implant to the gingival margin.

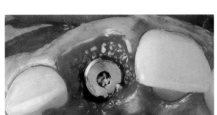
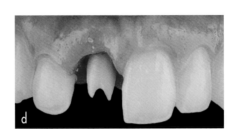

Fig 5-23c Xenograft is added in the gap between the implant and the buccal cortical plate.

Fig 5-23d The zirconia abutment is placed immediately after xenograft is added.

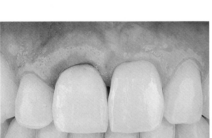
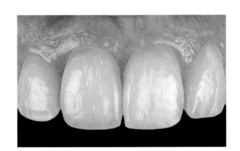

Fig 5-23e Placement of the provisional crown.

Fig 5-23f The definitive Procera restoration is placed 6 months later.

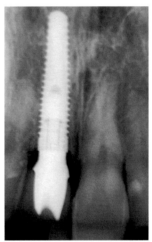

Fig 5-23g Postoperative radiograph showing bone at the same initial level. (Surgery and restoration by Dr M. Groissman, Rio de Janeiro, Brazil.)

Extraction and treatment planning recommendations

The clinician must be aware of the treatment limitations and should be able to predict the outcome prior to determining a final course of action when multiple anterior teeth are to be extracted. According to Spear,[48] the clinician should be prepared to encounter a few of the most common clinical situations.

In the first and most predictable situation, teeth are present and need to be removed but have no periodontal disease. The challenges in these patients are usually related to whether to use implants versus a fixed partial denture, and if implants are used, how many to use and where to place them. The answers generally depend upon which teeth are being removed.

If the maxillary central incisors are being removed and have good surrounding bone, adjacent implants can lead to a predictable and esthetic final result. Because the papilla between the central implants and the adjacent laterals will be excellent, the facial gingival margins can be easily augmented, if necessary; and the papilla between the central implants is likely to remain within 1 to 2 mm of the pre-extraction level, provided

Fig 5-24a Healed edentulous site 3 months postextraction, ready for flapless procedure.

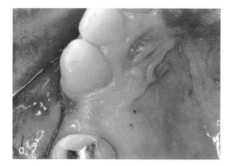
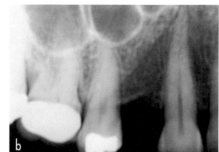

Fig 5-24b Radiograph of the site.

Fig 5-24c Cone guide with the drill to define the best implant position.

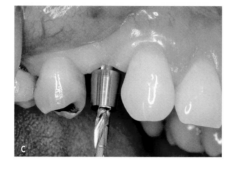
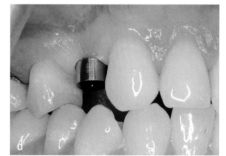

Fig 5-24d Tissue punch guide in position on the ridge.

Fig 5-24e Tissue punch over the guide.

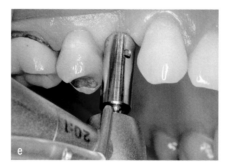
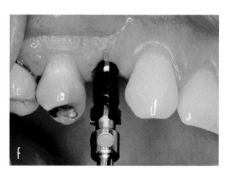

Fig 5-24f Bone drilling through the gingival punch.

Fig 5-24g Nobel Direct one-piece implant placement.

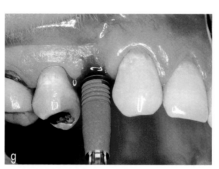
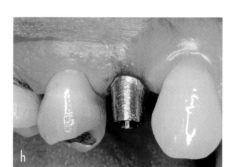

Fig 5-24h Supragingival preparation of the abutment.

Fig 5-24i Immediate provisionalization with no functional contact. (Restoration by Dr M. O'Reilly, Dublin, Ireland.)

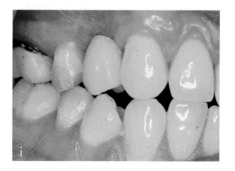

Restoring Dental Function and Esthetics

the implants are placed 4.5 mm apart and the interproximal crest of bone is maintained.

If the teeth to be removed involve a central and lateral incisor, or a lateral incisor and canine, however, the treatment choices are not quite as clear. It is difficult to place adjacent implants in a central and lateral position, or in a lateral and canine position, and have 3 mm between the platforms. This results in an increased risk of inter-implant bone loss over time, with subsequent loss of papilla height. In addition, if the papilla height between the central and lateral incisor is lost on one side while natural contralateral teeth are retained, the discrepancy in papilla height is much more noticeable than when there is a slight loss of papilla height between adjacent central incisor implants.

Another option for the missing central and lateral or missing lateral and canine is the use of soft tissue augmentation and a fixed prosthesis with pontic. When three or four adjacent anterior teeth with good periodontal support need to be removed, the preference is not to place adjacent implants but rather to separate them by one or two pontics. If both central incisors and a lateral incisor need to be removed, it is recommended to place a central incisor implant, pontic, and lateral incisor implant. This design allows excellent papilla height in all locations due to the predictability of the soft tissue augmentation in the pontic site.

If all four incisors need to be removed and good periodontal support exists, there are two acceptable options. The first is to place implants in both lateral incisor locations and use both central incisors as pontics. The second is to place the implants in both central locations and cantilever the lateral incisor pontics. Both options produce acceptable esthetic and structural results.

In the second situation, teeth are present and need removal but have periodontal disease. The new challenge in this scenario is that the papilla height in the areas of the periodontal disease becomes less predictable following tooth removal. Papillae are very likely to resorb, and a more apically placed contact in the restorations avoids an open gingival embrasure. The clinician can choose implant restorations that are functionally and structurally acceptable but esthetically more difficult, or soft tissue grafting and pontics that can produce significantly more soft tissue over the interproximal bone. If the adjacent teeth are unrestored, it might be preferable to choose the implants rather than prepare the unrestored teeth and live with esthetic compromise.

Forced eruption prior to extraction is another option to consider when it is necessary to remove multiple adjacent teeth with periodontal disease.[98] The eruption of a single tooth to be extracted does not alter the final papilla height because this is dictated by the bone on the adjacent teeth (see previous discussion of Forced Eruption). However, it is critical to apprise the patient that a perfect esthetic result is unlikely and that short

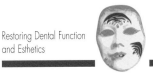

Restoring Dental Function and Esthetics

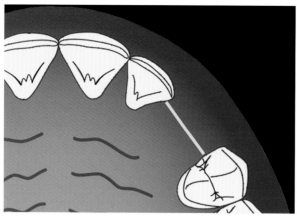

Fig 5-25a Crestal palatal incision.

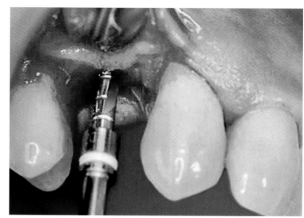

Fig 5-25b Envelope flap.

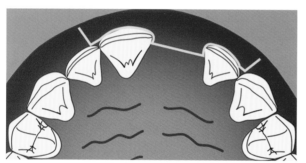

Fig 5-26a Palatal crestal incision with sulcular and vestibular divergent incisions.

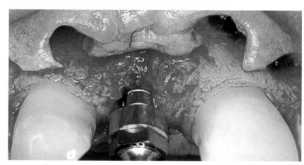

Fig 5-26b Same flap design for implant placement in conjunction with guided bone regeneration.

papillae, long contacts, and more rectangular definitive restorations should be expected.

The next clinical situation, when multiple teeth are missing, is the most difficult to manage esthetically because the teeth have already been removed. When this happens, the bony ridge flattens rapidly unless something is done to alter the process. This means that in cases where the teeth have been missing for a significant period of time, the interproximal crest of bone is completely gone, and it is difficult and unpredictable to re-create it through vertical bone augmentation. Accordingly, the use of adjacent implants invariably results in an inadequate papilla height. A connective tissue graft and pontics, however, can create and maintain significantly more soft tissue above the interproximal bone than is possible with adjacent implants. The patient must be informed that the best esthetic result may involve pontics instead of implants.

Flap design

Soft tissue handling is the most significant variable in the treatment outcome of any periodontal plastic procedure, particularly in the reduction of trauma.[99]

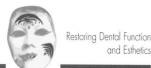

Restoring Dental Function
and Esthetics

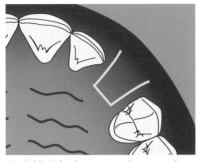

Fig 5-27 Palatal incision with two vestibular divergent incisions that leave the papillae tissue in place.

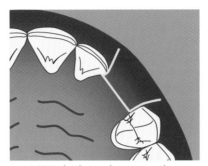

Fig 5-28 Palatal crestal incision with vestibular extension.

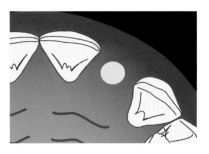

Fig 5-29 Slightly palatal tissue punch.

There are many types of flap design. The wide flap design may be an enveloped flap with a palatal crestal incision (Fig 5-25); a wide mobilized flap with sulcular buccal extension (Fig 5-26); or a buccopalatal pedicle flap with a vertical incision. The limited flap away from the papilla (Fig 5-27) consists of a limited flap design with sulcular buccal extension; palatal/lingual crestal incision with buccal extension if necessary (Fig 5-28); or a pedicle tissue punch with palatal/lingual crest orientation. Finally, the flapless approach uses a tissue punch (Fig 5-29) or pedicle tissue punch (Fig 5-30) to access the bone without the need to raise a usual large flap.

In a study comparing the wide mobilized flap approach including interproximal papillae with the limited flap design, which leaves a minimum width of 1 mm of the interdental papilla, the interproximal bone and crestal bone loss was more significant for the wide flap (1.2 mm) than the limited flap (0.2 mm). Therefore, it can be deduced that in a healed site, the limited flap design provides better interproximal esthetics through minimal bone loss and papilla recession.[100] All flaps that are apically repositioned and have a palatal incision will increase the amount of keratinized gingiva and the thickness of the gingival margin around the implant restoration.

Advantages of flap surgery

Visualization of anatomical structures is possible with an open flap procedure and is generally more predictable in cases with a lack of bone support or difficult bone anatomy. This approach allows correction of bone crest deformities and is indicated when buccal keratinized gingiva is limited or absent. The NobelGuide system (Nobel Biocare) is indicated in difficult situations (the limited or wide flap is raised earlier). A mucoperiosteal flap of less than 1 mm thick induces bone resorption.[69]

Fig 5-30a Tissue punch going into the crestal bone on the lingual.

Fig 5-30b Drilling is accomplished after a tiny pedicle flap is raised buccally.

Fig 5-30c The pedicle is rolled buccally during the insertion of the healing abutment.

Fig 5-30d Clinical photograph after removal of the healing abutment with the correct soft tissue height/thickness and a convex ridge.

Fig 5-30e Placement of implant-supported crown. (Restoration by Dr C. Raygot, Paris, France.)

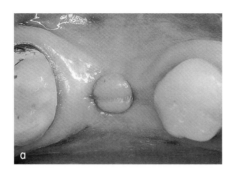
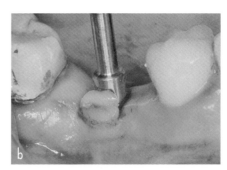
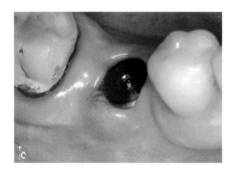
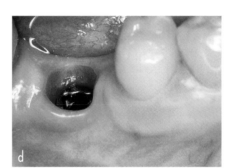
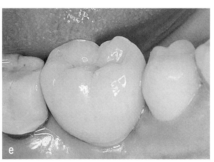

Advantages of flapless surgery

The tissue punch technique on healed sites offers several benefits and limitations.[21] This approach causes less trauma to bone and results in formation of a better blood clot. Because the soft tissue stability is undisturbed, there is less postoperative inflammation and, therefore, less pain. It is a difficult and sensitive technique with limited access visibility that requires an adequate amount of fibrous tissue but is often indicated in the esthetic zone on selected patients.

Bone resorption

Several studies suggest that flap elevation might result in 0.7 to 1.2 mm resorption in the alveolar ridge and recommend immediate implant placement using the flapless technique. Minimal buccal bone loss (0.5 mm) was experienced in the flapless approach.[101]

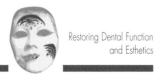

Postoperative pain

A recent study found a reduction of pain level in patients on whom the flapless approach had been performed.[102] The pain duration and use of pain medication was much lower than in flap surgeries: 43% of patients who had the tissue punch procedure reported no pain, compared with 25% of patients who underwent a flap elevation. Less bone resorption was seen, and no drying of the bone occurred.

Osseointegration

Becker et al[103] examined the question of whether the flapless approach was a problem for osseointegration. They found that no foreign body inclusion could occur with this approach. The rate of bone-to-implant contact was greater than with flap elevation. Accelerated osseointegration healing process saw no significant difference in marginal bone remodeling (0.7 mm). The higher the torque, the less stability at 3 months postoperatively; and the higher the initial implant stability quotient (ISQ), the more reduction of its value with time. Overall success rate was 97% to 98% at 28 months post–implant placement. When a flapless protocol was used, no autogenous bone or bone substitute that could interfere with the natural regeneration process was used to fill the gap between the implant and the residual alveolus. When biomaterial is used in the flap protocol, it may provide a false radiologic impression of fully formed bone.

Recently Binderman et al[104] found that P2X4, an ATP (adenosine 5'-triphosphate) receptor, is significantly upregulated in marginal gingival cells soon after flap surgery. It is hypothesized that local release of ATP signaling through P2X4 elicits activation of osteoclasts on the alveolar bone surface. Raising a flap has detrimental effects on facial bone,[105] and the radiographic analysis indicated that bone remodeling did not seem to stabilize until 1 year after the flap protocol, although bone remodeling occurred in the first 6 months after a flapless protocol.[25] In several flapless surgeries, dramatic bone regrowth of up to 3 mm on the exposed threads of two different implants (Mk III RP and NP Nobel Speedy Groovy RP [Nobel Biocare]) was seen.

3D Implant Position and Stability

The morphology of the bone defect is the basis for decision-making in implant treatment, but the emergence profile of the implant restoration determines the implant position, dictates the hard and soft tissue management procedures, and remains the key to esthetic success in the final prosthetic phase.[106–108] Restoration-driven implant placement must, therefore, develop and guide the harmonious peri-implant soft tissue profile with the contours and form of the restoration that imitate those of the adjacent natural teeth.[89,109]

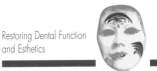

Restoring Dental Function and Esthetics

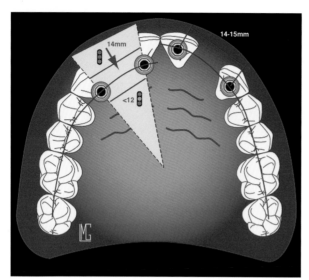

Fig 5-31 Anterior palatal ridge resorption limits the available normal interproximal distance for implants.

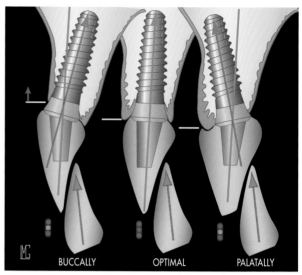

Fig 5-32 Diagram of the various buccopalatal options for orientation of the implant.

The bony housing should have a 3D configuration that permits optimal position and angulation of a restoration-driven implant of optimal length and diameter. It should also approximate the facial bone level on the adjacent and contralateral teeth and have interproximal surfaces of the adjacent teeth of adequate height to support the formation of the interproximal papillae.

When measured adjacent to the tooth and interdental papilla, the proximal supracrestal gingival mucosa should be 3 mm in type I biotypes and 5 mm in type II biotypes. In the midcervical area of the tooth, this distance should measure 2.7 and 3.0 mm, respectively, for the different biotypes.[110] Implants should be surrounded by 2 mm of bone to prevent outward bone resorption and to enable correct labiopalatal implant placement for the development of a peri-implant soft tissue collar. Therefore, it is necessary to have alveolar implant housing of sufficient dimension and quality (Fig 5-31). Any insufficiency or absence of bone should motivate the clinician to plan for bone reconstruction or augmentation prior to, or in conjunction with, implant placement. Hard and soft tissue augmentation enables the shift from a thin to a more favorable thick biotype.

3D implant position

Precise 3D orientation of the implant shoulder within the socket is a critical determinant for periodontal, functional, and esthetic success and minimal tissue recession.[82,111] Computer-based treatment planning enables clinicians to develop a comprehensive treatment plan that can be precisely executed in a timely matter.

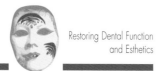

Restoring Dental Function and Esthetics

Complications

If the implant is angulated too buccally, this is an irreversible complication that causes the tooth to appear longer than the adjacent one. If the implant is angulated too palatally, the tooth will appear shorter than normal, with a saddle pontic.

Palatal positioning is a less critical complication (Fig 5-32). The thickness of soft tissue determines the available length for the emergence profile[112]; therefore, it is possible to correct the emergence profile only if the implant is located apically enough to manage a normal emergence profile.[113] Long-term peri-implant considerations, however, dictate that the sulcus should remain shallow. While soft tissue height of less than 2 mm makes esthetic restorations difficult and induces bone resorption to allow the formation of the biologic width, a height of more than 4 mm could cause long-term soft tissue complications.[114]

Rationale and rules for position

The mesiodistal position of the implant (Fig 5-33) determines the implant diameter selection, interproximal bone volume, and interproximal papilla predictability. The buccopalatal orientation determines the length of the implant crown restoration. The corono-apical location determines the emergence profile and the peri-implant sulcus depth.[6]

Minimum horizontal and vertical interproximal bone requirements should be respected between implants and adjacent teeth and between implants to obtain a predictable and stable esthetic result over time.

Buccopalatally, the external platform of the implant should be located 2 mm inside an imaginary line that connects the curve of the arch formed by the facial surfaces of the adjacent teeth. Alternatively, a distance of 2 mm plus the radius of the implant should exist from the center of the implant to this line and remain within a buccal cortical plate into an almost ideal relationship with the facial bone and adjacent teeth.[115]

The implant platform should be placed approximately 1.5 to 2.0 mm below the interproximal crest in a type I biotype and 3 to 4 mm below in a type II biotype. It should be slightly supracrestal to minimize the cervical bone resorption, and placed at a 2.5-mm depth from a free buccal (midcervical) gingival margin of the definitive restoration for a thick biotype, and at a 3.0-mm depth for a thin biotype.[114,116,117]

If the implant is placed apically within 1 mm of the facial bony crest of the tooth to allow for optimal facial gingival esthetics, the implant-abutment junction (IAJ) will inevitably be positioned below the interproximal bone, resulting in proximal bone loss. However, if the IAJ is placed above the bone on the proximal area to avoid or minimize the resorption process, the risk of exposing the implant collar at the facial area increases, thereby compromising esthetics.[118]

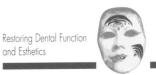

Restoring Dental Function and Esthetics

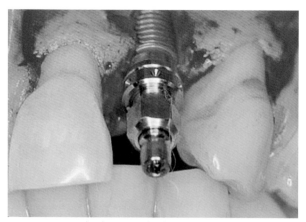

Fig 5-33a Mesiodistal position should leave adequate interproximal bone.

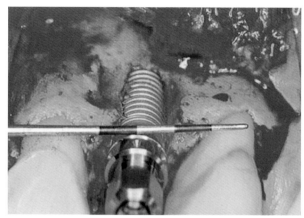

Fig 5-33b Corono-apical position at the bone level of the adjacent teeth.

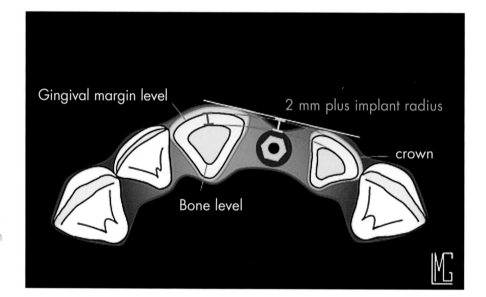

Fig 5-33c Buccopalatal position showing the implant collar 2 mm away from the line joining the enamel curve of contour of the adjacent teeth.

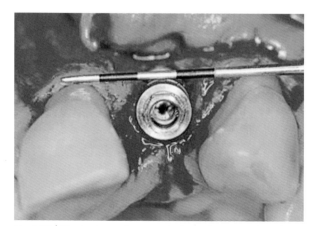

Fig 5-33d The implant collar is inside the probe joining the adjacent roots.

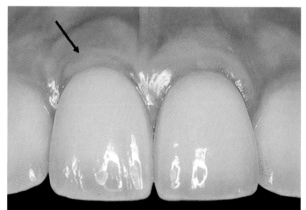

Fig 5-33e Esthetic Procera implant restoration on the right central incisor with harmonious gingival contour. *Arrow* denotes implant restoration. (Lab work by Mr M. Magne, Montreux, Switzerland. Restoration by Dr A. P. Saadoun, Paris, France.)

Restoring Dental Function
and Esthetics

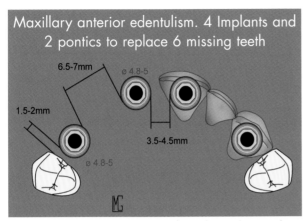

Fig 5-34a Horizontal biologic criteria for implant and pontic placement.

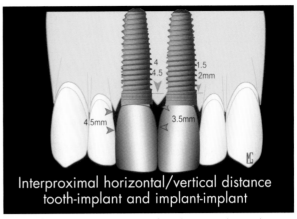

Fig 5-34b Vertical biologic criteria for adjacent implant and pontic placement.

Prerequisites for surgical papilla regeneration

The presence of intact papilla between anterior implants depends on whether the implant is placed according to horizontal and vertical biologic criteria (Fig 5-34).

Horizontal biologic criteria for implant placement

The "perfect papilla" between an implant and an adjacent tooth is when the interproximal bone height is within the normal bone range.[119] To achieve optimal papillae esthetics, it is appropriate to have at least 1.5 to 2.0 mm mesiodistal distance between an implant and an adjacent tooth (2.0 to 2.5 mm between an implant and central incisor), and at least 3 to 4 mm between two implants[60,114,116] (4.0 to 4.5 mm between two central incisor implants). Buccolingually, the implant should be placed 2 to 3 mm from the cervical height of contour of the adjacent teeth. Its corono-apical position should be 2.5 to 3.0 mm from the buccogingival margin depending on the biotype.

Vertical biologic criteria for implant placement [48,119,120]

- Bone crest to tooth-implant restoration contact point: 4.5 to 5.0 mm
- Bone crest to implant-implant restoration contact point: 2.3 to 4.0 mm
- Bone crest to implant-pontic restoration contact point: 5.5 to 6.0 mm
- Bone crest to pontic-pontic restoration contact point: 6.0 to 6.5 mm

In the case of single-tooth implant placement, the interproximal papilla levels are determined by the height of the interproximal bone on the adjacent natural teeth, not the interproximal bone on the implant.[46,121,122] As noted earlier, papilla height is normally 4.0 mm to 4.5 mm above the interproximal bone on natural teeth. Therefore, if the natural teeth had no bone loss, the papilla height would be similar after implant placement.[123,124] The facial gingival margin around the implant, however, is related to the facial bone levels and thickness on the implant, as well as the thickness and position of the free gingival margin prior to the tooth removal.[51,89] For a single anterior implant, the least predictable soft tissue outcome results when the adjacent natural teeth have interproximal bone loss, since management of the papilla can be difficult.

After soft tissue grafting, the amount of tissue above the interproximal bone between a pontic and a natural tooth, or between a pontic and an implant, averages 6.5 mm.[119] Therefore, it is important to place the implant with an ideal diameter for the existing mesiodistal distance in a correct buccopalatal and corono-apical location to maintain a buccal wall of hard and soft tissue equal to or thicker than that of a natural tooth and the adjacent proximal bone.[125]

In a case where two adjacent teeth are replaced with implants, it has been recommended that surgical and restorative procedures provide maximum support to the papillae.[126] Whenever placement of adjacent implants on central incisors is planned, it should be sequenced so that one tooth is extracted and replaced with an implant, and the adjacent tooth is extracted 6 months later and the second implant is placed. The idea is to maintain the interproximal dental bone adjacent to the integrated implant, which would be more likely to act as a stable scaffold for an inter-implant papilla peak. With adjacent implants placed simultaneously, coalescing lateral inter-implant bone remodeling could result in bone loss for that papilla support.

The most difficult areas in which to achieve this are between a maxillary lateral and central incisor or between a maxillary lateral incisor and canine because of the limited space. When the canine and the lateral incisor are missing, one canine implant and one lateral pontic should be placed; when a central incisor and lateral incisor are missing, one central implant and one lateral pontic should be placed to regenerate the papilla and achieve symmetry with the adjacent teeth.[48]

If the natural teeth adjacent to a single-tooth implant have bone loss due to trauma, periodontal disease, or other causes, soft tissue ridge augmentation followed by pontic placement can achieve greater coronal height of the papilla than a single-tooth implant could in the same situation.

When multiple implants are to be placed in the esthetic zone, the challenge of proper implant positioning increases. The use of implants with a smaller diameter may be beneficial to retain a minimum of 3 mm of inter-implant bone at the implant-abutment position. If this is not possible, it is recommended to decrease the number of implants and insert an implant with an ideal diameter in the correct 3D position, leaving adequate space for a pontic.

When the four maxillary incisors are missing, the choice to insert four implants to replace each tooth requires normal bone crest dimension

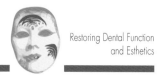

Restoring Dental Function and Esthetics

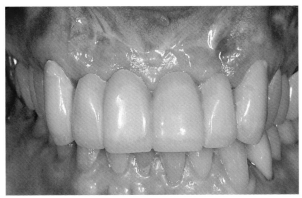

Fig 5-35a Initial consultation. Six-unit fixed provisional crowns to replace the four missing maxillary incisors.

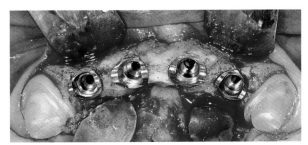

Fig 5-35b Four Nobel Perfect (Nobel Biocare) implants are placed with consideration of the horizontal biologic criteria.

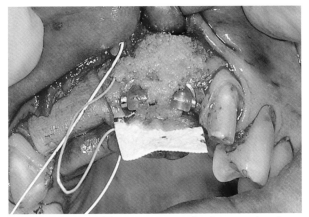

Fig 5-35c The bone dehiscence is covered with xenograft and bioresorbable membrane before the flap is sutured with horizontal mattress sutures.

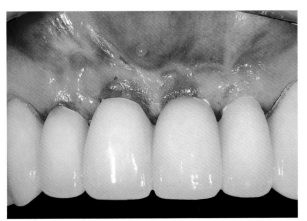

Fig 5-35d Provisional fixed bridge placed after exposure of the implants using the pedicle punch procedure.

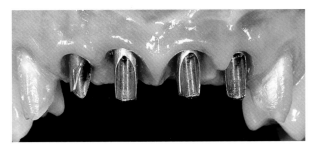

Fig 5-35e Maturation of the gingival and interdental papillae 3 months after provisionalization.

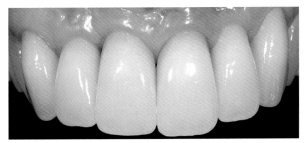

Fig 5-35f Four definitive single-unit implant restorations with two canine restorations. (Surgery and restoration by Dr P. Wöhrle, Newport Beach, CA.)

with limited bone resorption (Fig 5-35). Alternatively, two implants can replace the lateral incisors and a bone/membrane/connective tissue graft can be performed to maintain the soft tissue ridge at the central incisor region.[74] The final gingival contour of the missing central incisors will be obtained through the convex shape of the provisional pontic.

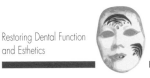

Restoring Dental Function and Esthetics

Fig 5-36a Scanning appliance with an occlusal bite and reference points.

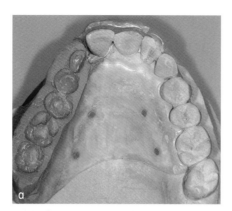

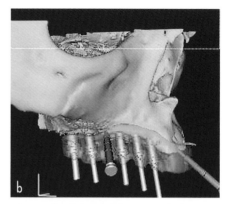

Fig 5-36b Simulated surgical guide with implants and anchor pins.

Fig 5-36c Surgical guide on the cast sent to the laboratory.

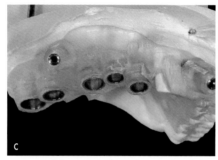

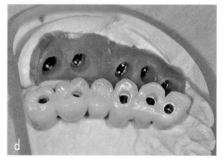

Fig 5-36d Six-unit provisional restoration received from the laboratory before the surgery. (Laboratory of Mr J. M. Etienne, Pulnoy, France.)

Fig 5-36e Surgical guide in place with a patient biting on the occlusal stent.

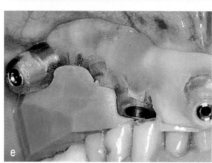

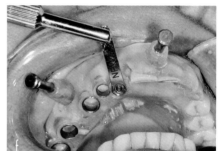

Fig 5-36f After placement of the anchor pins, the 2-mm-diameter guide pin is placed on the surgical guide.

Fig 5-36g Drilling is performed through the surgical guide.

Fig 5-36h After placement of the first implant, the drilling is performed for the second implant.

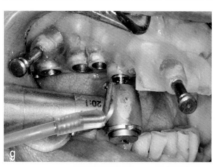

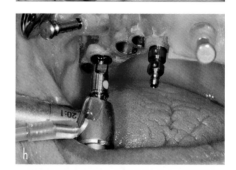

Fig 5-36i After final stabilization of the surgical guide with guided screws for anchorage, the three other implants are placed.

Fig 5-36j Provisional restoration placed on the five implants. Note the slight trauma at the base of the central papilla from the anchor pin and, more importantly, trauma to the lateral incisor from the punch drill that resulted from thin gingiva in the area. (Restoration by Dr B. Touati, Paris, France.)

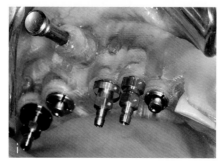

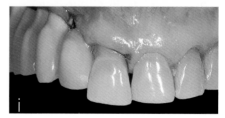

Restoring Dental Function and Esthetics

NobelGuide is an example of computer-based treatment planning software that can be used to successfully treat complex clinical cases (Fig 5-36).

Implant stability

The primary stability of an implant is a strictly biomechanical phenomenon, defined as the implant immobility after implant placement. This directly depends on bone quantity and density, implant site configuration, surgical protocol, and the implant design and surface.[127,128] These factors determine the quantity of dense bone in contact with the implant surface.[8]

Primary stability is a predictor of implant osseointegration, healing period, and success. It is a biomechanical result, assessed at each surgery and measured in terms of resistance to unscrewing and pull-out. The resistance is evaluated subjectively by tactile perception or objectively using the Periotest device (Medizintechnik Gulden) and/or the Ostell instrument. Prevention of implant micromotion depends on:

- The clinician's surgical skills
- Bone density/topography
- Implant design
- Surgical site preparation based on bone quality/implant design
- Torque; torque >35 Ncm causes elevated cortical bone resorption
- Maintenance of the stability during the first weeks in dense bone
- Radiographic control
- Absence of pain

Secondary stability has been identified as an implant's immobility following a predetermined healing period, prior to definitive prosthetic connection. It is a biomechanical and biologic result that may be assessed in the same way as primary stability or that may be evaluated with a sonic resonance frequency analysis (RFA) following implant exposure.[129]

The primary stability of a TiUnite implant remains throughout osseointegration.[31] Stable implants that exhibit maximum surface contact with the compact bone will be more rapidly osseointegrated and capable of handling loading. Implants that achieve less initial bone contact in poor-quality bone require an extended period to allow secondary stability after osseointegration.[130]

Resonance frequency analysis

The biomechanical aspects of implant stability can now be evaluated with a measurement of final torque at insertion (TI) or with the RFA method, the results of which are expressed in terms of its ISQ.[131] With values from 0 to 100, the ISQ yields the following decision in implant loading[132,133]:

- Less than 50: insufficient stability and no immediate loading
- 50 to 60: good stability and immediate loading but splinting is necessary
- 60 to 75: excellent stability and immediate loading/provisionalization
- Greater than 75: ischemia, risk of osteonecrosis

To achieve successful osseointegration, the TI must be at least 35 Ncm, and the quality of primary implant stability (as evaluated by RFA) should be at least 55 lSQ. These initial measurements allow the clinician to decide whether the implant should be loaded immediately or delayed, and whether this should be done less than 3 weeks post-placement or more than 5 weeks post-placement.

A recent study of RFA demonstrated that all bone types present the lowest value for implant stability at 3 weeks post–implant placement.[134] This effect was statistically significant and most pronounced in type 4 bone. After 5 weeks, however, there was no significant difference in the pattern of stability changes among different bone types. Therefore, it is imperative to place the final splinted restoration before or after this critical phase.

Radiographic and bone analysis performed during implant site evaluation allow the clinician to guide the surgical protocol, select the appropriate preparation techniques, improve the bone density, and increase implant stability. Type 1 or 2 bone requires pretapping with a normal-size implant. Type 3 bone calls for a normal preparation, with no pretapping. In type 4 bone, an undersized preparation with self-tapping implant is necessary.[3,127,135]

Stability versus load timing and bone density

A correlation has been shown between anatomical sites and bone density. The mandible's average mineral density is two times that of the anterior maxilla, and the posterior maxillary region is statistically the least mineralized zone.

Bone compression during implant surgery in soft-density bone is essential for obtaining the best stability. Use of thinner drills, osteotomes, and self-tapping implants of varying diameters ensures adequate primary stability.[127,135] It has been demonstrated that increased implant diameter is related to reduced stress transmitted to the cervical supporting bone.

A correlation exists between bone density and implant loading. For high-density bone, immediate loading (1 to 2 weeks) can result in biomechanical stability. Early loading (6 to 12 weeks) allows for biomechanical and biologic stability in low-density bone, and delayed loading (16 weeks or more) allows this stability in soft-density bone.[77,136]

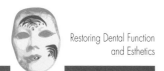

Restoring Dental Function and Esthetics

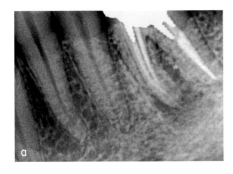

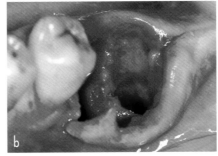

Fig 5-37a Initial radiograph of the mandibular first molar prior to extraction.

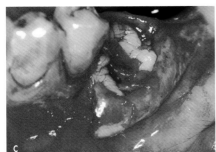

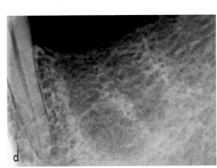

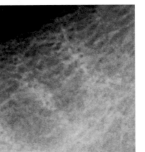

Fig 5-37b Extraction site after deep debridement.

Fig 5-37c Alveolar socket filled with platelet-rich fibrin (PRF) membrane.

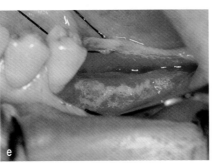

Fig 5-37d Radiograph of the extraction site 3 months postoperatively.

Fig 5-37e Surgical view of the ridge 6 months before implant placement. (Courtesy of Dr J. Choucroun, Nice, France.)

Platelet-rich plasma

The use of PRP is an extremely important consideration in implant therapy. This procedure enhances wound healing in extraction sites and improves clinical outcomes in alveolar ridge preservation for delayed implant placement, immediate implant placement, and hard and soft tissue grafting procedures (Fig 5-37).

It is recognized that stabilization and attachment of the blood clot to the surface of a dental implant facilitates the migration of bone cells to this surface, resulting in contact osteogenesis, a process that ultimately determines the percentage of bone-implant contact obtained. In addition, the growth factors contained within PRP enhance the maturation of bone and periodontal soft tissues.[137,138]

Platelet growth factors—along with their supposed healing benefits—have taken on a unique form: platelet-rich fibrin (PRF). Quite different from the other platelet concentrates used elsewhere in the world,[139] PRF can be considered to be an autologous healing biomaterial: a fibrin clot that concentrates the leukocytes, platelets, and a large majority of the molecules beneficial for immunity and healing into a single membrane.[140] Within the past 5 years, the use of PRF has developed enormously and has continued to demonstrate its great efficiency and its numerous potential applications in local/sinus bone grafting and mucogingival procedures, including the prevention of peri-implant gingival recession.[141]

Whether PRF functions by a purely mechanical action as a "standard resorbable membrane," or whether it acts in combination with the different factors captured by its fibrin network, thus transforming it into an "active" biologic membrane, it has been clinically proven that PRF enables the simple, effective, and predictable management of the gap between alveolar bone and implant. This, in turn, allows the prevention of secondary gingival recession by maintaining coronally the future level of the biologic space.

PRF can be used alone in a minimal bone-implant gap. In cases with a more substantial gap where bone augmentation is necessary, in the absence of one or more cortical walls, in dehiscence, or in an extraction site were immediate implantation is contraindicated, PRF can be combined with allogeneic bone or with allograft bone substitutes to minimize the number of surgeries. In fact, small bone defects may require secondary grafting procedures or become esthetically compromised because of contour defects in areas critical to the emergence profile.

In immediate implant placement, activated PRP need only be placed into the socket as the implant is delivered. When particulate bone grafts are used as part of the immediate placement protocol to occupy the voids existing between the implant body and the socket wall, the graft material can be mixed with PRP or directly with the PRF to facilitate the delivery of the graft.[140,142]

Once the PRP/particulate graft is delivered and condensed at the site, additional activated PRP is injected over the graft. This ensures the saturation of the implant body, graft material, and socket wall, and re-establishes the fibrin network within the graft that is disrupted during graft delivery and condensation.

When autologous particulate marrow bone grafts are used or combined with other graft materials, it is recommended that the autologous corticocancellous bone grafts be soaked in nonactivated PRP/PRF prior to delivery. This procedure allows for theoretical uptake of growth factors by the viable bone cells.

Histomorphometric analysis, however, indicates that the addition of PRP to the bone graft does not make a significant difference either in vital bone production or in interface bone contact on the test implants.[143] This was confirmed in a recent study showing that PRP does not exert additional effects on bone healing in bone defects created around dental implants and treated by guided bone regeneration.[144]

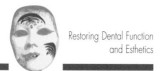

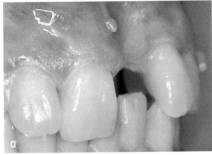

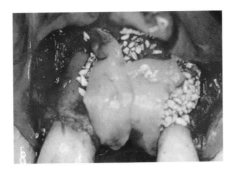

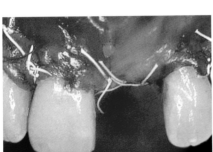

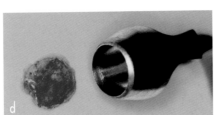

Fig 5-38a Ridge defect at the left maxillary central incisor site.

Fig 5-38b Implant placement in conjunction with xenograft mixed with PRF particulates and covered with PRF membrane.

Fig 5-38c Advanced coronal flap sutured without tension.

Fig 5-38d Three months later, a palatal connective tissue graft is harvested with a large tissue punch instrument.

Connective tissue grafting

In extremely difficult clinical situations, connective tissue grafting procedures have been very predictable for recession coverage and ridge augmentation. These procedures have enabled clinicians to restore the altered periodontal restorative interface to its original dimensions and to provide natural-looking crowns even in compromised sites. Moreover, this technique can be modified to optimize the soft tissue appearance.[145]

Connective tissue grafting is used to lower the risk of soft tissue recession in thin gingival biotypes through creation of a thicker zone of keratinized soft tissue, and for esthetic repair of existing recession. Thicker soft tissue allows a more stable and predictable situation when abutments are placed and loaded (Fig 5-38).

Achieving acceptable gingival esthetics around single anterior implants is a challenging procedure. Long-term maintenance can be an equally demanding task, especially if the teeth that had to be extracted initially showed gingival recession and/or absence of attached keratinized gingiva. In the esthetic zone, morphology of the soft tissues plays a central role in the achievement of satisfactory final results.[146]

Soft tissue procedures to ensure optimal esthetic reconstruction before implant placement, at implant placement, or at second-stage surgery can help to create ideal soft tissue profiles.[147] A buccal subperiosteal connective tissue graft could be placed at implant placement or during stage-two surgery at the time of abutment connection, once the recipient site is prepared with a split-thickness pouch extended beyond the adjacent teeth to ensure optimal vascular supply.[99]

Fig 5-38e This piece of connective tissue is submerged in the tunnel on the edentulous ridge.

Fig 5-38f Palatal curved incision performed 3 months later will allow the flap elevation to expose the implant.

Fig 5-38g Zirconia abutment with a concave submergence profile connected to the implant. Note the absence of the papilla.

Fig 5-38h Provisional restoration with a concave submergence profile.

Fig 5-38i Clinical aspect of the provisional crown 2 weeks later. Gingival disharmony and lack of interdental papilla are seen (arrow).

Fig 5-38j Gingival maturity after 3 months with gingival harmony.

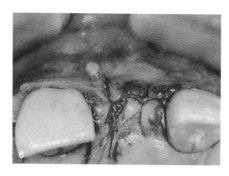

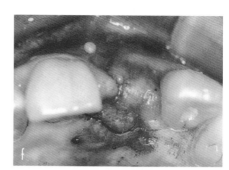

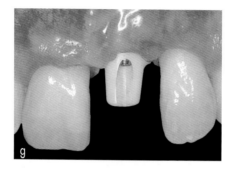

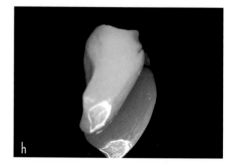

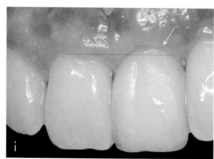

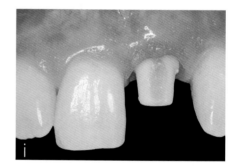

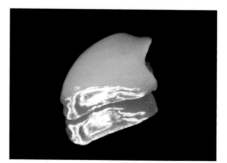

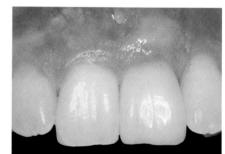

Fig 5-38k Definitive Procera restoration with concave submergence profile and slight buccal depression to reproduce the gingival profile of the adjacent incisor.

Fig 5-38l Definitive implant restoration 6 months after cementation with no more gingival disharmony and full interproximal papilla. (Laboratory work by Mr J. Wagner, Paris, France. Restoration by Dr C. Raygot and Dr A. P. Saadoun, Paris, France.)

Implants and connective tissue grafts

Regeneration of the bony crest and soft tissue should recreate ideal morphologic conditions and re-establish the contour as it existed before bone loss.[138,148]

Regardless of procedure, some tissue resorption occurs after implant exposure and restoration. The gingival margin at its highest point will lose 0.61 mm, and the interdental papillae will retract by an average of 0.37 mm.[122] The recession is most pronounced within the first 6 months. As noted earlier, type I gingival biotypes show less resorption. Implant materials also appear to influence tissue integration: aluminum/titanium abutment allows for normal soft tissue integration versus gold alloy, which results in tissue loss.

When site preservation is insufficient to maintain alveolar ridge anatomy in the esthetic zone, surgical restoration of the hard and soft tissue components is required at the site. An autogenous bone and xenograft with a membrane, combined with a connective tissue graft before or in conjunction with implant placement, are used to gain buccal thickness. A connective tissue graft placed on top of the cover screw increases the thickness as well as the vertical and buccal contour and prevents gingival recession and a visible shadow of the implant.[149,150]

To compensate for recession, the palatal tissue should always be positioned more coronally in the second-stage surgery to buccally increase the amount of keratinized gingiva.[122]

Several clinical complications (eg, bacterial colonization and infection) can occur and lead to failure of the implant when barrier membranes are used to close gaps of > 2 mm between the alveolar bone and implant. The connective tissue graft may prevent the complications induced by the use of synthetic barrier membranes, and at the same time, it improves the local metabolic environment of the superficial soft tissues to preserve and increase the keratinized tissues.[73,146]

Socket seal surgery

The re-formation of inter-implant papillae is a far more challenging clinical situation because current implant design may not permit the re-establishment of the collagen fibers as normally found between adjacent teeth or between a natural tooth and an implant. The inter-implant papillae rely mainly on crestal bone and the overlying soft tissue volume rather than on solid supracrestal functional soft tissue fibers.

The following are important considerations to predictably maintain inter-implant papillae with the socket seal procedure[78]:

Fig 5-39a Mobile first premolar surrounded by a natural canine with a post and core and an implant abutment in the site of the second premolar.

Fig 5-39b Following extraction, the alveolar socket is debrided and then filled with xenograft.

Fig 5-39c A palatal epithelio-connective tissue graft is sutured on top of the socket covering the bone graft.

Fig 5-39d Gingival aspect of the ridge 3 months later shows maintenance of the width.

Fig 5-39e One implant is placed in an optimal position using a flapless approach. (Surgery by Dr C. Landsberg, Tel Aviv, Israel.)

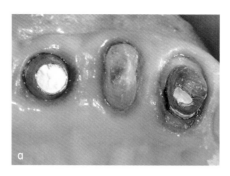
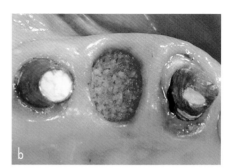
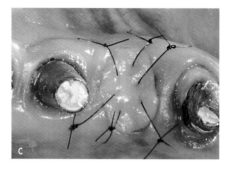
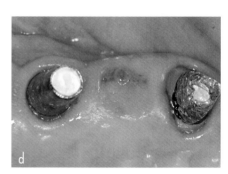
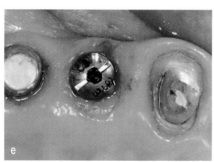

- Gingival biotype.
- Inflammation: healthy hard/soft tissue versus severe periodontal periapical inflammation or bony dehiscence.
- Radiographic evaluation: bone topography or pathology.
- Soft tissue donor site evaluation: intersocket implant placement labially versus papilla.
- Inter-implant distance: 3 mm between two implants allows only a thin peak of bone. A minimum distance of 4 mm is preferred to maintain a thick and wide crestal peak of bone to support the overlying papilla.
- Socket sealing with soft tissue graft: In addition to its wound-protective capacity, the soft tissue graft also augments the quality and quantity of the peri-implant soft tissue to be exposed at stage-two surgery or at implant placement using the tissue punch technique (Fig 5-39).

The osseointegration process is improved by protection against mechanical, chemical, and bacterial invasion and better clot stabiliza-

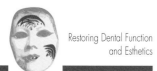

tion. Furthermore, soft tissue recession is minimized by increased width of the labial margins and the interproximal papillae, thereby enhancing the clinician's ability to design and sculpt the soft tissue contour around the implant.[73]

Pontics and connective tissue grafts

The use of pontics rather than adjacent implants to replace the central incisors poses its own challenge.[151] Just as it is between adjacent implants, the concern in this instance is the papillae between the adjacent pontics. The difference, however, is that when pontics are used, it is almost guaranteed that interproximal crestal bone between the extracted central incisors will resorb, creating a flat bony ridge and a subsequent loss of papillary height. Another difference is that it is possible to augment the soft tissue between pontics significantly more above the flattened osseous crest (ie, an average of 6.6 mm) as opposed to the typical tissue above interproximal inter-implant bone (ie, 3.0 to 3.5 mm). Ultimately, it becomes possible to have a papilla between central pontics 3 mm more coronal than that between adjacent implants for the same interproximal crest location and achieve optimal esthetic results.[48]

Implant-abutment considerations

Postrestorative reduction in crestal bone height around endosseous dental implants has long been acknowledged to be a normal consequence of implant therapy involving two-stage hexed implants.[152] This bone loss develops when an abutment is connected during stage-two surgery, when a two-stage implant is placed and connected to an abutment in a one-stage procedure, or when an implant is prematurely exposed to the oral environment and bacteria.[153]

When the diameter of the implant-platform surface matches that of the abutment, crestal bone loss typically occurs approximately 1.5 mm apical to the IAJ. This position appears to be constant regardless of where the IAJ is situated relative to the original level of the bony crest.[154] This connection design approximates the abutment inflammatory cell infiltrate with the crestal bone at the time of abutment connection.[155] Approximately 3 mm of peri-implant mucosa is required to create a mucosal barrier around a dental implant.[54] Crestal bone remodeling may occur to create space when soft tissue height is inadequate so that a biologic seal can be established to isolate the crestal bone and protect it from the oral environment.

Abutment placement with traditional divergent transmucosal profiles can have a negative effect whereby the transmucosal components create a centrifuge pressure at the internal side of the soft tissues, making them thinner and stretching the collagen bundles. This can result in

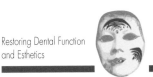

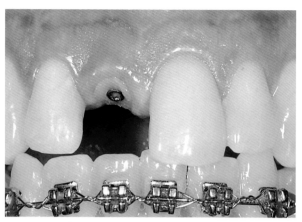

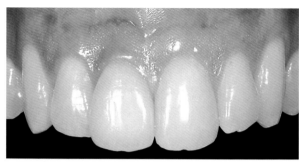

Fig 5-40b Definitive implant-supported restoration with optimal harmony in the gingival margin between the two central incisors. (Restoration by Dr P. Wöhrle, Newport Beach, CA.)

Fig 5-40a Scalloped NobelPerfect implant with healing abutment placed at the maxillary right central incisor site.

recession at the buccal aspect of 80% of the implants with a mean recession value of 0.88 mm. Alternatively, a convergent narrow and concave transmucosal profile induces thicker, more stable, and tighter peri-implant mucosa.

Several other approaches are currently being researched to resolve this loss of the interproximal/buccal crest of bone between implants. They include scalloped implants, platform switching, altered coronal implant surface design, and microgap location.

Available implants

NobelPerfect

The scalloped NobelPerfect implant presents many advantages[156] (Fig 5-40):

- Supports the natural anatomy of the alveolar crest
- Preserves interproximal bone through the increased interproximal design/TiUnite surface
- Maintains the natural, harmonious gingival contour through an anatomically designed machined collar for soft tissue apposition.[157]

In comparative studies between NobelPerfect implants with machined surfaces and NobelPerfect Groovy implants with TiUnite surfaces, at 6 months, there was no significant difference in interproximal recession (1 mm bone loss) between the two types of implants. There was, however, a greater incidence of completed papilla fill and papilla harmony on the scalloped Nobel Perfect Implant.[158–160]

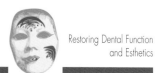

Restoring Dental Function and Esthetics

The marginal bone level was a major determinant of the optimal PES. A nearly equal proportion of patients have been shown to experience an improvement, a slight decrease, or no change in PES. During an observation period of up to 27 months, the interproximal bone was preserved for single-tooth or adjacent implants, but bone was not regularly maintained around the scalloped area of the implants.[161]

After 3 months of function, no significant changes to the mean papilla index score were observed. Only minor overall mean (SD) marginal bone change (–0.1 mm) around the scalloped implants was noted 1 year after immediate provisional restoration. This was well below the mean marginal bone loss observed in delayed loaded implants with a flat platform and indicates a favorable implant success rate and peri-implant tissue response after placement of immediate provisional restorations for scalloped implants.[118]

Curvy zirconium one-piece implant
- This Nobel Biocare implant is not yet available on the market
- Straight: no implant abutment connection
- Angulated: no implant abutment connection
- Titanium/zirconium[162]

NobelActive

Although the NobelActive (Nobel Biocare) implant is a one-piece design, it maintains the flexibility of a two-piece implant, with the ability to change direction during surgery with total control over placement (Fig 5-41). The implant features a variable thread profile and an obtuse, rather than acute, cutting edge angle. This innovative self-tapping design condenses bone for higher primary stability. It also allows preparation of narrower and shallower osteotomies, which is beneficial when implants are to be placed near vital structures or in atrophic ridges. These aspects result in potentially fewer drilling steps and a quicker surgical procedure, which also promotes soft tissue preservation and growth. The external abutment connection allows extraoral cementation of the definitive restoration, and the internal conical abutment connection potentially eliminates microgap and includes automatic platform shifting.[163,164]

Available abutments

The behavior of the soft tissues can be dramatically improved through the use of transmucosal components with an altered design. A tight biologic seal at the implant component's level is mandatory to protect the underlying bone crest from the external environment. To retain soft and hard tissues around the IAJ, the transmucosal aspect should not be oversized and divergent but rather shifting from wide and divergent to a narrow and concave shape.

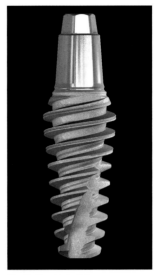

Fig 5-41a Nobel Active one-piece implant design.

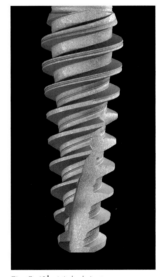

Fig 5-41b Nobel Active two-piece implant design.

Restoring Dental Function and Esthetics

The abutment should provide maximum space to the soft tissue and clearly avoid a flared geometry. Its submergence profile needs to be negative to avoid compression on the soft tissue and allow maximum thickness so the biologic space has more room, and to immobilize the circular soft tissue around the connection.[165]

Curvy

The concave transmucosal profile of the Curvy abutment (Nobel Biocare) demonstrates the following features (Fig 5-42a):

- Depth of macrogroove: 0.45 mm
- Distance from abutment shoulder to implant level: 2 mm
- Total length of concave profile in contact with soft tissue: 3 mm
- Two macrogroves: 0.05 mm deep and 0.25 mm apart

Positive soft tissue behavior with this abutment is linked to a combination of three factors:

1. The circumferential macrogroove creates a chamber in which a blood clot forms that provides space for nonsurgical soft tissue regeneration comparable to a localized connective tissue graft.
2. Curved profile allows for increased length of the soft tissue-to-implant interface, meaning that a biologic seal of 3 mm can be obtained despite only a 2-mm crown-to-implant distance.[166]
3. After maturation of the soft tissues, a ring-like seal is created that could stabilize the connective tissue adhesion and, to some degree, functionally mimic the effect of the Sharpey fiber attachment to teeth.

With the concave profile at the transmucosal level, 87% of implant sites demonstrated limited gingival recession (less than 0.5 mm in 13% of the cases), 33% showed facial soft tissue stability, and 53.7% experienced a mean vertical facial soft tissue gain of 0.34 mm. These results remain stable during the 12- to 24-month period until definitive restoration placement.[162]

After the regenerated connective tissue has matured into the empty chamber delineated by the implant's concave profile, a ring of tissue is formed. The connective tissue ring increases the soft tissue thickness barrier; therefore, in the esthetic zone, the reduced crown-to-implant distance of 2 mm has a positive effect and does not warrant placement of the implant at an infrabony level that will then induce additional bone remodeling.[162] This design also establishes a mechanical interlocking of the mucosa three-dimensionally and stabilizes the mucosa, giving long-term protection to the biologic seal against tearing upon strain and trauma (Figs 5-42b to 5-42f).

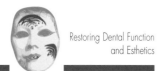

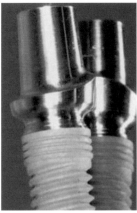

Fig 5-42a Curvy abutment screwed on the internal implant connection.

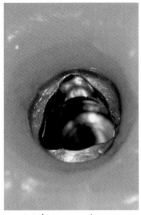

Fig 5-42b O-ring soft tissue thickness created nonsurgically by the concavity of the Curvy abutment. (Courtesy of Dr B. Touati, Paris, France.)

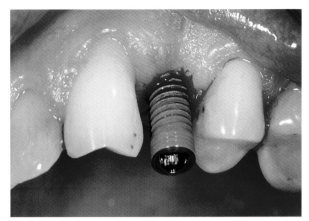

Fig 5-42c Flapless surgery is performed to place a TiUnite implant with grooves to top of platform.

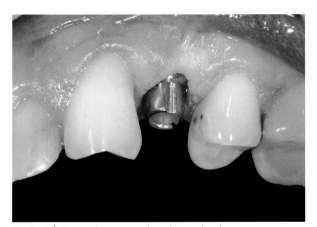

Fig 5-42d Curvy abutment is placed immediately postoperative.

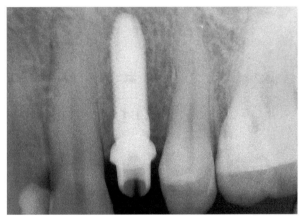

Fig 5-42e Radiograph 6 months postoperative showing perfect maintenance of the interproximal bone.

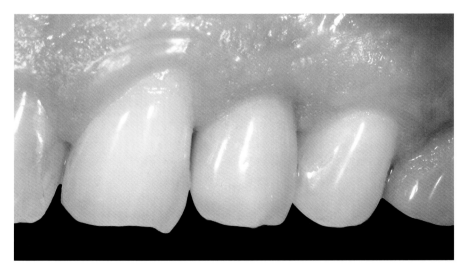

Fig 5-42f Procera restoration in place showing no gingival recession. (Surgery and restoration by Dr B. Touati, Paris, France.)

The Curvy abutment has grooves up to its top that preserve the bone level after final loading takes place. This bone is preserved despite being in direct contact with the IAJ, which demonstrates the absence of any detrimental effect of the so-called microgap IAJ on bone remodeling. Overall, the features of the Curvy abutment improve outcomes in the esthetic zone.[21]

Ankylos

The long-term support of the bone and peri-implant gingival contour is obtained by the stabilization of the cervical crestal bone and its low resorption with the Ankylos abutment (Dentsply) in comparison with the traditional abutment connection. The Ankylos system features a tight seal and high resistance to wear and stress on the flat IAJ. With a superior Morse taper connection and platform switching,[167] it is able to protect hard and soft tissue at a mechanical, bacterial, and biologic level (Fig 5-43). Its resistance to micromotion is a prerequisite for the stability of the peri-implant tissue. In the microgap between an implant and an abutment with parallel walls, micromotion limits the healing around the abutment and creates a favorable environment for bacterial colonization that induces junctional epithelium apicalization below the IAJ and is responsible for resorption of the cervical bone to the first thread.

The undersized diameter of the usual Ankylos abutment, compared with the implant platform, will medially push away the junctional zone (between the implant platform and the abutment) from the IAJ between the implant and the bone. This configuration allows the regeneration of the biologic width partially on the horizontal free platform of the implant and the vertical wall of the abutment.[168]

Ong et al[169] showed that the Ankylos implant system is highly successful in maintaining the crestal bone at its initial height after implant healing and loading. The esthetic outcomes were good not only from clinical assessment but also reflected in the high level of patients' satisfaction.

Platform switching

The ability to reduce or eliminate crestal bone loss results in significant esthetic and clinical benefits. The platform switching technique refers to the use of a smaller-diameter abutment on a larger-diameter implant collar; this connection shifts the perimeter of the IAJ inward toward the central axis of the implant. This inward movement causes a shift in the inflammatory cell infiltrate inward and away from the adjacent crestal bone, which limits the bone resorption that occurs around the implant's coronal aspect.[153] The biologic space can then re-form partially on the remaining horizontal platform of the implant. The relatively expanded collar of the implant can provide better engagement of the bone crest, better sealing in extraction sockets, and better primary stability. The

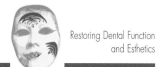

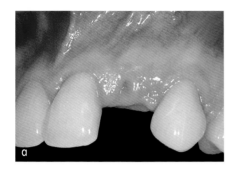

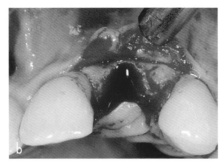

Fig 5-43a Initial consultation. Missing left lateral incisor with normal ridge thickness.

Fig 5-43b Broken submerged root is extracted.

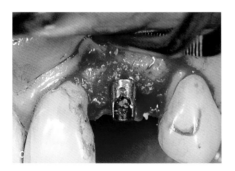

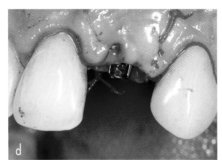

Fig 5-43c Ankylos implant in the extraction site with immediate abutment connection.

Fig 5-43d Connective tissue graft is placed over the bone graft prior to flap closure.

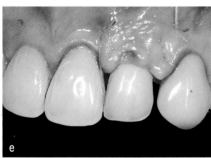

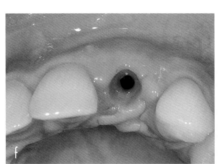

Fig 5-43e A provisional restoration is placed immediately on the abutment.

Fig 5-43f Clinical photograph of the subgingival soft tissue thickness around the abutment 3 months later.

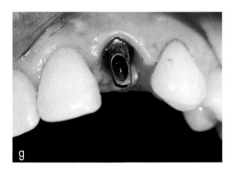

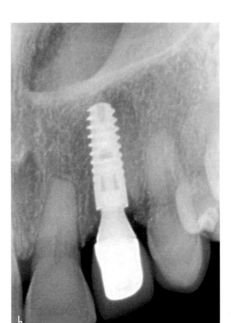

Fig 5-43g Final cone of Morse tapered titanium abutment is connected.

Fig 5-43h Radiograph showing bone on the implant platform.

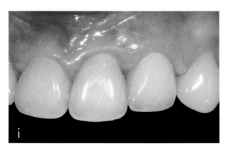

Fig 5-43i Zirconia implant restoration with normal gingival height and thick gingival margins and papillae. (Surgery and restoration by Dr A. Pinto, Paris, France.)

Restoring Dental Function and Esthetics

collar then bevels back at a 15-degree angle to provide a color-coded restorative platform with a 4.1-mm-diameter prosthetic component that shifts the IAJ inward. The typical pattern of crestal bone resorption has not been observed radiographically in cases where platform switching was utilized.

Platform shifting

According to Nobel Biocare, *platform shifting* is the "concept of 'stepping down' the size of an implant platform to increase the volume of soft tissue around the implant platform during implant treatment." In practice, platform shifting adapters convert regular platform (RP) implants into narrow platform (NP) implants, and wide platform (WP) implants into RP implants.

Platform shifting is currently a method to restore teeth with more predictable results than before, especially on immediate implant treatments. When shifting to a narrower interface, the space increases and the soft tissue becomes more stable with better esthetic results.[170] The undercontour of the prosthetic abutment has the potential to change the vertical biologic space into a horizontal and a vertical component, keeping the same total biologic dimension. The bone located away from the implant prosthetic abutment connection should not resorb as usual because the biologic width is regenerated.

In implants where a microgap is present, microbial leakage could lead to inflammation and marginal bone loss. Thus, it is important to minimize the bacterial presence in and around the IAJ. The seal provided by a locking-tapered design abutment has been demonstrated to be airtight.[171]

Use of any of these abutments requires that the switch be in place from the day the implant is uncovered or platform shifting exposed to oral cavity in a single- or two-stage approach. It cannot be used after the biologic width is established around a conventional IAJ configuration to regain crestal bone height.[172]

Abutment connection

To obtain predictable implant esthetics and soft tissue integration, repeated connections of an abutment are not recommended, but one reconnection should not affect the tissue support and preserved hard and soft tissue.[173] The peri-implant mucosa variation during repeated connections is highly deleterious. The tearing of the hemidesmosome of the basal lamina of the epithelial attachment occurs with microbleeding and induces a new phase of healing of the protective junctional epithelium. The disruption of the biologic width causes additional resorption. Consequently, a layer of 1 mm of connective tissue and the junctional epithelium tend to migrate and re-form more apically beyond the IAJ

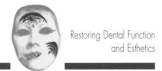

Restoring Dental Function and Esthetics

until they can adhere again, which frequently results in marginal bone loss, often at the expense of the bone crest and soft tissue, particularly in a thin gingival biotype.

As multiple reconnections of the abutment to the implant induce soft and hard tissue resorption, the final ceramic or titanium abutment should be screwed at the earliest stage into the implant during the surgical phase and left in place during the restorative phase. Installation of the final abutment at the time of implant placement transforms a two-unit into a single-unit implant. The rationale for this transformation is the knowledge that soft tissue instability after implant placement may jeopardize the seal around the implant and affect esthetics.

It is also recommended to use sterilized or decontaminated healing abutments after each necessary disconnection to limit bacterial proliferation and apical migration of the hard and soft tissues.[117]

Model-guided and computer-guided techniques are gaining ground in implant dentistry. They allow the implant abutment to be prepared in the laboratory before surgery and its design to be scanned (or impressed) before connection. Thus, after soft tissue maturation, a simple pick-up impression can be used to fabricate a crown without harming the mucosal seal or causing injury to the crestal bone, particularly in the case of thin soft tissue.

The total immobilization of the prosthetic abutment prevents any micromotion also responsible for cervical bone resorption and maintains the horizontal component of the biologic width, thickening the connective tissue and ensuring a better microgap isolation. This concept achieves and potentially enhances crestal bone preservation, decreases the amount of peri-implant cervical bone resorption, and may achieve a more predictable soft tissue level stability and a significant esthetic result.

Abutment biomaterials

Biomaterials for prosthetic components should be limited to titanium, alumina, or zirconium oxides, which are the only materials that are biocompatible and allow adhesion to the implant surface of junctional epithelium hemidesmosomes and connective tissue fibroblasts. Other materials (eg, gold or glazed ceramic) should be avoided because they are not biocompatible and induce the resorption of the mucosal seal on the implant neck, often at the expense of the bone.[30,174]

Zirconium abutments offer sufficient stability to support single-tooth restorations in anterior and premolar regions. In thin and moderate biotypes, the mucosal seal formed by biocompatible materials is essential to prevent bone remodeling and soft tissue esthetic repercussions. The newer concave transmucosal design for implant abutments made entirely of biocompatible materials allows cell adhesion.

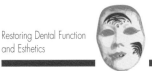

The use of all-ceramic abutments might be beneficial over the use of titanium abutments when the soft tissue thickness labial to the implant is equal to or less than 2 mm.[175] This abutment material, especially customized digitally generated or preplanned zirconia, influences the shape of the provisional restorations and the timing of connection and insertion of the final abutment. It results in harmonious healing of the tissues with guided soft tissue growth and papilla regeneration and minimizes the discrepancies between the anatomical emergence profile of a natural tooth and an implant.[176]

Provisional and definitive restorations

A natural tooth has never displayed a convex or divergent contour below the CEJ but rather a flat emergence. Conventional abutments that displayed a transmucosal design with divergent walls were an incorrect prosthetic interpretation of the emergence profile for implant restoration.

With regard to the cervical concept, vertical criteria and the restoration form are restorative prerequisites to achieve esthetic results with an optimal PES/papilla index score (PIS).

Cervical contouring concept

The cervical aspect of the abutment plays an important role in the final vertical level of the soft tissue. When overcontoured, pressure on the soft tissue mechanically causes apicalization. The subgingival aspect of provisional and definitive crowns should avoid a convex and flared profile except when one wishes to more apically relocate the free gingival margin around implants.

Two weeks postoperatively, reshaping provisional crowns and adding self-curing acrylic resin chairside induces minimum pressure on the buccal margin, optimal pressure on the adjacent papilla, and apicalization of the proximal contacts.

This cervical pressure concept is only valid proximally (not facially), where soft tissue and collagen bundles should be stretched or compressed for papilla stimulation.[177] On the buccal aspect, the emergence profile of the provisional and definitive restoration should be flat (undercontoured) for type I biotypes and concave for type II biotypes, which keeps the free gingival margin more coronal (Fig 5-44). Any increased bulk is detrimental to the vertical level of the peri-implant soft tissue and is responsible for gingival recession.

Vertical biologic criteria

As stated above, the presence of the papilla and the maintenance of the gingival margin for anterior implant restoration depend not only on the

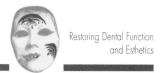

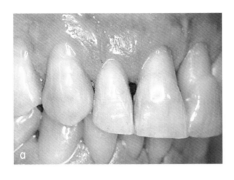

Fig 5-44a Patient with advanced periodontal disease involving the anterior maxillary teeth.

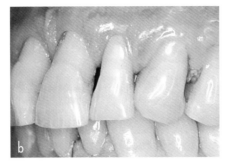

Fig 5-44b Left three-quarters view of the same patient showing class IV gingival recession.

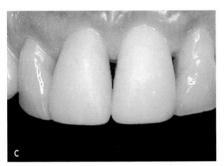

Fig 5-44c Following extraction of the central incisors, implants and provisional crowns were placed during the same session.

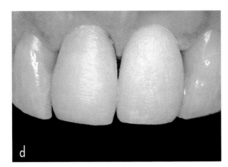

Fig 5-44d Flattening of the buccal margins of the provisional restoration and apicalization of the proximal contacts regenerate the interproximal papilla.

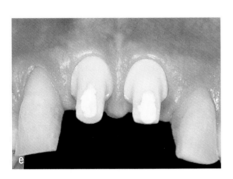

Fig 5-44e Zirconia abutments with concave submergence profiles connected to the implants.

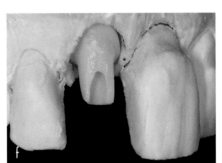
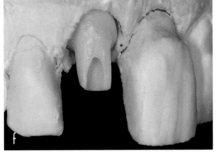

Fig 5-44f Flat emergence profile created with ceramic paste on the cast.

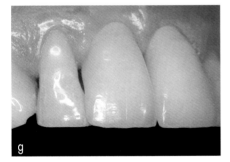

Fig 5-44g Definitive Procera restorations, right side.

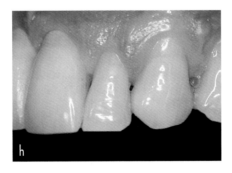

Fig 5-44h Definitive Procera restorations, left side. This is an acceptable esthetic result for such a periodontally advanced case. (Laboratory work by Mr J. M. Etienne Pulnoy, France. Provisional and final restorations by Dr A. Saadoun, Paris, France.)

implant placement parameters (see previous discussion of Implant Placement) but also on the implant restoration parameters. Early placement of single-tooth implants may be preferable to the delayed implant placement technique in terms of early generation of interproximal papilla, gingival margin level, and the achievement of an appropriate clinical crown height. In one report, no difference in papilla dimension was seen 1.5 years after placement of the implant crown.[178]

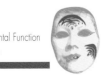

Implant restoration form

Tooth form in natural dentition is classically described as square, elliptical, or triangular. Even if the original interproximal bone height and interdental papilla height are successfully maintained, the supracrestal height of the inter-implant papilla may rarely exceed 3.0 mm. Therefore, typical implant-supported restorations have their contact area lengthened 2.0 mm or more to meet the reduced papilla. If the above parameters are respected, a decreased distance from the interproximal bone peak to the apical point of the contact surface between the implant restoration and the adjacent tooth or between adjacent implant restorations results in a squarer tooth form, which compensates for the loss of a portion of the interdental papilla. This is particularly true in the type II gingival biotype and may necessitate some type of restorative work on the adjacent tooth.[179]

Pink esthetic score and papilla index score

The final esthetic result of the implant restoration can be verified objectively using the seven anatomical determinants[180] of the PES (see chapter 4). If the initial PES is acceptable, immediate implantation and restoration can be performed. If initial PES is poor, alternative treatment methods should be considered.[180] The PIS introduced by Jemt[181] is a series of values defined as follows:

0 =   no papilla
1 =   less than half the height of the papilla
2 =   at least half the height of the papilla is present, but not all the
        way to the contact point
3 =   papilla fills the entire proximal space
4 =   hyperplastic papilla

Occlusal trauma

Implant osseointegration depends on a variety of factors, such as bone quality and type of implant surface. It is also subject to adaptation in response to changes in bone metabolism or transmission of masticatory forces. Understanding of long-term physiologic adjustment is critical to prevent potential loss of osseointegration, especially because excessive occlusal forces are a major factor in peri-implant bone loss and implant failure.[182]

Excessive pressure on the bone around titanium implants can cause fracture of the bone and can also induce bone resorption in an aseptic environment.[183] The biologic response of the bone to mechanical tension around dental implants is similar.[184] The shear stress force that can appear at the bone-implant interface upon occlusal loading can have a major impact on the success of osseointegration.

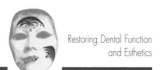

Restoring Dental Function
and Esthetics

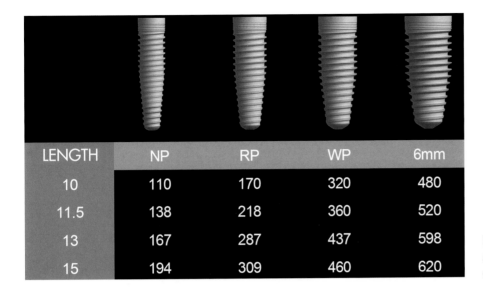

LENGTH	NP	RP	WP	6mm
10	110	170	320	480
11.5	138	218	360	520
13	167	287	437	598
15	194	309	460	620

Fig 5-45a TiUnite tapered implant surface in various lengths and diameters.

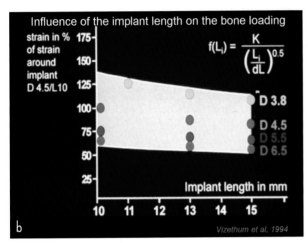

Influence of the implant length on the bone loading

$$f(L_i) = \frac{K}{\left(\frac{L_i}{dL}\right)^{0.5}}$$

strain in % of strain around implant D 4.5/L10

D 3.8
D 4.5
D 5.5
D 6.5

Implant length in mm

Vizethum et al, 1994

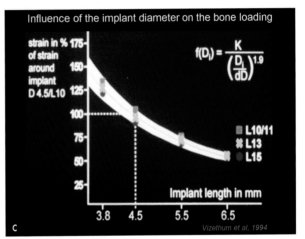

Influence of the implant diameter on the bone loading

$$f(D_i) = \frac{K}{\left(\frac{D_i}{dD}\right)^{1.9}}$$

strain in % of strain around implant D 4.5/L10

L10/11
L13
L15

Implant length in mm

Vizethum et al, 1994

Fig 5-45b The cervical stress does not significantly decrease when the implant length is increased.

Fig 5-45c The cervical stress decreases significantly when the implant diameter is increased.

During the first year of function, bone loss around implants in poorly adapted bone follows a contour similar to that of the zone of tension.[185] The control of horizontal occlusal forces during the first months of function is a determining factor in reduced stress in the crestal zone, bone adaptation, and minimal crestal bone loss. Therefore, marginal bone remodeling occurs after the placement of the definitive restoration in zones where no effective 3D interlocking between bone and the implant abutment surface exists, while the chances of preserving intact bone level increase when retention elements extend to the top of the implant.[44]

Several factors influence the occlusal forces on implant restorations: (1) bone density; (2) the available bone volume topography; (3) implant size, design, position, and number; and (4) direction of forces in patient function or parafunction.[186] Rough-surface tapered implants decrease the dispersion of stress on the implant away from the collar. Their design allows a better distribution of forces along the body of the implant, which indirectly minimizes cervical bone resorption (Fig 5-45).

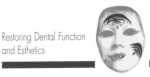

This increases the primary stability and accelerates osseointegration. Depending on the collar position, a change in the osseous microgap level may occur.

Bone resorption close to the first thread of osseointegrated implants is frequently observed during initial loading. Bone resorption at the implant neck area, however, is not inevitable because some clinical observations have indicated that bone preservation is possible with platform switching. Platform switching may also alter the microgap location or the stress concentration area between the abutment and implant.[187] This configuration has the biomechanical advantage of shifting the stress concentration area away from the cervical bone-implant interface. The disadvantage, however, is that it may increase stress on the abutment or abutment screw.

Factors in peri-implant bone loss

In the presence of healthy peri-implant mucosa, overloading of implants in the dog model increased bone-to-implant contact percentage and slightly reduced marginal bone level. However, resorption did not progress beyond the implant neck. Overloading aggravated the plaque-induced bone resorption when peri-implant inflammation was present. Nevertheless, the control of both plaque accumulation and occlusal load is essential for implant longevity.[188]

A recent study showed that the 5-year mean bone level change amounted to 0.4 mm for axially positioned implants and 0.5 mm for nonaxially positioned implants. Correlation analysis revealed lack of statistically significant correlation between inter-implant inclination and 5-year bone level change. The study failed to support the hypothesis that implant inclination has an effect on peri-implant bone loss.[189]

Effect of length and diameter

The length and diameter of the implant influence the implant cervical bone stress. By increasing the length of a 4.5-mm-diameter implant from 10 to 15 mm, the maximum cervical bone load or bone loss decreases by only 10% (see Fig 5-45a). The length of the implant should be adequate to ensure a favorable implant-restoration ratio. An increase in implant diameter from 3.8 to 6.5 mm results in a 60% decrease in the maximum cervical bone load (see Fig 5-45c). Larger-diameter implants should be selected with consideration to the characteristics of the interproximal bone buccopalatal position.

Adjacent bone density may be influenced by implant diameter, perhaps due to differences in force dissipation. Bone density in proximity to wide implants was decreased in comparison to narrower sizes when all other parameters remained similar. Force distribution is more

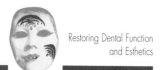

Restoring Dental Function
and Esthetics

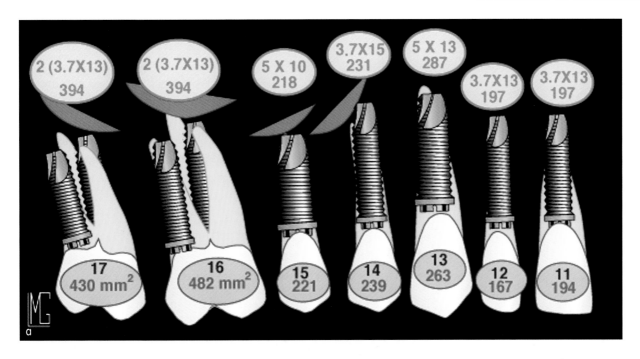

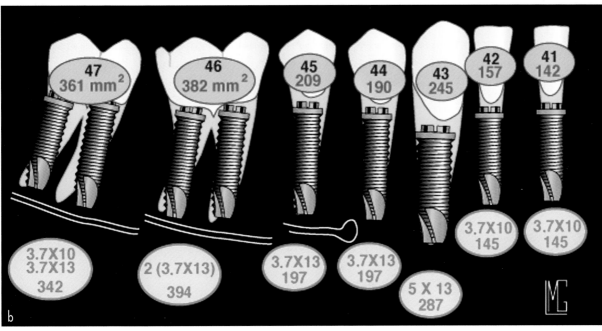

Figs 5-46a and 5-46b Maxillary teeth- and implant-bearing surfaces in square mm (a). Mandibular teeth- and implant-bearing surfaces in square mm (b). (Courtesy of Dr M. LeGall, Lorient, France.)

diluted when wider implants with a greater surface area are placed. The clinical consequence may be long-term maintenance of osseointegration.[182]

The occlusal surface of the tooth to be replaced can be used as reference for the choice of diameter and length of the implant (Fig 5-46), particularly for an immediate placement and/or loading, where the implant dimensions directly influence its immediate stability.[190]

Restoring Dental Function and Esthetics

Conclusion

Implant surgery, perhaps more than other aspects of dentistry, demands predictability and longevity. While ideal treatment decisions must be determined on a case-by-case basis, it is important to recognize in advance the various potential outcomes to ensure that realistic treatment plans are made for each patient. Fortunately, new trends in implant therapy decrease the length of treatment, enhance implant survival rates, preserve soft tissue contours, decrease functional stress, and improve the psychologic aspects of treatment.

When implants are to be placed in the esthetic zone, the surgeon and restorative dentist must include a cohesive functional, periodontal, and esthetic evaluation of the implant site and adjacent natural dentition in their pretreatment assessment. Soft tissue esthetics is essential for successful esthetic implant treatment. Biologic considerations must guide clinicians' prosthetic decisions. Harmonious soft tissue integration depends on *(1)* the architecture and density of the underlying bone, *(2)* the gingival biotype, *(3)* the thickness of the gingiva, and *(4)* the presence of sound interproximal bone at the level of the adjacent teeth. The condition of keratinized gingiva, facial bone level, and surface topography of transmucosal implant components can influence the soft tissue interface and gingival recession at implant components.

Successful treatment also involves the design and surface of the implant, the 3D position at the implant head, the horizontal distance between the implant and the adjacent structures, and the vertical distance between the interproximal bone and the apical implant contact restoration.

Understanding the periodontal implications, the physiology of the biologic space and its re-formation around implants, and the biocompatibility of the prosthetic components is essential for the selection of appropriate prosthetic procedures.[10,191] Peri-implant bone remodeling is mainly driven by the establishment of the biologic width and is influenced by several factors.[192] Consideration of these principles has improved the predictability of implant procedures and, therefore, the functional and esthetic results.

To establish an optimal esthetic implant restoration and to achieve esthetic predictability with a successful outcome, the prerequisites should always be a precise, comprehensive, biologic, and prosthetic diagnosis, combined with the most conservative, appropriate, and least traumatic treatment for the patient (Table 5-2).

Advances in surgical techniques and implant materials have moved implant treatment beyond functional integration toward restoratively driven principles with a heightened awareness that favorable results will also depend on biologically driven therapy.[10] Several changes need to be implemented in materials and procedures to reduce or prevent tissue remodeling, stabilize the volume of the soft tissues, and improve esthetics.

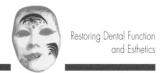

Restoring Dental Function
and Esthetics

Table 5-2 Esthetic predictability criteria: favorable versus unfavorable factors

Parameters	Favorable criteria	Unfavorable criteria
Level of free gingival margin	Identical or more coronal to the margin of the adjacent teeth	More apical than the gingival margin of the adjacent teeth
Periodontal biotype	Thick and flat biotype	Thin and scalloped biotype
	Rectangular teeth	Triangular teeth
Proximal bone sounding of the teeth adjacent to the implant	Presence of bone at 3.0-mm distance from the buccal side and 4.5-mm maximum distance from the proximal side	Bone architecture with more than 3.0 mm on the buccal side and more than 4.5 mm on the proximal side
Location of the tooth-implant restoration contact point	Less than 4.5 mm to the peak of the bone with the adjacent teeth	More than 5 mm to the peak of bone with the adjacent teeth
	Less than 3.5 mm between two implants	More than 3.5 mm between two implants
Mesiodistal length of the edentulous crest	Enough bone (> 2 mm) between implant and natural teeth and ≥ 3 mm between two implants	Less than 1 mm between the natural teeth and the adjacent implant or < 3 mm between two implants
Buccopalatal width of the edentulous crest	More than 6 mm, leaving > 2 mm of buccal bone from the implant	Less than 6 mm, leaving < 1 mm of buccal bone from the implant
Timing of the procedure	Immediate implant placement within a short time following the extraction (< 1 week)	Delayed implant placement (> 8 weeks)
Surgical technique	Flapless procedure preserving the papilla	Flap elevation with incision affecting the papilla
Provisionalization	> 6 months allows stability of the peri-implant hard and soft tissue	< 4 months causes recession of the peri-implant hard and soft tissue

Material developments include tapered implants with microthreads, rough-surface implants, and new abutment designs and biomaterials (eg, titanium, zirconia, and alumina) for prosthetic components.[30] Model-guided and computer-guided techniques allow customized abutments and accurate surgical templates to be prepared and provisional restorations created in the laboratory prior to any surgical procedure.

Procedural developments include noninvasive surgical approaches (flapless) and immediate placement of implants after extraction.[193,194] When flap elevation is mandatory, soft tissue grafting is favorable to improve the biotype and create a certain level of soft tissue "auto-stability."

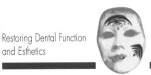

Restoring Dental Function and Esthetics

Avoidance of soft tissue recession, especially in thin and moderate biotypes, requires several criteria to be respected. Procedures that avoid multiple connections of prosthetic components should be favored for additional maintenance of soft tissues.

Since peri-implant stability is a complex multifactorial issue, summarizing the "ideal procedure" is not easy. The optimal management of esthetic perio-implant dentistry cases results from the following:

- An understanding and application of biologic factors
- Management of bone, soft tissue, and prosthetic contours
- A multidisciplinary approach with the surgeon, laboratory technician, and restorative dentist in agreement on the biologic concerns and trends

All of these factors play a key part in the esthetic outcome and the long-term stability of the soft tissue esthetics.[175]

The art is in the details, and in esthetic dentistry the objective is the same: Perfection is the only option.[195]

Acknowledgments

I would like to thank my friend and colleague Dr Marcel Le Gall (Lorient, France) for the quality of his drawings used in this chapter and also all the other colleagues who gave clinical documentation to illustrate this chapter.

References

1. Ericsson I, Nilner K. Early functional loading using Brånemark dental implants. Int J Periodontics Restorative Dent 2002;2(1):9–19.
2. Renouard F, Rangert B. Facteurs de Risque et Traitements Implantaires. Evaluation Clinique et Approche Rationelle. Paris: Quintessence International, 1999.
3. Abbou M. Primary stability and osseointegration: Preliminary clinical results with a tapered diminishing-thread implant. Pract Proced Aesthet Dent 2003;15(2):161–168.
4. Van Dooren E. Optimizing esthetics at the periodontal-restorative interface. In: Romano R, Bichacho N, Touati B (eds). The Art of the Smile: Integrating Prosthodontics, Orthodontics, Periodontics, Dental Technology, and Plastic Surgery in Esthetic Dental Treatment. Chicago: Quintessence, 2005:321–340.
5. Ahmad I. Geometric considerations in anterior dental aesthetics: Restorative principles. Pract Periodontics Aesthetic Dent 1998;10:813–822.
6. Saadoun AP, Le Gall M, Touati B. Selection and ideal tridimensional implant position for soft tissue aesthetics. Pract Periodontics Aesthet Dent. 1999;11(9):1063–1072.
7. Palacci P. Esthetic Implant Dentistry: Soft and Hard Tissue Management. Chicago: Quintessence, 2001.
8. Sennerby L, Rasmusson L. Implant stability. Inf Dent 2002:270–272.
9. Schuler RF, Roberts FA. Advanced surgical techniques to enhance implant success in the maxilla. Pract Proced Aesthet Dent 2005;17(10):697–704.

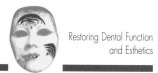

Restoring Dental Function and Esthetics

10. Touati B. Biologically driven implant treatment. Pract Proced Aesthet Dent 2003;15(10):734.
11. Salama H, Jundslalys G. Immediate implantation and soft tissue reaction. Clin Oral Implants Res 2003;14(2):144–149.
12. Hermann JS, Cochran DL, Nummikoski PV, Buser D. Crestal bone changes around titanium implants. A radiographic evaluation of unloaded nonsubmerged and submerged implants in the canine mandible. J Periodontol 1997;68:1117–1130.
13. Hermann JS, Buser D, Schenk RK, Cochran DL. Crestal bone changes around titanium implants. A histometric evaluation of unloaded non-submerged and submerged implants in the canine mandible. J Periodontol 2000;71:1412–1424.
14. Glauser R, Ruhstaller P, Windisch S, et al. Immediate occlusal loading of Branemark System TiUnite implants placed predominantly in soft bone: 4-year results of a prospective clinical study. Clin Implant Dent Relat Research 2005;7(suppl 1):52–59.
15. Small PN, Tarnow DP, Cho SC. Gingival recession around wide-diameter versus standard-diameter implants: A 3- to 5-year longitudinal prospective study. Pract Proced Aesthet Dent 2001;13(2):143–146.
16. Small PN, Tarnow DP. Gingival recession around implants: A 1-year longitudinal prospective study. Int J Oral Maxillofac Implants 2000;15:527–532.
17. Oates TW, West J, Jones J, Kaiser D, Cochran DL. Long-term changes in soft tissue height on the facial surface of dental implants. Implant Dent 2002;11:272–279.
18. Adell R, Lekholm U, Rockler B, et al. Marginal tissue reactions at osseointergrated titanium fixtures (I). A 3-year longitudinal prospective study. J Oral Maxillofac Surg 1986;15:39–52.
19. Ekfeldt A, Ericsson A, Johansson LA. Peri-implant mucosal level in patients treated with implant-supported fixed prostheses: A 1-year follow-up study. Int J Prosthodont 2003;16:529–532.
20. Albrektsson T, Zarb G, Worthington P, Eriksson AR. The long-term efficacy of currently used dental implants: A review and proposed criteria of success. Int J Oral Maxillofac Implants 1986;1(1):11–25.
21. Rompen E, Domken O, Degidi M, Pontes AE, Piattelli A. The effect of material characteristics, of surface topography and of implant components and connections on soft tissue intergration: A literature review. Clin Oral Implants Res 2006;17(suppl 2):55–67.
22. Rasmusson L, Kahnberg KE, Tan A. Effects of implant design and surface on bone regeneration and implant stability: An experimental study in the dog mandible. Clin Implant Dent Relat Res 2001;3:2–8.
23. Widmark G, Friberg B, Johansson B, Sindet-Pedersen S, Taylor A. Mk III: A third generation of the self-tapping Bränemark System implant, including the new Stargrip internal grip design. A 1-year prospective four-center study. Clin Implant Dent Relat Res 2003; 5(4):273–279.
24. Siepenkothen T. Clinical performance and radiographic evaluation of a novel single-piece implant in a private practice over a mean of seventeen months. J Prosthet Dent 2007;97(6, suppl):69S-78S.
25. Villa R, Rangert B. Immediate and early function of implants placed in extraction sockets of maxillary infected teeth: A pilot study. J Prosthet Dent 2007;97(6, suppl): 96S-108S.
26. Park SE, Da Silva JD, Weber HP, Ishikawa-Nagai S. Optical phenomenon of peri-implant soft tissue. Part I. Spectrophotometric assessment of natural tooth gingiva and peri-implant mucosa. Clin Oral Implants Res 2007;18:569–574.
27. Ishikawa-Nagai S, Da Silva JD, Weber HP, Park SE. Optical phenomenon of peri-implant soft tissue. Part II. Preferred implant neck color to improve soft tissue esthetics. Clin Oral Implants Res 2007;18:575–580.
28. Saadoun AP, Le Gall MG, Touati B. Current trends in implantology: Part II— Treatment planning, aesthetic considerations, and tissue regeneration. Pract Proced Aesthet Dent 2004;16(10):707–714.

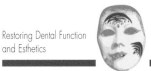

29. Leziy SS, Miller BA. Replacement of adjacent missing anterior teeth with scalloped implants: A case report. Pract Proced Aesth Dent 2005;17(5):331–338.

30. Abrahamsson I, Berglundh T. Tissue characteristics at microthreaded implants: An experimental study in dogs. Clin Implant Dent Relat Res 2006;8(3):107–113.

31. Schüpbach P, Glauser R, Rocci A, et al. The human bone-oxidized titanium implant interface: A light microscopic, scanning electron microscopic, back-scatter scanning electron microscopic, and energy dispersive x-ray study of clinically retrieved dental implants. Clin Implant Dent Relat Res 2005;7(suppl 1):36–43.

32. Souza A. Histometric analysis of bone implant contact with 4 different implant surfaces. Int J Oral Maxillofac Implants 2000;17:337–353.

33. Albrektesson T, Johansson C, Lundgren A, Sul Y, Gottlow J. Experimental studies on oxidized implants. A histomorphometrical and biomechanical analysis. Appl Osseo Res 2000;1:21–24.

34. Friberg B, Dahlin C, Widmark G, Östman P, Billström C. One-year results of a prospective multicenter study on Brånemark System Implants with a TiUnite surface. Clin Implant Dent Relat Res 2005;7(suppl 1):70–75.

35. Glauser R, Schüpbach P, Gottlow J, Hämmerle CH. Peri-implant soft tissue barrier at experimental one-piece mini-implants with different surface topography in humans: A light-microscopic overview and histometric analysis. Clin Implant Dent Relat Res 2005;7(Suppl 1):44–51.

36. Cochran D, Hermann J, Schenk R, Higginbottom F, Buser D. Biologic width around titanium implants. A histometric analysis of the implanto-gingival junction around unloaded and loaded nonsubmerged implants in the canine mandible. J Periodontol 1997;68:186–198.

37. Abrahamsson I, Berglundh T, Moon IS, Lindhe J. Peri-implant tissues at submerged and non-submerged titanium implants. J Clin Periodontol 1999;26:600–607.

38. Aalam AA, Nowzari H. Clinical evaluation of dental implants with surfaces roughened by anodic oxidation, dual acid-etched implants, and machined implants. Int J Oral Maxillofac Implants 2005;20:793–798.

39. Alomrani AN, Hermann JS, Jones AA, Buser D, Schoolfield J, Cochran DL. The effect of a machined collar on coronal hard tissue around titanium implants: A radiographic study in the canine mandible. Int J Oral Maxillofac Implants 2005;20:677–686.

40. Shin YK, Han CH, Heo SJ, Kim S, Chun HJ. Radiographic evaluation of marginal bone level around implants with different neck designs after 1 year. Int J Oral Maxillofac Implants 2006;21:789–794.

41. Berglundh T, Gotfredsen K, Zitzmann NU, Lang NP, Lindhe J. Spontaneous progression of ligature induced peri-implantitis at implants with different surface roughness: An experimental study in dogs. Clin Oral Implants Res 2007;18:655–661.

42. Jansen CE, Weisgold A. Presurgical treatment planning for the anterior single-tooth implant restoration. Compend Contin Educ Dent 1995;16:746.

43. Hurzeler M. New tendency in esthetic implantology. Société Française de Dentisterie Esthétique (SFDE) meeting. Achieving Ultimate Aesthetics with Implants in the Aesthetic Zone, Paris, France, Oct 2006.

44. Schropp L, Isidor F, Kostopoulos L, Wenzel A. Optimizing anterior esthetics with immediate implant placement and single-implant treatment. Int J Periodontics Restorative Dent 1999;19(1):21–29.

45. Rompen E, Touati B, Van Dooren E. Factors influencing marginal tissue remodeling around implants. Pract Proced Aesthet Dent 2003;15(10):754–761.

46. Kan JY, Rungcharassaeng K, Lozada J. Immediate placement and provisionalization of maxillary anterior single implants: 1-year prospective study. Int J Oral Maxillofac Implants 2003;18:31–39.

47. Park C, Kim S, Choi Y. Modification of gum biotype to prevent midfacial gingival recession. [Proceedings of the Sixteenth Annual Scientific Meeting of the European Association for Osseointegration, 25–27 Oct 2007, Barcelona.] Barcelona: European Association for Osseointegration, 2007.

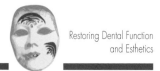

Restoring Dental Function
and Esthetics

48. Spear FM. The use of implants and ovate pontics in the esthetic zone. Compend Contin Educ Dent 2008 Mar;29(2):72–74.

49. Kan JY, Rungcharassaeng K, Lozada J. Immediate placement and provisionalization of maxillary anterior single implants: 1-year prospective study. Int Oral Maxillofac Implants 2003;18:31–39.

50. Kois JC. The restorative-periodontal interface: Biological parameters. Periodontol 2000 1996;1:29–38.

51. Kois J. Predictable single-tooth peri-implant esthetics: Five diagnostic keys. Compend Contin Educ Dent 2004;25:895–900.

52. Linkevicus T, Apse P, Grybauskas S, Puisys A. The influence of soft tissue thickness on crestal bone changes around implants. [Proceedings of the Sixteenth Annual Scientific Meeting of the European Association for Osseointegration, 25–27 Oct 2007, Barcelona.] Barcelona: European Association for Osseointegration, 2007.

53. Gargiulo AW, Wentz FM, Orban B. Mitotic activity of human oral epithelium exposed to 30 per cent hydrogen peroxide. Oral Surg Oral Med Oral Pathol 1961;14:474–492.

54. Berglundh T, Lindhe J. Dimension of the periimplant mucosa. Biological width revisited. J Clin Periodontol 1996;23(10):971–973.

55. Gottlow J, Johansson C, Albrektsson T, Lundgren A. Biomechanical and histologic evaluation of the TiUnite and Osseotite implant surfaces in rabbits after 6 weeks of healing. Appl Osseo Res 2000;1:25–27.

56. Ericsson I, Nilson H, Lindh T, Nilner K, Randow K. Immediate functional loading of Brånemark single tooth implants. An 18 months' clinical pilot follow-up study. Clin Oral Implant Res 2000;11:26–33.

57. Schupbach P, Glauser R. The defense architecture of the human peri-implant mucosa: A histological study. J Prosthet Dent 2007;9(6, suppl)7:15S–25S.

58. Listgarten MA, Buser D, Steinemann SG, Donath K, Lang NP, Weber HP. Light and transmission electron microscopy of the intact interfaces between non-submerged titanium-coated epoxy resin implants and bone or gingiva. J Dent Res 1992;71:364–371.

59. Glauser R, Lundgren AK, Gottlow J, et al. Immediate occlusal loading of Branemark System TiUnite implants placed predominantly in soft bone: 1-year results of a prospective clinical study. Clin Implant Dent Relat Res 2003;5 (suppl 1):47–56.

60. Elian N, Jalbout ZN, Cho SC, Froum S, Tarnow DP. Realities and limitations in the management of the interdental papilla between implants: Three case reports. Pract Proced Aesthet Dent 2003;15(10):737–744.

61. Saadoun AP, Le Gall MG, Touati B. Current trends in implantology: Part I— Biological response, implant stability, and implant design. Pract Proced Aesthet Dent 2004;16(7):529–535.

62. Tarnow DP, Cho SC, Wallace SS. The effect of inter-implant distance on the height of inter-implant bone crest. J Periodontol 2000;71:546–549.

63. Azzi R, Etienne D, Takei H, Fenech P. Surgical thickening of the existing gingiva and reconstruction of interdental papillae around implant-supported restorations. Int J Periodont Rest Dent 2000;22(1):71–77.

64. Ingber J. Forced eruption. I. A method of treating isolated one and two wall infrabony osseous defects—Rationale and case report. J Periodontol 1974; 45:199–206.

65. Salama H, Salama M. The role of orthodontic extrusive remodeling in the enhancement of soft and hard tissue profiles prior to implant placement: A systematic approach to the management of extraction site defects. Int J Periodontics Restorative Dent 1993;13(4):312–333.

66. Tarnow DP. When to extract or save a tooth in the esthetic zone. [Proceedings of the AAID Fifty-Sixth Annual Meeting, 7–11 Nov 2007, Las Vegas]. Chicago: American Academy of Implant Dentistry, 2007.

67. Esposito M, Worthington HV, Coulthard P, Jokstad A. Interventions for replacing missing teeth: Maintaining and re-establishing healthy tissue around dental implants. Cochrane Database System Rev 2002;(3):CD003069.

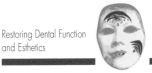

68. Schropp L, Wenzel A, Kostopoulos L, Karring T. Bone healing and soft tissue contour changes following single-tooth extraction: A clinical and radiographic 12-month prospective study. Int J Periodont Restorative Dent 2003;23:313–323.

69. Botticelli D, Berglundh T, Lindhe J. Hard tissue alterations following immediate implant placement in extraction sites. J Clin Periodontol 2004;31:820–828.

70. Hämmerle C. Augmenting bone plus soft tissue. News Geistlich 2005;1:10–11.

71. Saadoun AP, Landsberg CJ. Treatment classifications and sequencing for post-extraction implant therapy: A review. Pract Periodontics Aesthet Dent 1997;9(8):933–941.

72. Buser D. Good prognosis with early implantation. News Geistlich 2005;1:12–14.

73. Landsberg CJ. Socket seal surgery combined with immediate implant placement. A novel approach for single-tooth replacement. Int J Periodontics Restorative Dent 1997;17(2):140–149.

74. Elian N, Cho SC, Froum S., Smith RB, Tarnow DP. A simplified socket classification and repair technique. Pract Proced Aesthet Dent 2007;19(2):99–104.

75. Araujo M, Lindhe J. Dimensional ridge alterations following tooth extraction. An experimental study in the dog. J Clin Periodontol 2005;32:212–218.

76. Nevins M, Camelo M, De Paoli S, et al. A study of the fate of the buccal wall of extraction sockets of teeth with prominent roots. Int J Periodontics Restorative Dent 2006;26:19–29.

77. Testori T, Bianchi F. Ideal implant positioning in a maxillary anterior extraction socket. Academy News 2003;14(2):1–13.

78. Landsberg C. Preservation of the interimplant papilla in the esthetic zone. In: Romano R, Bichacho N, Touati B (eds). The Art of the Smile: Integrating Prosthodontics, Orthodontics, Periodontics, Dental Technology, and Plastic Surgery in Esthetic Dental Treatment. London: Quintessence, 2005:297–320.

79. Araujo M, Sukekava F, Wennstrom J, Lindhe J. Ridge alterations following implant placement in fresh extraction sockets: An experimental study in the dog. J Clin Periodontol 2005;32(6):645–652.

80. Botticelli D, Berglundh T, Persson LG, Lindhe J. Bone regeneration at implants with turned or rough surfaces in self-contained defects. An experimental study in the dog. J Clin Periodontol 2005;32:448–455.

81. Botticelli D, Persson LG, Lindhe J, Berglundh T. Bone tissue formation adjacent to implants placed in fresh extraction sockets: An experimental study in dogs. Clin Oral Implants Res 2006;17:351–358.

82. Chen ST, Darby IB, Reynolds EC. A prospective clinical study of non-submerged immediate implants: Clinical outcomes and esthetic results. Clin Oral Implants Res 2007;18:552–562.

83. Hurzeler M, Weng D, Akimoto K, Becker W, Persson R. Peri-implant tissue management: Optimal timing for functional and esthetic outcome. Int J Periodontics Restorative Dent 1999;19:36–43.

84. Simion M, Jovanovic SA, Trisi P, Scarano A, Piattelli A. Vertical ridge augmentation around dental implants: Esthetic tissue principles. Pract Periodontics Aesthet Dent 2000;12(9):837–841.

85. Becker W, Hujoel P, Becker BE. Effect of barrier membranes and autologous bone grafts on ridge width preservation around implants. Clin Implant Dent Relat Res 2002;4:143–149.

86. Wilson TG Jr, Buser D. Advances in the use of guided tissue regeneration for localized ridge augmentation in combination with dental implants. Tex Dent J 1994;111(7):5,7–10.

87. Jemt T, Lekholm U, Adell R. Osseointegrated implants in the treatment of partially edentelous patients: A preliminary study on 876 consecutively placed fixtures. Int J Oral Maxillofac Implants 1989;4(3):211–217.

88. Maiorana C, Beretta M, Salina S, Santoro F. Reduction of autogenous bone graft resorption by means of bio-oss coverage: A prospective study. Int J Periodontics Restorative Dent 2005;25:19–25.

89. Smukler H, Castellucci F, Capri D. The role of the implant housing in obtaining aesthetics: Generation of peri-implant gingivae and papillae—Part 1. Pract Proced Aesthet Dent 2003;15(2):141–149.

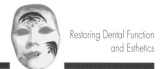

Restoring Dental Function and Esthetics

90. Araujo M, Wennstrom JL, Lindhe J. Modeling of the buccal and lingual bone walls of fresh extraction sites following implant installation. Clin Oral Implants Res 2006;17:606–614.

91. Paolantonio M, Dolci M, Scarano A, et al. Immediate implantation in fresh extraction sockets. A controlled clinical and histological study in man. J Periodontol 2001;72(11):1560–1571.

92. Wörhle P. Single-tooth replacement in the esthetic zone with immediate provisionalization: Fourteen consecutive case reports. Pract Periodont Aesthet Dent 1998;10(9):1107–1114.

93. Wöhrle P. Immediate implant placement and provisionalization: 36-month statistical results. [Proceedings of the Fifteenth Annual Meeting of the Academy of Osseointegration, 9–11 Mar 2000, New Orleans]. Arlington Heights, IL: Academy of Osseointegration, 2000.

94. Grunder U. Immediate functional loading of immediate implants in edentulous arches: Two-year results. Int J Periodontics Restorative Dent 2001; 21:545–551.

95. Schwartz-Arad D, Chaushu G. Placement of implants into fresh extraction sites: 4 to 7 years retrospective evaluation of 95 immediate implants. J Periodontol 1997;68:1110–1116.

96. Ericsson I, Nilson H, Nilner K. Immediate functional loading of Branemark single tooth implants. A 5-year clinical follow-up study. Appl Osseo Res 2001;2:12–26.

97. Garber DA, Salama MA, Salama H. Immediate total tooth replacement. Compend Contin Educ Dent 2001;22(3):210–218.

98. Salama H, Salama M, Kelly J. The orthodontic-periodontal connection in implant site development. Pract Periodontics Aesthet Dent 1996;8:923–932.

99. Wachtel HC, Hûrzeler MB, Zuhr O, Bolz W. Soft tissue management around teeth and implants: A microsurgical approach. In: Romano R, Bichacho N, Touati B (eds). The Art of the Smile: Integrating Prosthodontics, Orthodontics, Periodontotics, Dental Technology, and Plastic Surgery in Esthetic Dental Treatment. London: Quintessence, 2005:341–361.

100. Gomez-Roman G. Influence of flap design on peri-implant interproximal crestal bone loss around single-tooth implants. Int J Oral Maxillofac Implants 2001;16(1):61–67.

101. Cardaropoli G, Monticelli F, Osorio R, et al. Healing following tooth extraction and immediate implant installation with flapless surgery. [Proceedings of the Sixteenth Annual Scientific Meeting of the European Association for Osseointegration, 25–27 Oct 2007, Barcelona]. Barcelona: European Association for Osseointegration, 2007.

102. Fortin T, Bosson J, Isidori M, Blanchet E. Effect of flapless surgery on pain experienced in implant placement using an image-guided system. Int J Oral Maxillofac Implants 2006;21:298–304.

103. Becker W, Goldstein M, Becker BE, Sennerby L. Minimally invasive flapless implant surgery: A prospective multicenter study. Clin Implant Dent Relat Res 2005;7(1, suppl):21S–27S.

104. Binderman I, Bahar H, Jacob-Hirsch J, et al. P2X4 is up-regulated in gingival fibroblasts after periodontal surgery. J Dent Res 2007;86(2):181–185.

105. Cardaropoli G, Lekholm U, Wennstrom JL. Tissue alterations at implant-supported single-tooth replacements: A 1-year prospective clinical study. Clin Oral Implants Res 2006;17:165–171.

106. Garber D, Salama M, Salama H. Immediate total tooth replacement in the external root resorption case. World Dentistry 2000;1:1–5.

107. Kois J. Altering gingival levels: The restorative connection. I: Biologic variables. J Esthet Dent 1994;6:3–9.

108. Grunder U, Gracis S, Capelli M. Influence of the 3-D bone-to-implant relationship on esthetics. Int J Perio Rest Dent 2005;25(2):113–119.

109. Garber DA, Belser UC. Restoration-driven implant placement with restoration-generated site development. Compend Contin Educ Dent 1995;16:796–804.

110. Becker W, Ochsenbein C, Tibbett L, Becker BE. Alveolar bone anatomic profiles as measured from dry skulls: Clinical ramifications. J Clin Periodontol 1997;24(10):727–731.

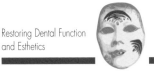

Restoring Dental Function and Esthetics

111. Saadoun AP, Le Gall MG. Implant positioning for periodontal, functional and esthetic results. Pract Periodontics Aesthet Dent 1992;4(7):43–54.

112. Saadoun AP, Sullivan DY, Krichek M, Le Gall M. Single tooth implant: Management for success. Pract Periodontics Aesthet Dent 1994;6(3):73–82.

113. Arnoux J, Weisgold A, Lu J. Single-tooth anterior implant: A word of caution. Part I. J Esthet Dent 1997;9:225–233.

114. Saadoun AP, Sebbag P. Immediate implant placement and temporization: Literature review and case studies. Compend Cont Educ Dent 2004;25(4):277–286.

115. Hebel KS, Gajjar R. Achieving superior aesthetic results: Parameters for implant and abutment selection. Int J Dent Symp 1997;4(1):42–47.

116. Esposito M, Ekestubbe A, Grondahl K. Radiological evaluation of marginal bone loss at tooth surfaces facing single Branemark implants. Clin Oral Implants Res 1993;4(3):151–157.

117. Jovanovic S. Anterior esthetic implant therapy. Société Française de Dentisterie Esthétique (SFDE) meeting. Achieving Ultimate Aesthetics with Implants in the Aesthetic Zone, Paris, France, 2003.

118. Kan JY, Rungcharassaeng K, Liddelow G, Henry P, Goodacre CJ. Periimplant tissue response following immediate provisional restoration of scalloped implants in the esthetic zone: A one-year pilot prospective multicenter study. J Prosthet Dent 2007;97(6, suppl):109S–118S.

119. Salama H, Salama M, Garber D, Adar P. The interproximal height of bone: A guidepost to predictable aesthetic strategies and soft tissue contours in anterior tooth replacement. Pract Periodontics Aesthet Dent 1998;10:1131–1141.

120. Tarnow DP, Malevez C. Clinical and radiographic evaluation of soft and hard tissue periodontal defects. Am J Dent 2002;15(5):339–345.

121. Choquet V, Hermans M, Adriaenssens P, Daelemans P, Tarnow DP, Malevez C. Clinical and radiographic evaluation of the papilla level adjacent to single-tooth dental implants. A retrospective study in the maxillary anterior region. J Periodontol 2001;72:1364–1371.

122. Grunder U. Stability of the mucosal topography around single-tooth implants and adjacent teeth: 1-year results. Int J Periodontics Restorative Dent 2000;20:11–17.

123. Tarnow D, Magner AW, Fletcher P. The effect of the distance from the contact point to the crest of the bone on the presence or absence of the interproximal dental papilla. J Periodontol 1992; 63:995–996.

124. Van der Velden U. Regeneration of the interdental soft tissues following denudation procedures. J Clin Periodontol 1982;9:455–459.

125. Saadoun AP. Immediate implant placement and temporization in extraction and healing sites. Compend Contin Educ Dent 2002;23(4):309–318.

126. Rungcharassaeng K, Kan J. Aesthetic implant management of multiple adjacent failing anterior maxillary teeth. Pract Proced Aesthet Dent 2004;16(5):365–369.

127. O'Sullivan D, Sennerby L, Meredith N. Measurements comparing the initial stability of five designs of dental implants: A human cadaver study. Clin Impl Dent Relat Res 2000;2(2):85–92.

128. Rompen E, DaSilva D, Lundgren AK, Gottlow J, Sennerby L. Stability measurements of a double-threaded titanium implant design with turned or oxidized surfaces. An experimental resonance frequency analysis study in the dog mandible. Appl Osseo Res 2000;1:18–20.

129. Meredith N, Book K, Friberg B, Jemt T, Sennerby L. Resonance frequency measurements of implant stability in vivo. A cross-sectional and longitudinal study of resonance frequency measurements on implants in the edentulous and partially dentate maxilla. Clin Oral Implants Res 1997;8:226–233.

130. Mori H, Manabe M, Kurachi Y, Nagumo M. Osseointegration of dental implants in rabbit bone with low mineral density. J Oral Maxillofac Surg 1997;55 (4):351–361.

131. Friberg B, Sennerby L, Meredith N, Lekholm U. A comparision between cutting torque and resonance frequency measurements of maxillary implants: A 20-month clinical study. Int J Oral Maxillofac Surg 1999;28:297–303.

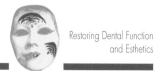

Restoring Dental Function and Esthetics

132. Meredith N, Alleyne D, Cawley P. Quantitative determination of the stability of the implant-tissue interface using resonance frequency analysis. Clin Oral Implants Res 1996;7:261–267.

133. Sennerby L, Meredith N. Resonance frequency analysis: Measuring implant stability and osseointegration. Compend Contin Educ Dent 1998;19(5):493–502.

134. Barewal RM, Oates TW, Meredith N, Cochran DL. Resonance frequency measurement of implant stability in vivo on implants with a sandblasted and acid-etched surface. Int J Oral Maxillofac Implants 2003;18(5):641–651.

135. Saadoun AP, Le Gall MG. Implant site preparation with osteotomes: Principles and clinical application. Pract Periodontics Aesthet Dent 1996;8(5):453–463.

136. Ericsson I, Randow K, Nilner K, Peterson A. Early functional loading of Brånemark dental implants: 5-year clinical follow-up study. Clin Implant Dent Relat Res 2000;2(2):70–77.

137. Marx RE. Platelet concentrate: A strategy for accelerating and improving bone regeneration. In: Davies JE (ed). Bone Engineering. Toronto: Em Squared, 2000:447–453.

138. Poitras Y. Reformer les limites du traitement implantaire au-delà des zones anatomiques défavorables. Inf Dent 2003;5:273–274.

139. Marx RE. Platelet-rich plasma: A source of multiple autologous growth factors for bone grafts. In: Lynch SE, Genco RJ, Marx RE (eds). Tissue Engineering: Applications in Maxillofacial Surgery and Periodontics. Hanover Park, IL: Quintessence, 1999:71–82.

140. Choukroun J, Adda F, Schoeffler C, Vervelle A. Une opportunité en paro-implantologie: le PRF. Implantodontie 2001;42:55–62.

141. Morioussef G. PRF et chirurgie muco-gingivale. Implantologie 2004;2:69–75.

142. Petrungaro P. Bone grafting at the time of extraction. A new technique for achieving natural bone and tissue contours in esthetic tooth replacement. AACD J 2000;16(1):30–43.

143. Froum SJ, Wallace SS, Tarnow DP, Cho SC. Effect of platelet-rich plasma on bone growth and osseointegration in human maxillary sinus grafts: Three bilateral case reports. Int J Periodontics Restorative Dent 2002;22(1):45–53.

144. De Vasconcelos Gurgel BC, Gonçalves PF, Pimentel SP, et al. Platelet-rich plasma may not provide any additional effect when associated with guided bone regeneration around dental implants in dogs. Clin Oral Implants Res 2007;18:649–654.

145. Allen EP. Use of mucogingival surgical procedures to enhance esthetics. Dent Clin North Am 1988;32:307–330.

146. Covani U, Marconcini S, Galassini G, Cornelini R, Santini S, Barone A. Connective tissue graft used as a biologic barrier to cover an immediate implant. J Periodontol 2007;78(8):1644–1649.

147. Sonick M. Periodontal plastic surgery: Enhancing the esthetic outcome of implant dentistry through addition and subtraction procedures. [Proceedings of the AAID Fifty-Sixth Annual Meeting, 7–11 Nov 2007, Las Vegas]. Chicago: American Academy of Implant Dentistry, 2007.

148. Kan JY, Rungcharassaeng K, Lozada JL. Bilaminar subepithelial connective tissue grafts for immediate implant placement and provisionalization in the esthetic zone. J Calif Dent Assoc 2005;33:865–871.

149. Mathews D. Soft tissue management around implants in the esthetic zone. Int J Periodontics Restorative Dent 2000;20:141–149.

150. Jovanovic SA, Paul SJ, Nishimura RD. Anterior implant-supported reconstructions: A surgical challenge. Pract Periodontics Aesthet Dent 1999;11(5):551–558.

151. Spear FM. Maintenance of the interdental papilla following anterior tooth removal. Pract Periodontics Aesthet Dent 1999;11(1):21–28.

152. Lekholm U, Sennerby L, Roos J, Becker W. Soft tissue and marginal bone conditions at osseointegrated implants that have exposed threads: A 5-year retrospective study. Int J Oral Maxillofac Implants 1996;11:599–604.

153. Lazzara RJ, Porter SS. Platform switching: A new concept in implant dentistry for controlling post-restorative bone levels. Int J Periodontics Restorative Dent 2006;26(1):9–17.

154. Hermann J, Schoolfield J, Nummiloski P, et al. Crestal bone changes around titanium implants: A methodologic study comparing linear radiographic with histometric measurements. Int J Oral Maxillofac Implants 2001;16(4):475–485.

155. Ericsson I, Persson LG, Berglundh T, Marinello CP, Lindhe J, Klinge B. Different types of inflammatory reactions in peri-implant soft tissues. J Clin Periodontol 1995;22(3):255–261.

156. Wörhle P. Nobel Perfect esthetic scalloped implant: Rationale for a new design. Clin Implant Dent Relat Res 2003;5(suppl 1):64–73.

157. Wöhrle P, Jovanovic S. NobelPerfect—A biologic approach to predictable natural esthetics. Appl Osseo Res 2004;4:49–54.

158. Kan JY, Rungcharassaeng K, Liddelow G, Henry P, Goodacre C. Periimplant tissue response following immediate provisional restoration of scalloped implants in the esthetic zone: A one-year pilot prospective multicenter study. J Prosthet Dent 2007;97(6, suppl):109S–118S.

159. McGehee J, Greenwell H, Hill M, Martin E, Scheetz J. A comparison of maxillary anterior soft tissue esthetics for immediately placed scalloped and standard platform implants. [Proceedings of the AO 2007 Annual Meeting, 8–10 Mar 2007, San Antonio]. Arlington Heights, IL: Academy of Osseointegration, 2007.

160. Rocci A, Gottlow J. Esthetic outcome of immediately loaded scalloped implants placed in extraction sites using flapless surgery. A 6 months report of 4 cases. Appl Osseo Res 2004;4:55–62.

161. Noelken R, Morbach T, Kunkel M, Wagner W. Immediate function with NobelPerfect implants in the anterior dental arch. Int J Periodontics Restorative Dent 2007;27(3):277–285.

162. Rompen E, Raespsaet N, Domken O, Touati B, Van Dooren E. Soft tissue stability at the facial aspect of gingivally converging abutments in the esthetic zone: A pilot clinical study. J Prosthet Dent 2007;97(6, suppl):119S–125S.

163. Bichacho N, Fromovitch O. The active implant: The implant solutions for every indication. Nobel BioCare Review. September 2007.

164. Karmon B, Fromovich O. Solutions for patients with compromised dentition utilizing a new implant design—An application demonstration. [Proceedings of the AAID Fifty-Sixth Annual Meeting, 7–11 Nov 2007, Las Vegas]. Chicago: American Academy of Implant Dentistry, 2007.

165. Touati B. Biologically driven prosthetic options in implant dentistry. Pract Proced Aesthet Dent 2004;16(7):517–520.

166. Touati B, Rompen E, van Dooren E. A new concept for optimizing soft tissue integration. Pract Proced Aesthet Dent 2005:17(10):712–715.

167. Norton MR. A short-term clinical evaluation of immediately restored maxillary TiOblast single-tooth implants. Int J Oral Maxillofac Implants 2004;19:274–281.

168. Pinto A, Dersot J. Remplacements implantaires unitaires: Critères et strategies esthétiques. Implantologies 2005;1:98–107.

169. Ong S, Chye M, Quake P. Crestal level and esthetics in maxillary anterior single-tooth implants. [Proceedings of the Sixteenth Annual Scientific Meeting of the European Association for Osseointegration, 25–27 Oct 2007, Barcelona.] Barcelona: European Association for Osseointegration, 2007.

170. Gamborenas I. Platform shifting: Gingival beauty to the next level. Nobel BioCare Review 2007:1–11.

171. Dibart S, Warbington M, Su MF, Skobe Z. In vitro evaluation of the implant-abutment bacterial seal: The locking taper system. Int J Oral Maxillofac Implants 2005;20(5):732–737.

172. Baumgarten H, Cocchetto R, Testori T, Meltzer A, Porter S. A new implant design for crestal bone preservation: Initial observations and case report. Pract Proced Aesthet Dent 2005;17(10):735–740.

173. Abrahamsson I, Berglundh T, Lindhe J. Soft tissue response to plaque formation at different implant systems. A comparative study in the dog. Clin Oral Implants Res 1998;9:73–79.

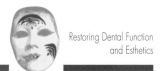

Restoring Dental Function
and Esthetics

174. Touati B, Guez G. Immediate implantation with provisionalization: From literature to clinical implications. Pract Proced Aesthet Dent 2002;14(9):699–707.

175. Fischer J, Jung R, Frost C, Mankoo T. Interdisciplinary management of implants in the esthetic zone: Data on strategy, systematic outcome and complications. [Proceedings of the Sixteenth Annual Scientific Meeting of the European Association for Osseointegration, 25–27 Oct 2007, Barcelona]. Barcelona: European Association for Osseointegration, 2007.

176. Jovanovic S. New advances in tissue management and esthetic implant treatment. [Proceedings of the AAID Fifty-Sixth Annual Meeting, 7–11 Nov 2007, Las Vegas]. Chicago: American Academy of Implant Dentistry, 2007.

177. Bichacho N, Landsberg CJ. A modified surgical/prosthetic approach for an optimal single implant-supported crown. Part II. The cervical contouring concept. Pract Periodontics Aesthet Dent 1994;6(4):35–41.

178. Schropp L, Isidor F, Kostopoulos L, Wenzel A. Interproximal papilla levels following early versus delayed placement of single-tooth implants: A controlled clinical trial. Int J Oral Maxillofac Implants 2005;20:753–761.

179. Garber DA, Salama H, Salama MA. Two-stage versus one-stage—Is there really a controversy? J Periodontol 2001;72(3):417–421.

180. Fürhauser R, Florescu D, Benesch T, Haas R, Mailath J, Watzek J. Evalution of soft tissue around single-tooth implant crowns: The pink esthetic score. Clin Oral Implants Res 2005;16:639–644.

181. Jemt T. Regeneration of gingival papillae after single-implant treatment. Int J Periodontics Restorative Dent 1997;17:326–333.

182. Brink J, Meraw SJ, Sarment D. Influence of implant diameter on surrounding bone. Clin Oral Implants Res 2007;18(5):563–568.

183. Frost HM. Bone's mechanostat: A 2003 update. Anat Rec A Discov Mol Cell Evol Biol 2003;275(2):1081–1101.

184. Misch CE, Suzuki JB, Misch-Dietsh FM, Bidez MW. A positive correlation between occlusal trauma and peri-implant bone loss: Literature support. Implant Dent 2005;14:108–116.

185. Kitamura E, Stegaroiu R, Nomura S, Miyakawa O. Biomechanical aspects of marginal bone resorption around osseointegrated implants: Considerations based on a three-dimensional finite element analysis. Clin Oral Implants Res 2004;15:401–412.

186. Misch CE. Efficient sequencing for prosthetic success—A 10-year perspective. [Proceedings of the AAID Fifty-Sixth Annual Meeting, 7–11 Nov 2007, Las Vegas]. Chicago: American Academy of Implant Dentistry, 2007.

187. Maeda Y, Miura J, Taki I, Sogo M. Biomechanical analysis on platform switching: Is there any biomechanical rationale? Clin Oral Implants Res 2007;18(5):581–584.

188. Kozlovsky A, Tal H, Laufer BZ, et al. Impact of implant overloading on the peri-implant bone in inflamed and non-inflamed peri-implant mucosa. Clin Oral Implants Res 2007;18(5):601–610.

189. Koutouzis T, Wennström JL. Bone level changes at axial- and non-axial-positioned implants supporting fixed partial dentures. A 5-year retrospective longitudinal study. Clin Oral Implants Res 2007;18(5):585–590.

190. Le Gall M, Saadoun A. Quelle surface portante pour un implant? J Periodont 1996;4:317–334.

191. Saadoun AP, Le Gall M. Periodontal implications in implant treatment planning for aesthetic results. Pract Periodontics Aesthet Dent 1998;10(5):655–664.

192. Cosyn G, Sabzevar MM, De Wilde P, De Rouck T. Two-piece implants with turned versus microtextured collars. J Periodontol 2007;78:1657–1663.

193. Saadoun AP, Touati B. Soft tissue recession around implants: Is it still unavoidable?—Part I. Pract Proced Aesthet Dent 2007;19(1):55–62.

194. Saadoun AP, Touati B. Soft tissue recession around implants: Is it still unavoidable?—Part II. Pract Proced Aesthet Dent 2007;19(2):81–87.

195. Romano R, Bichacho N, Touati B (eds). The Art of the Smile: Integrating Prosthodontics, Orthodontics, Periodontics, Dental Technology, and Plastic Surgery in Esthetic Dental Treatment. Chicago: Quintessence, 2005.

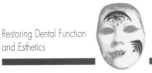

Single-Tooth Implants in the Esthetic Zone–Contemporary Concepts

6

Tidu Mankoo, BDS

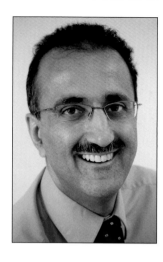

Tidu Mankoo, BDS

Tidu Mankoo is in private and referral practice in Windsor, UK. He treats implant, restorative, and esthetic cases, with particular emphasis on complex cases. He is the current president (2009–2010) of the European Academy of Esthetic Dentistry.

Email: tidu@advanceddentistry.co.uk

As discussed in earlier chapters, the placement of dental implants is now a mainstream procedure in esthetic and restorative dentistry. Because of currently available ceramics and technical expertise, the creation of an appropriate restoration that mimics the natural tooth in form, esthetics, and function is no longer considered the greatest challenge in implant dentistry. In cases where missing and failing teeth in the esthetic zone are to be restored, the dental implant restoration frequently is the first treatment modality considered. However, clinical experience and the literature indicate that the soft tissue esthetics remain a challenge, particularly with regard to maintenance of stability of labial soft tissue contours, the papillae between implants and teeth, and the inter-implant papillae.

Although clinicians now more fully understand the limitations in these areas, which leads to stronger treatment planning for implant restorations in the esthetic zone, many questions remain unanswered. The plethora of implant systems available today demands that treating clinicians have a clear appreciation and understanding of the response of the soft and hard tissues around various implant restorations, as there is no doubt that this response plays a key role in the esthetic outcome and determines the stability and predictability of the result over time. In the past, successful soft tissue esthetics in implant treatment were largely achieved by luck rather than by design. The contemporary approach to implant treatment planning anticipates the biologic response of the bone and the soft tissues once implants and prosthetic components are placed and uses this knowledge to attain optimal esthetic outcomes.

Key Factors in Soft Tissue Esthetics

Influences on the bone remodeling process

It is now generally accepted that bone and soft tissue remodeling occurs around all dental implant restorations, irrespective of the system used. This remodeling has been attributed to a number of factors, the most commonly accepted of which would seem to be the concept of the establishment of a biologic seal, described as a *biologic width*, between the free gingival margin and the crest of the peri-implant alveolar bone.[1–3] From a clinical perspective, this concept can be described as the three-dimensional remodeling of bone to create space for a connective tissue compartment between the bone and the epithelium. The extent of this remodeling is potentially influenced by several factors[2–16]:

- Three-dimensional position of the implant-abutment interface relative to the bone crest
- Presence of an inflammatory infiltrate in connective tissue adjacent to the microgap
- Design of the implant-abutment connection
- Repeated removal and replacement of prosthetic components
- Material of the transmucosal components (ie, titanium, alumina, zirconia, acrylic resin composite, gold, or porcelain)
- Shape and contours of the transmucosal components
- Thickness of the soft tissues
- Genetically predetermined normal wound healing in the individual host

Clinicians in contemporary clinical practice attempt to anticipate and compensate for the hard and soft tissue changes that result from this remodeling through proper treatment planning and procedures. Regardless of the reason for the remodeling, a certain dimension of soft tissue is required to house the necessary components of this biologic seal.

Traditionally, a great deal of emphasis has been placed on the volume of bone around implants in the esthetic zone. Some authors have advocated the creation of certain dimensions of peri-implant bone by means of extensive grafting procedures.[3,17] More recently, the tissue quality, tissue thickness, and tissue biotype have been given more credence.[9,18,19] The author believes that a paradigm shift needs to occur within the dental implant community in recognition that the relationship between bone and soft tissue is a more reciprocal one than previously thought—that is, bone is not the only key, but soft tissue quality and thickness influence bone remodeling and may even be more important than bone when it comes to long-term esthetics and stability of the peri-implant mucosa.

Implant component design

New concepts for component designs have been proposed for the head of the implant, the implant-abutment connection, and the form of the transmucosal abutment contour levels.[13–15,20–23] These proposals mainly serve the same purpose of creating a transmucosal undercontour, which logically should increase the available volume of peri-implant soft tissue and effectively thicken the soft tissue cuff around the implant-abutment connection. Four main ideas are commonly suggested today:

1. Creation of vertical or, more commonly, horizontal offset (*platform switching*) to reduce the vertical remodeling of the bone and soft tissues
2. Use of an abutment connection that incorporates a conical seal, which may reduce the micromotion of the components and/or bacterial contamination at the microgap

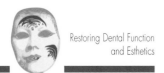

Restoring Dental Function and Esthetics

3. Use of an undercontoured or concave transmucosal form for the abutment and prosthetic components
4. Placement of the final abutment at the time of surgery or within a short time frame before soft tissues fully heal, and subsequently not removing it again

It has not been demonstrated conclusively that any of these individual concepts holds the key to bone remodeling; more likely, it is a combination of factors relating to the bone, the soft tissue, and indeed the design of the components used in treatment. In addition, the clinician should always consider the individual biologic variability in host response.

However, the majority of the newer implant-abutment designs effectively narrow or undercontour the transmucosal components, thereby increasing the room available to create a thicker cuff of soft tissue around the neck of the transmucosal components. Certainly, this increased thickness of soft tissue could be key factor for successful esthetic results in terms of longer-term soft tissue stability. It is logical to presume that if 3 to 4 mm of tissue is required to house the dimension of the peri-implant tissues, then ensuring that this dimension of soft tissue is present at the time of implant abutment placement may preclude the need for bone to remodel vertically to create the necessary dimension for the biologic seal. This may also prevent the gingival recession that is commonly reported to follow restoration of single-tooth implants in the esthetic zone.

In recent years, immediate implant placement using flapless procedures has gained popularity, as these procedures offer a minimally invasive and often virtually atraumatic surgery. While this has obvious benefits for the patient in terms of the surgical experience and perhaps treatment acceptance, it may not be advantageous from the standpoint of long-term clinical outcome. Both gingival recession and labial bone volume loss are accepted risks when using this technique,[24–29] prompting many clinicians to advocate a number of additional surgical steps such as grafting of biomaterials and tissue grafting in an attempt to increase the predictability and stability of the soft tissue outcomes.[18,19,30–36]

The goal of any implant therapy in the esthetic zone is to produce a lasting restoration that blends inconspicuously into the patient's smile. Factors such as a high lip line, a thin gingival biotype, and the number of adjacent teeth to be replaced can present significant hurdles to achieving of a lasting esthetic outcome. It is commonly accepted that in most cases with a single missing or single failing tooth, this goal is more easily achieved than in cases that require the restoration of multiple adjacent missing or failing teeth.[37–39] Box 6-1 lists the key factors necessary to achieve optimal results with implants in the esthetic zone. The relationship between these key points and clinical management are demonstrated in the case presentations later in this chapter.

> **Box 6-1 Key factors in the management of implants in the esthetic zone**
>
> - Adequate stable bone volume and architecture
> - Correct three-dimensional positioning of the implant
> - Adequate soft tissue thickness
> - Timing of final abutment connection
> - Transmucosal material, form, and contours of the abutment and prosthesis
> - Development and maintenance of appropriate soft tissue contours

Single-Tooth Restorations in the Esthetic Zone

The single-tooth restoration in the esthetic zone is a common application of dental implant therapy and in many ways represents the most demanding clinical management, particularly when it comes to long-term soft tissue esthetics. There are generally two situations where implants are indicated in the restoration of a single tooth in the esthetic zone: *(1)* in an existing edentulous site, and *(2)* in the replacement of a failing tooth.

In terms of the healed edentulous site, a site that has a mature healed edentulous ridge with good remaining bone volume and adequate soft tissue thickness in a patient with a thick tissue biotype is significantly different from a site where there has been significant damage to bone, soft tissue, or both through infection or trauma, or where there has been a large amount bone resorption and the soft tissue quality and biotype are unfavorable. Established protocols are well documented and effective, and in the favorable sites, good results can be achieved relatively easily. The compromised sites pose a greater challenge,[39–41] especially when it comes to achieving stable soft tissue esthetics that stand the test of time.

Similarly, management of a failing tooth with healthy intact tissues and a thick biotype is vastly different from management of one with thin tissue and prominent roots or with significant damage to the tissues through infection or trauma. In the case of a failing tooth with potential for immediate implant placement or immediate provisionalization, the challenges relate mainly to the preservation and maintenance of the interdental papillae and, more significantly, the labial soft tissue volume and contours. Significant bone and tissue damage, however, invariably require delayed loading, socket preservation, or a regenerative approach.[34,40–42]

Addressing the Clinical Challenge

The clinician should consider a few main factors that can be used to address the challenge to create or preserve and, more importantly, main-

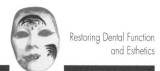

Restoring Dental Function
and Esthetics

tain the appropriate soft tissue contours around a restoration that allow them to blend inconspicuously with the patient's natural dentition and smile. First, it is necessary to have a stable bone scaffold to house the implant and support the soft tissue. In a healed edentulous site with adequate bone width, this is not a critical issue. In a site with inadequate bone, however, augmentation techniques must be employed to create a stable bone volume. Second, soft tissue procedures such as connective tissue grafts and rolled flaps may be necessary to augment the thickness of peri-implant soft tissue and establish the necessary 3 to 4 mm required for the biologic seal at the time of transmucosal component connection. Finally, soft tissue thickness in the transmucosal zone can be maximized through the use of biocompatible materials and, more importantly, components that possess the appropriate narrow contours (undercontours) near the implant level, with a concave form that flares late to the margin of the restoration.

Bone augmentation

In more compromised sites, whether edentulous or with failing teeth, effective protocols are essential if one is to obtain predictable results. In the past, autogenous bone grafting often has been presented as the gold standard, either as a block graft prior to implant placement or as particulate graft in combination with guided bone regeneration techniques. Although these techniques have proved valuable in the creation of sufficient bone volume for correct implant placement, the longer-term esthetic results of such grafts are questionable.[43–46] Indeed, a lack of stability may create esthetic problems resulting from a flattened or thinned labial aspect of the implant restorations. This leads to labial tissue recession, discoloration, or dark shadowing of the tissue labial to the implant. Such outcomes are unacceptable to many of today's patients.

The current trend is to employ bone augmentation materials that better support and maintain volume to obtain stable soft tissue esthetics. Materials such as bovine anorganic bone mineral, used in conjunction with resorbable or nonresorbable membranes, seem to offer this benefit of greater volumetric stability because the graft material is incorporated into newly formed bone with less resorption.[46–51]

Hard and soft tissue factors

As previously mentioned, the two key factors to consider in evaluation and management of a proposed implant site from the perspective of soft tissue esthetics are the interproximal and the labial hard and soft tissues. Generally, the interproximal bone level of the adjacent teeth, combined with the distance from the contact point to the bone crest, determines adequate papilla length. It is thought that this distance should

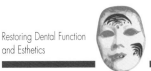

Restoring Dental Function
and Esthetics

be 4.5 mm or less for a papilla to fill the space.[37,38,52] The literature also indicates that the distal papilla may be shorter than the mesial and that both papillae will improve with time if the prosthetic contours are appropriate.[53]

The literature has suggested that some labial recession of 1.0 to 1.5 mm should be expected after a definitive restoration has been placed.[1,8,54,55] However, much of the generally accepted data on this issue was published several years ago, and ideas have evolved since then. One of the greatest shortcomings in the literature pertaining to the labial soft tissue response is the tendency to attribute this response to a single factor (eg, the labial bone thickness or bone height). It has been said time and again that "the bone sets the tone," but this seems without doubt to be only a small part of the story. Contemporary thinking encompasses broader concepts, noting that the bone, the soft tissue quality and thickness, the implant, and the restorative components likely all influence the host biologic response and, therefore, the remodeling process of the tissues.

Transmucosal elements

The shape and contours of the transmucosal components are also considered important factors that influence the biologic response and subsequent stability and form of the soft tissues. The component design, the type of implant-abutment connection, the transmucosal materials used (eg, zirconia, titanium, gold, or feldspathic porcelain), and the timing of the connection of the final abutment all play a role. The late 1990s and the early part of the 2000s saw a tendency for convex, broad transmucosal components to be used, in contrast to more contemporary concepts that suggest narrow, flat, or even concave labial transmucosal contours with the goal to create more space for the tissue and therefore allow increased soft tissue thickness on the labial side of the restoration. In the author's opinion, the latter approach is essential to attain and maintain soft tissue contours. Clinical experience has demonstrated that it leads to improved stability and esthetics. These concepts form the basis of the approach to implant restoration in the esthetic zone today.

The presence of labial bone is important, but it is questionable whether the thickness of this bone has any bearing on the soft tissue stability. Frankly, there is no evidence to suggest that the thickness of bone is maintained over time and, in fact, personal experience may even suggest that the bone continues to remodel despite implant placement. Implants can remain in healthy functional and esthetic situations with very thin labial bone or even a labial dehiscence. The often-cited paper by Spray et al,[17] which justifies the thinking that 2 mm of labial bone is required for stability, evaluates only short-term changes to bone

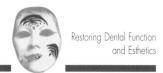

contours between implant placement and uncovering in a conventional two-stage approach. It does *not* provide any information on the behavior of the soft tissues over a long period of time, particularly subsequent to transmucosal restoration.

In fact, many clinicians and authors working in the esthetic zone advocate the use of bone grafting techniques that incorporate materials to improve the volume and stability of the labial contours over time, in addition to augmentation of the soft tissue thickness on the labial aspect of the restoration by means of connective tissue grafting or by a roll flap if the latter gives adequate soft tissue thickness. These protocols are considered routine and are an important factor in achieving adequate labial soft tissue thickness and stability. When combined with the use of narrow undercontoured or even concave transmucosal components that create increased room for labial soft tissue, these techniques result in a thicker labial connective tissue cuff that seems to be more resistant to recession over time. It is the contention of this author that the establishment of an adequate thickness of soft tissue at the time of transmucosal component connection, such that the biologic width of 3 to 4 mm is already established, may reduce the bone remodeling necessary to create the tissue required for a biologic seal.

The application of the factors described above are examined in the management of the following two challenging clinical cases, where all of these factors come into play and provide a better understanding of the key clinical steps. Box 6-2 summarizes the key steps to optimize the soft tissue esthetics of single-tooth implants in the esthetic zone.

Box 6-2 Key steps to optimize soft tissue esthetics with implants in the esthetic zone

1. Perform orthodontic extrusion prior to tooth extraction where possible.
2. If bone augmentation is required, use bovine anorganic bone mineral versus autogenous bone for better stability of volume and contours.
3. Position implant-abutment connection 3 mm apical and 2 mm palatal to final gingival margin.
4. Thicken labial tissues (ie, boost biotype through connective tissue graft or roll flap).
5. Use undercontoured or concave transmucosal components.
6. Use more biocompatible materials for the transmucosal components or abutment: zirconia, alumina, or titanium versus gold, feldspathic porcelain, or acrylic resin composite.
7. Avoid repeated disconnection and reconnection of abutments and components, ie, early or immediate placement of definitive abutment.
8. Develop contours with provisional restorations.
9. Control and remove cement excess at final cementation.

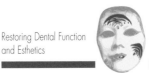

Case 1: The Compromised Single-Tooth Site

Management of compromised sites, whether previously edentulous or with a failing tooth, is always a challenge, particularly if optimal esthetics are to be achieved.[41,56] While it must be stressed that the "perfect" result is not always achievable in these cases due to the compromised biology and damage to the site, nonetheless much can be learned and gained from the management of these cases. The clinician can subsequently apply this learning so as to provide better management and greater predictability for simpler cases that require implant treatment in the esthetic zone. The reader is encouraged to look into the articles referenced in this chapter for more information regarding the approaches to management of compromised sites.

Presentation and evaluation

Case 1 provides a useful situation to demonstrate the key aspects in the management of implants in the esthetic zone. A 48-year-old man was referred to the practice in 2004 after the loss of his maxillary left central incisor (Figs 6-1a to 6-1g), which had been extracted about 2 months before his referral. The tooth had been endodontically treated and restored with a post crown. This had failed due to root fracture and was subsequently extracted after the patient's general dentist attempted antibiotic therapy of the infection. The patient was then provided with a removable partial denture.

Careful evaluation of the patient reveals a number of challenges and prognostic factors that may influence the likely outcome:

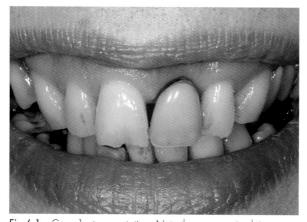

Fig 6-1a Case 1 at presentation. Note the compromised tissue esthetics.

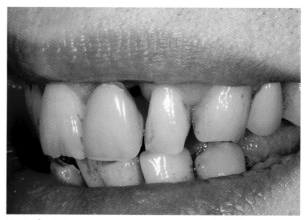

Fig 6-1b Oblique view at presentation reveals the deficient tissue volume.

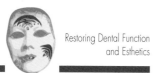

Restoring Dental Function and Esthetics

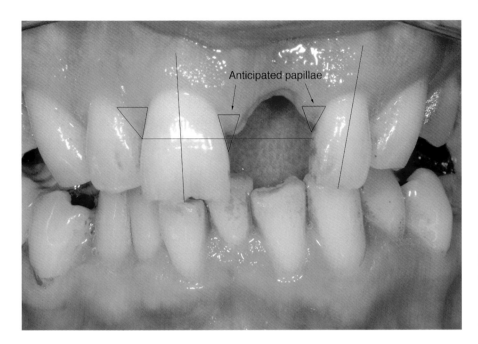

Fig 6-1c Preoperative anterior view. Note the thin tissue, triangular tooth form, blunt papillae, and unfavorable mesial angulation of the lateral incisor.

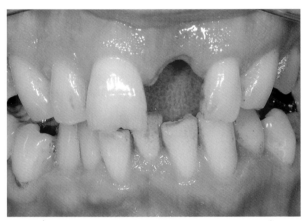

Fig 6-1d Analysis of some of the diagnostic and prognostic factors in this case.

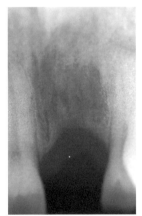

Fig 6-1e Preoperative radiograph.

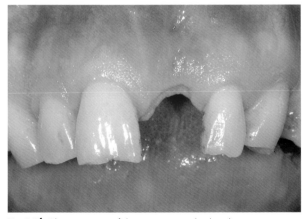

Fig 6-1f Close-up view of the compromised edentulous site.

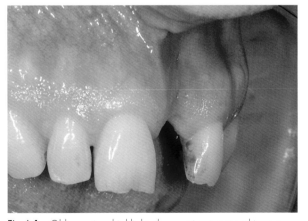

Fig 6-1g Oblique view highlights the prominent root architecture and extent of the defect.

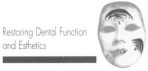

- Poor oral hygiene is evident.
- The patient has a high lip line (see Fig 6-1a).
- A thin scalloped biotype is combined with prominent roots and thin labial bone and tissue (see Figs 6-1c and 6-1g).
- A triangular tooth form (see Fig 6-1c) means the contact points are likely to be more coronal, therefore complete papilla fill is more difficult or unlikely to achieve, creating unless the crowns are recontoured a more apical contact point (see Fig 6-1d).
- The papilla on the mesial aspect of the left lateral incisor is already compromised. Due to the angulation of the tooth, the proximal bone level, and the tooth form, it is unlikely that an ideal distal papilla will be achievable on the future implant crown (see Fig 6-1d).
- A large volume of bone and soft tissue is missing, and there is significant damage to the site (see Figs 6-1b and 6-1f). The defect is a broad U shape rather than a narrow V shape (see Fig 6-1g).
- The state of the patient's mouth at presentation indicates an apparent lack of concern for ideal esthetics. The patient also stated that his primary concern was function and not optimal esthetics.

In a case like this, a clinician should expect to see a large defect in the bone and possibly an inadequate volume of keratinized gingiva and soft tissue. As mentioned above, assessment of the patient shows an unfavorable gingival biotype with a high scalloping, triangular tooth form and a low frenum attachment. The papilla on the distal aspect of the tooth to be restored is already deficient. This is partly due to some bone loss on the mesial aspect of the lateral incisor but also because the triangular tooth form is combined with a mesial tilt and rotation of the lateral incisor, thereby leading to inadequate proximal support of the soft tissues. These issues will affect the likely esthetic outcome and need to be discussed in detail with the patient. Ideally, considerations could include orthodontic treatment to upright the right lateral incisor or addition of some resin composite to the mesial aspects of the adjacent incisors, which would help create a contour that produces a less triangular tooth form and likely prevents black triangles in the final proximal embrasures. In this case, the patient did not wish to undergo orthodontic treatment, so a compromise was agreed upon whereby the distal papilla was expected to remain slightly deficient. Discussion of these types of issues with the patient ensures that expectations are realistic, particularly in heavily compromised cases such as this one.

 Diagnostic study models and a wax-up allow for a better visualization and evaluation of the missing tissue contours (Fig 6-1h). In cases like this, it unlikely that any immediate provisionalization of the implant can be considered, so it is preferable to provide a fixed provisional restoration such as a Rochette bridge whenever possible. A Rochette bridge can be easily cemented with a resin-ionomer cement (Fuji II LC,

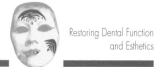

Restoring Dental Function
and Esthetics

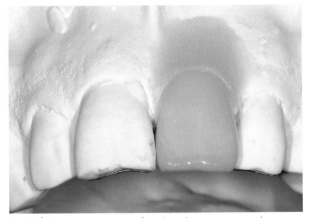

Fig 6-1h Diagnostic wax-up of tooth and tissue to restored.

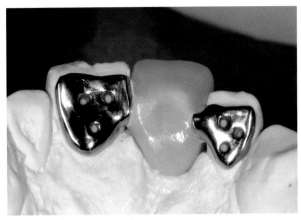

Fig 6-1i Rochette provisional restoration.

GC America) (Fig 6-1i), which provides adequate retention without complex isolation or etching of the teeth, and allows for simple removal and replacement during the various stages of surgical treatment. The fit surface of the pontic can easily be hollowed and adjusted to fit over any healing abutment if necessary. If there is insufficient room in the occlusion to allow placement of the retentive wings, then a removable partial denture can be used. If this is done, it is important to ensure that the adjacent teeth support the prosthesis well; that is, the prosthesis should sit passively on the edentulous ridge, particularly after any ridge augmentation has been completed, and should not place inadvertent pressure on the area when the patient occludes.

Decision-making in bone augmentation for ideal esthetics

Wherever a significant bone graft or regeneration is expected, a full thickness flap is raised using a sulcular incision around the adjacent teeth and at the palatal aspect of the ridge. This approach was used in this patient, and a large three-dimensional defect was revealed in the bone (Fig 6-1j). Periosteal releasing incisions, which allow easy advancement of the flap, were created early in the procedure to help reduce postoperative bleeding and swelling. Remote vertical releasing incisions, which allow the tissue to have sufficient mobility to cover any expanded volume created by grafting, also were made.

At this point, the clinician has two options to consider: (*1*) to complete bone grafting and augmentation at this stage and place the implant at a later stage after suitable healing; or (*2*) to place the implant in the ideal three-dimensional position if there is adequate stability and perform simultaneous bone augmentation. Both approaches have been advocated, but it should be stressed that the latter option is more demanding and requires a higher degree of surgical skill. Furthermore, consideration should be given to which bone grafting technique and

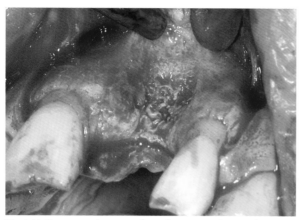

Fig 6-1j Osseous architecture after a flap is raised. Note the extent of the defect and the volume of missing bone.

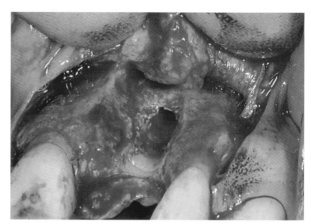

Fig 6-1k The prepared implant osteotomy.

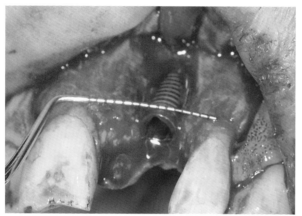

Fig 6-1l Ideal position of the implant is 3 mm apical and 2 mm palatal to the desired final gingival margin.

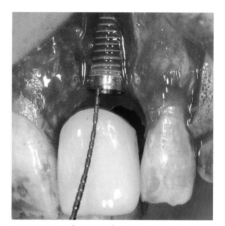

Fig 6-1m Verification of the implant head position against the provisional restoration.

material will be used. The current general trend leads away from autogenous block grafting and towards particulate grafts with biomaterials such as anorganic bovine bone material, which maintain better long-term volume. Ultimately, the goal is to create a volume of bone that produces a lasting result in terms of soft tissue contours and maintainable gingival esthetics.

Clinical experience would suggest that one approach may have advantages over the other in terms of results, and in the majority of cases the second option is the author's preference, as it produces consistent results that have stood the test of time. The premise of this concept is that the simultaneous implant placement reduces the volume of bone to be regenerated, because the implant itself occupies much of the space.

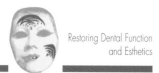

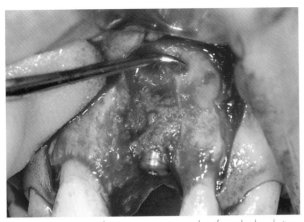

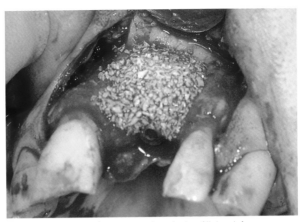

Fig 6-1n Autogenous bone scrapings are taken from the local site to cover the exposed threads.

Fig 6-1o Anorganic bone mineral grafted to fill the defect.

All bone grafting and regenerative techniques result in some degree of subsequent bone volume shrinkage during the bone remodeling process. Anorganic bovine bone mineral seems to demonstrate a smaller percentage of overall shrinkage than other materials. Therefore, it seems logical that earlier placement of the implant reduces the overall volume to be grafted and, subsequently, the total shrinkage, since the shrinkage only occurs in the small amount of regenerated bone covering the implant. For example, if 20% volume loss is expected, then shrinkage of 20% of 1 to 2 mm of bone (0.2 mm to 0.4 mm) has far less of an impact than 20% of 10 mm of bone (2 mm).[33,46–51]

Case 1 illustrates this concept well. In Figs 6-1k and 6-1l, a significant volume of bone would have to be regenerated if the implant is not placed. Simultaneous implant placement also shortens the overall treatment time, although this may not necessarily be a priority for the patient.

Steps 1 and 2: Correct implant placement and bone augmentation

After the implant osteotomy was performed, it was established that an implant could be placed with adequate primary stability. The head of the implant must be placed in the ideal three-dimensional position, which is usually 3 mm apical and 2 mm palatal to the desired final gingival margin of the definitive restoration (see Figs 6-1l and 6-1m). In this type of case, where the implant is buried and bone augmentation is performed, it is always necessary to take a two-stage approach. The augmentation was completed using autogenous bone scrapings harvested from the apical aspect of the site, with a goal to bring some potential bone-forming cells close to the implant surface (Fig 6-1n). A layer of anorganic bovine bone mineral (Bio-Oss [Geistlich]) was placed over this (Fig 6-1o) and covered with resorbable collagen

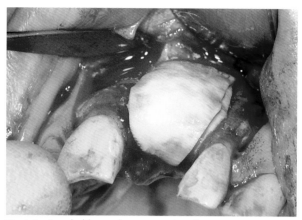

Fig 6-1p Resorbable membranes are placed.

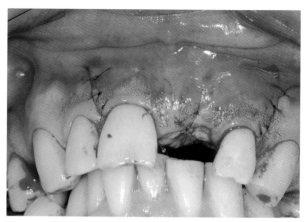

Fig 6-1q Good primary closure is achieved, and the flap is sutured using 6-0 monofilament polypropylene sutures.

membranes in two layers (Bio-Gide [Geistlich]). Care was taken to ensure the membranes did not come into contact with the adjacent roots (Fig 6-1p). In cases like this, the goal should be to have slightly more labial tissue volume than required to allow for some degree of inevitable shrinkage as the graft heals. In simpler cases, simultaneous connective tissue grafting can be considered. When bone grafting results in significant augmentation of bone volume, however, it is better to delay soft tissue grafting until later (before or possibly during stage 2 surgery when the implant or healing abutment is uncovered or abutment placement is performed) so that good primary closure of the wound can be achieved passively. In this patient, the flap was sutured using 6-0 monofilament polypropylene sutures, and the fixed partial denture was recemented after the pontic was adjusted to fit passively against the augmented ridge (Figs 6-1q and 6-1r).

Step 3: Soft tissue augmentation

As expected, after 6 months the bone augmentation was sufficiently mature for reentry (Fig 6-1s). The site can be reopened with a sulcular incision on the adjacent teeth and a U-shaped incision on the palatal aspect of the implant that preserves the palatal blood supply to the papillae on both sides (Fig 6-1t). This can usually be done without vertical releasing incisions and with a split thickness flap that tunnels under the tissue labial to the implant and recipient site for creation of additional connective tissue. In Case 1, vertical releasing incisions were made so that the regenerated bone could be clearly visualized and the success of the graft confirmed.

It is suggested that at least 3 mm of tissue be retained coronal to the bone on the labial aspect of the implant to establish the necessary biologic seal, and a thicker tissue biotype will maintain a greater thick-

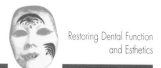

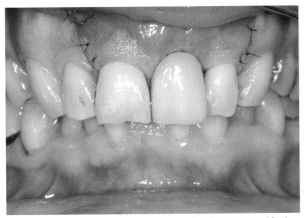

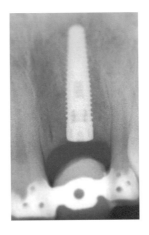

Fig 6-1r Provisional restoration is cemented with a resin-modified glass-ionomer cement. Note that the soft tissue contours are still inadequate.

Fig 6-1s Radiograph of the implant and graft in place shows good restoration of bone contours before stage 2 surgery.

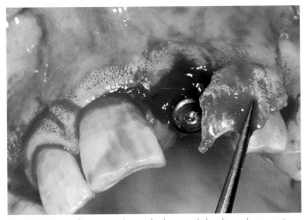

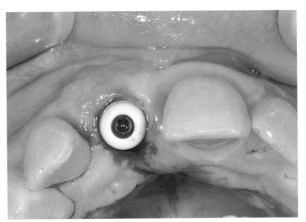

Fig 6-1t Stage 2 surgery 6 months later with healing abutment in place. A split-thickness dissection of labial flap creates the recipient site for a connective tissue graft, which will thicken the labial peri-implant tissue.

Fig 6-1u Example of an alternate approach where simple small roll flap at stage 2 surgery after a connective tissue graft has been completed at stage 1 surgery to thicken the tissue. A small U-shaped incision is made and the tissue surface is de-epithelialized. The small tissue is then rolled under the labial gingival margin to increase the tissue volume labial to the healing abutment.

ness of peri-implant tissue (ie, the thicker the tissue, the less recession observed). Therefore, it is essential to augment the connective tissue.

It is often noted that at stage 2 surgery, the tissue overlying the regenerated bone is relatively thin. If the implant were to be uncovered and the transmucosal component placed at this stage, and if the tissue were only 1 mm thick, then the bone would have to remodel apically to establish the sufficient thickness to create the necessary biologic seal that comprises a sulcus, an area of junctional epithelium, and a connective tissue zone above the bone. However, the need is reduced for this remodeling (see Fig 6-1t) if an adequate volume of tissue is present at stage 2 surgery, created either by *(1)* connective tissue grafting at stage 2 surgery

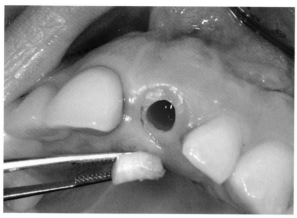

Fig 6-1v Example of a tissue punch procedure, which is appropriate only when the tissue thickness is sufficient, eg, when a previous graft has already been completed.

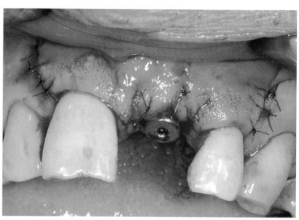

Fig 6-1w Flap and graft are sutured.

or *(2)* connective tissue grafting prior to uncovering of the implant followed by a simple roll flap (Fig 6-1u), or tissue punch procedure if the tissue over the implant already has sufficient thickness (Fig 6-1v). In any case, good passive adaptation of the tissues to the components and precise suturing of incisions is important to minimize creation of scars (Fig 6-1w).

Step 4: Transmucosal component design and material

As discussed earlier, the transmucosal components should be kept narrow near the implant level with a concave form that flares late to the tooth contour. This will help to maximize the thickness of tissue around the neck of the implant restoration (Fig 6-1x). If a healing abutment is used, it should be narrow, and abutment placement should be followed by placement of narrow transfer impression copings (Figs 6-1y and 6-1z) to maintain the maximum tissue thickness on the labial aspect of the tooth.

Evidence increasingly suggests that zirconia offers advantages as the material of choice in the transmucosal zone (ie, for the abutment or for the transmucosal aspect of a screw-retained restoration) in terms of its color and influence on tissue color,[57] its biocompatibility, and its influence on tissue adaptation and health.[10–12]

Step 5: Provisionalization

Ideally, a custom zirconia abutment is fabricated to allow for a crown margin that is positioned approximately 1 mm below the final desired gingival margin. The ideal transmucosal contours can be developed on the cast and then transferred to the mouth with a provisional crown that

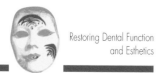

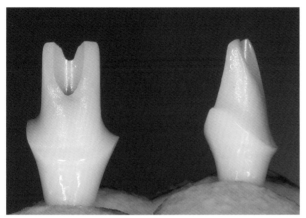

Fig 6-1x Example of the ideal contours for the abutment from the facial *(left)* and lateral *(right)* views highlights the maintenance of a narrow or undercontour at the level of the implant head that flares late to the full contour of the crown. This maximizes the available space for soft tissue.

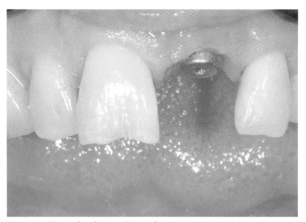

Fig 6-1y Tissue healing at 3 months.

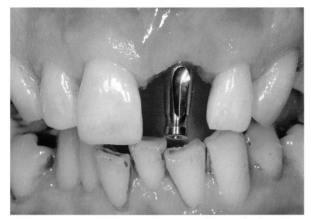

Fig 6-1z A narrow impression coping is used to transfer the implant position to the model.

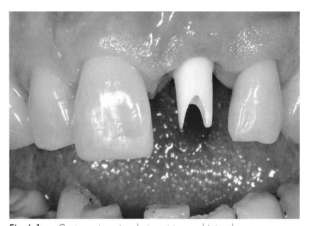

Fig 6-1aa Custom zirconia abutment torqued into place.

can be modified as necessary to develop the appropriate soft tissue contours (Fig 6-1aa). A concave labial profile is maintained for the abutment as much as possible to allow for slight undercontour on the labial transmucosal area, which prevents apical migration of the tissue.

Step 6: Careful cementation

The use of retraction cord during cementation of the crown (whether provisional or definitive) is essential to ensure that no excess cement travels into the submucosal area, because this can lead to peri-implantitis and therefore compromise the result.

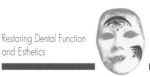

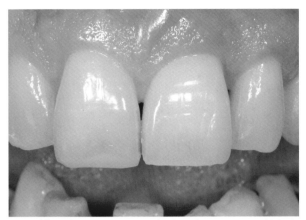

Fig 6-1bb Definitive restoration at loading shows position of labial tissue and proximal tissue contours.

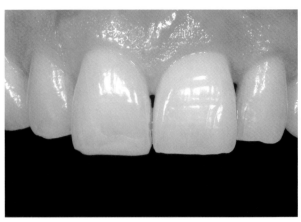

Fig 6-1cc Definitive restoration at 5 years postoperatively. Note the stability of the labial tissue, which is contrary to what is commonly anticipated and, if anything, is now in a more coronal position, while the papillae remain slightly deficient as expected.

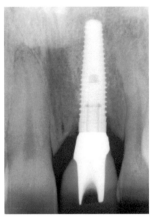

Fig 6-1dd Follow-up radiograph 3 years postoperatively.

Figure 6-1bb shows the final crown at cementation. The adjacent central incisor has been restored with resin composite. The patient was instructed to maintain optimal plaque control, and the clinician should explain that continued maturation of the tissues, particularly the papillae, will take place over time.

This case and others previously published by the author (see References) demonstrate that the approximately 1 mm of labial recession that is commonly reported can be avoided if clinicians follow the protocols described. The 3- and 5-year follow-ups (Figs 6-1cc and 6-1dd) shows that the labial gingival margin has not receded and, if anything, is now in a slightly more coronal position than at the crown placement. As expected, the papillae have somewhat improved, but because of the triangular form of the teeth and the various issues discussed in the evaluation of this case, the papillae are not complete. However, because there was no evidence of the original natural papillae positions, the end result may be as good as what was there previously.

Case discussion

In review, the successful restoration of an implant in the esthetic zone is not reliant on any single feature but rather on a number of factors that combine and interact to create the desired result. The synergy of bone, soft tissue, and implant components, combined with a clear understanding of the key steps in the case management, are essential if stable esthetic outcomes are to be created, particularly in relation to the stability of the soft tissue contours.

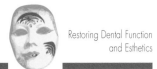

Case 2: Failing Teeth in the Esthetic Zone

While the overriding principles of clinical management of failing teeth remain largely the same as the management of the edentulous site, it is important to make some significant distinctions in the goal of the treatment. In the restoration of an edentulous site, the goal is to reconstruct and restore the appropriate soft tissue contours around the final crown. Management of the failing tooth, however, can be broken into two distinct kinds of cases: *(1)* the failing tooth where the bone and/or soft tissues are already significantly compromised; and *(2)* the failing tooth with intact labial and interproximal bone and an ideal or slightly compromised soft tissue contour. Case 2 presents a challenging example of the latter situation for possible implant treatment.

Treatment approaches

In patients with significantly compromised tissues, a clinician is likely to perform either a delayed implant approach—where the tooth is extracted, soft tissues are allowed to heal, and the site is treated in more or less the same manner as the edentulous site above—or perhaps a socket preservation technique. Both approaches have been described in detail.[34,35,40,58] In patients with intact bone and intact or only slightly compromised soft tissues, the goal of treatment is to preserve the existing soft tissue contours or perhaps improve them if necessary. Typically, this slight compromise would be in the form of minor labial recession or discrepancy in the labial gingival margins.

Immediate implant placement using a flapless technique has been shown to offer a viable esthetic alternative for the replacement of failing maxillary anterior teeth in the esthetic zone. As previously mentioned, recession and labial volume loss are challenges that should be addressed in these cases, and additional treatment and surgical steps may be required (eg, orthodontic extrusion, grafting of biomaterials, and tissue grafting) to ensure the ideal soft tissue outcomes.[18,19,59–61] Orthodontic extrusion (see Chapter 5) is often recommended as a way to bring the labial gingival tissue to a more coronal position and then allow for remodeling to take place after the implant is placed at the correct level. However, the main drawback of this technique is that it is not always feasible to extrude a tooth—for example, if there is a failing endodontic treatment, vertical root fracture, or ankylosis. In addition, the technique may not be the best option for thin gingival biotypes. These additional steps require a higher degree of surgical skill and are by no means easy when working in a small site such as an extraction socket. In addition, it is not possible to say at this time that cases with a thin tissue biotype have reliable predictability. These cases certainly present a greater challenge, and the clinician may be wise to take a more cautious route, using either a socket preservation or delayed implant placement approach.

From a biologic perspective, the challenge in these cases is the same as in the compromised site—ie, that the clinician needs to establish a stable bone contour, soft tissues of adequate thickness for the biologic seal, and final gingival contours that are stable and esthetically appropriate.

Presentation and evaluation

A 33-year-old woman was referred to the practice with a failing maxillary left central incisor. Both central incisors had been crowned for years, and a recent attempt had been made to remake the crowns. The left central incisor, however, although asymptomatic, presented with a fracture that the referring clinician estimated extended some 5 mm subgingivally. The general dentist placed provisional restorations and subsequently referred the patient to us. The patient was extremely nervous and found it very difficult to undergo dental treatment.

Once again, the patient should be evaluated carefully to examine the main challenges and prognostic factors that may influence the likely outcome:

- The patient has a large smile and a high lip line (Fig 6-2a), and demands a high level of esthetics.
- The maxillary central incisors are prominent and dominate the smile.
- Thin tissue over the failing root is determined by the way the dark underlying tooth structure shows through in Figs 6-2a and 6-2b, and by the prominent root architecture (Fig 6-2c).
- The position of the labial gingival margin is slightly higher on the failing tooth than on the contralateral central incisor.
- The presence of a deep root fracture in the distal aspect of the tooth means probable loss of bone in the interproximal area. The papilla is puffy and inflamed on the distal aspect of the left central incisor (see Figs 6-2b and 6-2d).
- The radiograph shows that the interproximal bone between the central and lateral incisors is in a fairly apical position (Fig 6-2e). This may be due to the root proximity or to resorption because of the fracture. However, the interdental papilla here is in a markedly coronal position (see Fig 6-2a), well outside of the Tarnow 5 mm rule (see Chapter 5), so it is unlikely that an ideal distal papilla can be achieved on the future implant restoration.
- The central incisors are a little long relative to the lateral incisors. There is evidence of altered passive eruption on the lateral incisors, as the gingival margins are in a more coronal position than is desirable (see Fig 6-2a).

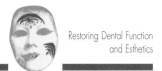

Restoring Dental Function
and Esthetics

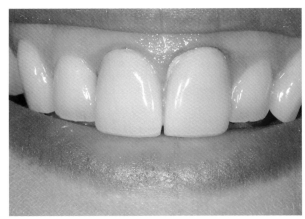

Fig 6-2a Case 2 at presentation. Note high lip line on the smile and discoloration of gingival tissue above the failing incisor.

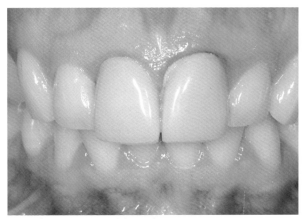

Fig 6-2b Anterior view of the teeth at presentation.

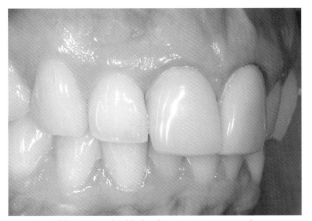

Fig 6-2c Oblique view highlights the prominent root architecture and vestibular concavity.

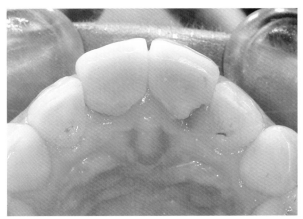

Fig 6-2d Occlusal view shows the inflamed tissue distal to the left central incisor.

In this case, it would be ideal to complete some orthodontic extrusion of the failing root. This would improve the level of the labial gingiva (although not the thickness) and may bring the interproximal bone crest to a more coronal position to help create a "perfect" papilla on the distal aspect of the failing incisor. However, as is often the case, there was concern about the extent of the root fracture and possible increased bone loss from infection.

An impression was made of the right central incisor to make an immediate provisional restoration in the form of a cantilevered fixed partial denture with a hollow pontic for the failing tooth. This type of provisional restoration is useful because it allows the clinician to extract the failing tooth and decide whether to place an immediate implant once a clear view of the socket is gained and the situation can be appropriately assessed. In some cases it may be feasible to place a provisional restoration

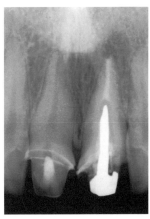

Fig 6-2e Preoperative radiograph shows the apical position of the bone distal to the failing incisor.

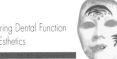

Restoring Dental Function and Esthetics

on the implant at the time of immediate placement. In this type of situation, however, the possibility of immediate placement is never certain because of the risk that important labial bone has been damaged by infection. It is important to have an alternate provisional restoration in the event that the clinician is unable to place the implant or feels that immediate provisionalization of the implant is not possible or advisable. This "backup" restoration can either be a Rochette-type partial denture, a fixed partial denture (used here), or a removable partial denture.

The basic principles in the management of Case 2 are very similar to those in Case 1. The application may vary slightly with the individual case parameters, nevertheless the concept remains the same.

Step 1: Careful extraction and evaluation of the site

After the crown was removed, the extent of the fracture could be fully realized (Figs 6-2f to 6-2h). It is important to remove the tooth in a manner that minimizes trauma to the bone and tissues. The use of magnification is particularly helpful in these cases, and the author routinely uses 4.8× magnification loupes. Once the tooth is successfully removed, the socket is carefully debrided under magnification, and the bone is evaluated to ensure that the labial plate is intact. Patients are given prophylactic antibiotics (eg, penicillin V 250 mg 4 times a day, cephalexin 500 mg 2 times a day, or clindamycin 150 mg 4 times a day) for 5 days, with the initial dose given just prior to surgery.

Figures 6-2i and 6-2j show the socket immediately after tooth removal. The distal aspect reveals the inflammation and ingrowth of tissue and the likely bone loss in this area. At this point, a decision must be made whether to continue with an immediate implant placement or to pursue a delayed approach of some kind.

The main complication here is the loss of distal proximal bone. However, it is important to realize that regardless of the treatment plan chosen, it is unlikely that complete maintenance of the distal papilla can be achieved on this tooth. To date there are no techniques available that can guarantee complete regeneration of this proximal bone. In fact, the flapless approach may better maintain the integrity and blood supply to the papilla and thereby offer the best possible result considering the circumstances. This is done through careful degranulation of the tissue below the bone level (or at least where the bone should be) while maintaining the superficial papilla integrity, grafting the area with anorganic bone mineral, and applying some enamel matrix protein (Emdogain, Straumann) to the adjacent root exposed by bone loss below the gingival tissues.

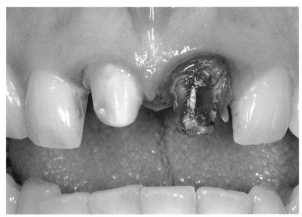

Fig 6-2f The extent of the fractures is evident after removal of the provisional crowns.

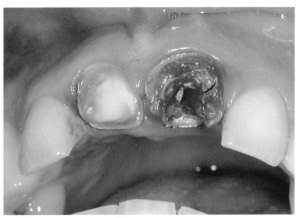

Fig 6-2g Occlusal view of fractured tooth.

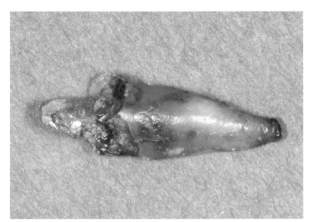

Fig 6-2h The extent of the vertical fracture can be seen on the distal aspect of the root of the extracted tooth.

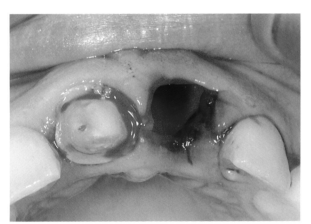

Fig 6-2i Occlusal view of the extraction socket. Note the inflammation and invagination of tissue on the distal aspect of the socket.

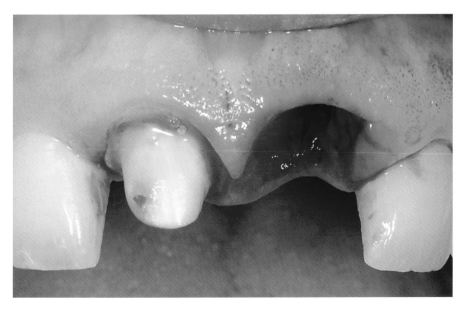

Fig 6-2j Anterior view of socket.

Restoring Dental Function and Esthetics

Step 2: Correct implant placement

The next step in a case like this is to place the implant using commonly accepted protocols. The pilot hole should be prepared in the palatal wall of the apical third of the socket and the osteotomy performed so that implants are placed in the palatal aspect of the socket and lined up with the incisal edge. Any apical granuloma or defect should be thoroughly curetted and debrided through the socket. The implant is usually placed palatal to any apical defect, and depending on the size of the defect, it can be either left to heal spontaneously or packed through the socket with anorganic bone mineral (Bio-Oss) prior to implant placement. The implant head should be placed 3 mm apical and 2 mm palatal to the desired final gingival margin of the final restoration. A transfer impression of the implant can then be made for the laboratory to fabricate the abutment and provisional restoration, and a narrow healing abutment should be seated on the implant.

Steps 3 and 4: Bone augmentation and soft tissue augmentation

Although there will be some remodeling of the bone contours regardless of what is done, the key is to reduce this as much as possible and compensate for the bone flattening by means of soft tissue augmentation. A space of approximately 2 mm should be left labial to the implant in the sockets, and anorganic bone mineral (Bio-Oss) or nonresorbable bone substitute should be packed firmly into the void between the implant and the labial bone to the level of the implant head (Fig 6-2k). This is necessary to minimize the shrinkage of labial bone volume during subsequent remodeling and helps to optimize the esthetic outcome. Because augmentation of the connective tissue is an extremely important step both to establish the necessary biologic seal and to maintain a greater thickness of peri-implant tissue, a labial connective tissue graft is then harvested from the palate and sandwiched between the healing abutment or the abutment and labial gingiva. This can be placed into a pouch produced by careful tunneling under the labial gingiva or, more commonly, between the abutment and labial tissue. The inner aspect of the labial tissue should be de-epithelialized and the graft secured into position with 6-0 or 7-0 monofilament polypropylene sutures (Figs 6-2l and 6-2m).

At this stage, the provisional restoration is tried in, and the pontic is adjusted, relined, and adapted to the healing abutment using provisional fixed partial denture material and flowable resin composite to create the appropriate contours to support the interproximal tissues (Fig 6-2n). The fixed partial denture is provisionally cemented on the adjacent incisor and sits passively on the healing abutment. It is slightly undercontoured and short on the labial aspect to allow space for the soft tissue graft (Fig 6-2o).

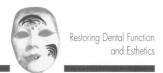

Restoring Dental Function
and Esthetics

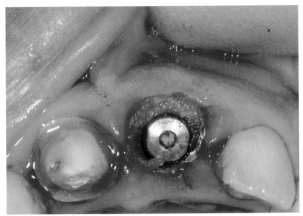

Fig 6-2k Implant correctly placed with space for the graft material, which is packed into the labial socket space between the implant and labial bone. A narrow healing abutment is placed.

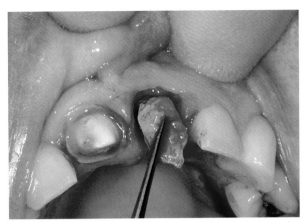

Fig 6-2l A connective tissue graft is harvested from the palate to be placed between the healing abutment and the labial tissue after de-epithelialization of the inner aspect of the labial tissue.

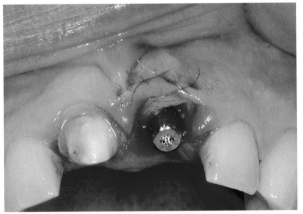

Fig 6-2m The graft is sutured precisely into place.

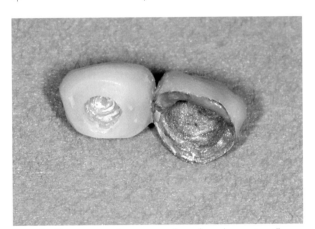

Fig 6-2n The provisional restoration shows how the pontic will adapt to the healing abutment.

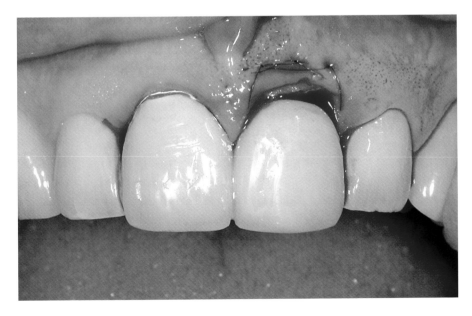

Fig 6-2o Provisional restoration cemented in position immediately after surgery. Note the undercontour to allow space for soft tissue.

Restoring Dental Function and Esthetics

The patient was seen 1 week postoperatively for suture removal (Fig 6-2p). The postoperative radiograph (Fig 6-2q) shows a narrow (or, in this case, platform-switched) healing abutment, and one can see the graft material attempting to regenerate as much as possible the lost bone on the distal aspect of the implant.

Step 5: Transmucosal component design and material

The labial aspects of the abutment and restoration should be undercontoured in the transmucosal area to allow additional room for thicker soft tissue. If the implant is stable enough, then the abutment and provisional restoration can be placed a few weeks or even a few days after surgery. If the primary stability of the implant is uncertain, it is better to wait for at least 6 weeks. In Case 2, the abutment and provisional crowns were fitted at 3 months. The final abutment is preferably a custom zirconia abutment that is shaped to the appropriate contours as previously discussed (Fig 6-2r).

Step 6: Provisionalization

The provisional crown is cemented with provisional cement at the same time as placement of the final abutment. It is imperative that retraction cord be placed prior to cementation to facilitate complete removal of excess cement and ensure that no cement is trapped in the subgingival area of the implant. Crown lengthening of the adjacent lateral incisors was performed by means of a simple gingivoplasty to determine the correct gingival contours (Fig 6-2s). The labial bone on these teeth was recontoured to establish the correct biologic width and labial contours, using a simple tunneling technique to gain access to the bone without the need to raise a flap. The tissues were left to mature and remodel, and the provisional crowns were refined over the next few months until the desired result was achieved (Fig 6-2t). At this stage, final impressions of the tooth and the abutment are made using conventional crown impression techniques.

Step 7: Careful cementation

After impressions have been taken, the definitive restorations can then be fabricated using the appropriate bisque try-ins and adjustments until the desired outcome is achieved. Once again, retraction cord is essential when the crown is cemented on the implant to ensure that no excess cement travels into the submucosal area, especially where the concave form of the abutment would make removal difficult.

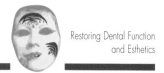

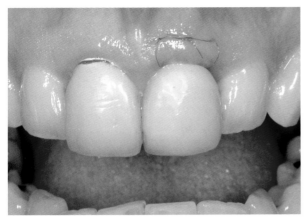

Fig 6-2p Healing 1 week postoperatively. Note the volume of tissue now present, although there is still some swelling.

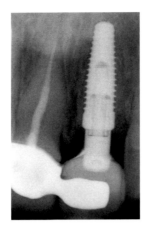

Fig 6-2q Postoperative radiograph of implant shows the bone graft filling any voids and the narrow platform-switched abutment.

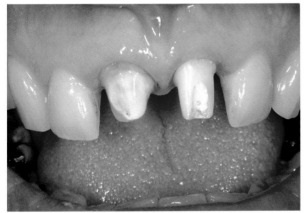

Fig 6-2r Custom zirconia abutment is fitted; the healed tissue is well adapted to the abutment.

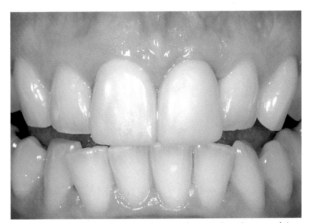

Fig 6-2s Provisional crowns in place and crown lengthening of the lateral incisors.

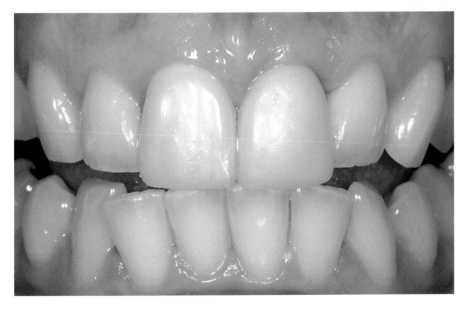

Fig 6-2t Maturation of tissue after 3 months.

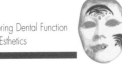

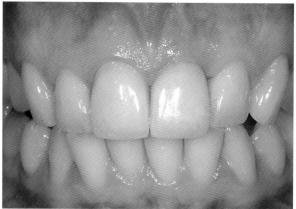

Fig 6-2u Definitive crowns at 1 year.

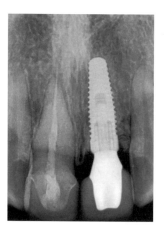

Fig 6-2v Follow-up radiograph at 1 year demonstrates the undercontoured abutment used with the platform switching technique. Note the good bone levels and the apparent regeneration of bone in the distal proximal area.

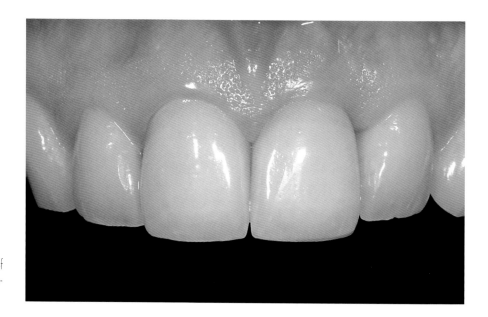

Fig 6-2w Close-up at 1 year demonstrates excellent stability of the labial tissue and slightly compromised distal papilla.

Case discussion

Figures 6-2u to 6-2w show the final crowns at approximately 1 year postoperatively. As expected, the distal papilla is not ideal, but the radiograph (see Fig 6-2v) reveals good apparent regeneration of the bone in this area. Since maturation and remodeling of the papilla continues for as long as 3 years, further improvement of the papilla should be expected over time.

This case reinforces the author's view that the reported 1 mm or so of labial recession seen in the first year after implant restoration can indeed be avoided, even in immediate placement cases, by following the protocols described.

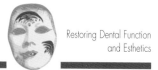

Restoring Dental Function
and Esthetics

Conclusion

Contemporary implant dentistry aims not only to restore function but also to create a lasting esthetic outcome. This is particularly important in the esthetic zone, where single-tooth replacement is frequently indicated. While optimal results can be accomplished predictably in simple cases, the achievement of ideal results is difficult in complex cases, which usually present with significant obstacles. Nevertheless, the protocols described in this chapter serve to highlight contemporary concepts that can maximize the outcomes in these cases. These principles, and the key steps described, form a sound basis for the successful restoration of single teeth with implants in the esthetic zone.

References

1. Bengazi F, Wennström JL, Lekholm U. Recession of the soft tissue margin at oral implants. A 2-year longitudinal prospective study. Clin Oral Implants Res 1996;7:303–310.
2. Saadoun AP, LeGall M, Touati B. Selection and ideal tridimensional implant position for soft tissue aesthetics. Pract Periodontics Aesthet Dent 1999;11:1063–1072.
3. Grunder U, Gracis S, Capelli M. Influence of the 3-D bone-to-implant relationship on esthetics. Int J Periodontics Restorative Dent 2005;25:113–119.
4. Abrahamsson I, Berglundh T, Glantz PO, Lindhe J. The mucosal attachment at different abutments. An experimental study in dogs. J Clin Periodontol 1998;25:721–727.
5. Abrahamsson I, Berglundh T, Lindhe J. The mucosal barrier following abutment dis/reconnection. An experimental study in dogs. J Clin Periodontol 1997;24:568–572.
6. Hermann JS, Buser D, Schenk RK, Higginbottom FL, Cochran DL. Biologic width around titanium implants. A physiologically formed and stable dimension over time. Clin Oral Implants Res 2000;11:1–11.
7. Hermann JS, Buser D, Schenk RK, Schoolfield JD, Cochran DL. Biologic width around one- and two-piece titanium implants. Clin Oral Implants Res 2001;12:559–571.
8. Grunder U. Stability of the mucosal topography around single-tooth implants and adjacent teeth: 1-year results. Int J Periodontics Restorative Dent 2000;20:11–17.
9. Kan JYK, Rungcharassaeng K, Umezu K, Kois JC. Dimensions of peri-implant mucosa: An evaluation of maxillary anterior single implants in humans. J Periodontol 2003;74:557–562.
10. Degidi M, Artese L, Scarano A, Perrotti V, Gehrke P, Piattelli A. Inflammatory infiltrate, microvessel density, nitric oxide synthase expression, vascular endothelial growth factor expression, and proliferative activity in peri-implant soft tissues around titanium and zirconium oxide healing caps. Periodontol 2006;77:73–80.
11. Rimondini L, Cerroni L, Carrassi A, Torricelli P. Bacterial colonization of zirconia ceramic surfaces: An in vitro and in vivo study. Int J Oral Maxillofac Implants 2002;17:793–798.
12. Welander M, Abrahamsson I, Berglundh T. The mucosal barrier at implant abutments of different materials. Clin Oral Implants Res 2008;19:635–641.
13. Baumgarten H, Cocchetto R, Testori T, Meltzer A, Porter S. A new implant design for crestal bone preservation: Initial observations and case report. Pract Proced Aesthet Dent 2005;17:735–740.

14. Lazzara RJ, Porter SS. Platform switching: A new concept in implant dentistry for controlling postrestorative crestal bone levels. Int J Periodontics Restorative Dent 2006;26:9–17.

15. Shin YK, Han CH, Heo SJ, Kim S, Chun HJ. Radiographic evaluation of marginal bone level around implants with different neck designs after 1 year. Int J Oral Maxillofac Implants 2006;21:789–794.

16. Nowzari H, Yi K, Chee W, Rich SK. Immunology, microbiology, and virology following placement of NobelPerfect scalloped dental implants: Analysis of a case series. Clin Implant Dent Relat Res 2008;10:157–165.

17. Spray JR, Black CG, Morris HF, Ochi S. The influence of bone thickness on facial marginal bone response: Stage 1 placement through stage 2 uncovering. Ann Periodontol 2000;5:119–128.

18. Bianchi AE, Sanfilippo F. Single-tooth replacement by immediate implant and connective tissue graft: A 1-9-year clinical evaluation. Clin Oral Implants Res 2004;15:269–277.

19. Kan JY, Rungcharassaeng K, Lozada JL. Bilaminar subepithelial connective tissue grafts for immediate implant placement and provisionalization in the esthetic zone. J Calif Dent Assoc 2005;33:865–871.

20. Wöhrle PS. Nobel Perfect esthetic scalloped implant: Rationale for a new design. Clin Implant Dent Relat Res 2003;5(suppl 1):64–73.

21. Chou CT, Morris HF, Ochi S, Walker L, DesRosiers D. AICRG, Part II: Crestal bone loss associated with the Ankylos implant: Loading to 36 months. J Oral Implantol 2004;30:134–143.

22. Norton MR. Multiple single-tooth implant restorations in the posterior jaws: Maintenance of marginal bone levels with reference to the implant-abutment microgap. Int J Oral Maxillofac Implants 2006;21:777–784.

23. Rompen E, Raepsaet N, Domken O, Touati B, Van Dooren E. Soft tissue stability at the facial aspect of gingivally converging abutments in the esthetic zone: A pilot clinical study. J Prosthet Dent 2007;97(6, suppl):119S–125S[erratum 2008;99(3):167].

24. Schropp L, Kostopoulos L, Wenzel A, Isidor F. Clinical and radiographic performance of delayed-immediate single-tooth implant placement associated with peri-implant bone defects. A 2-year prospective, controlled, randomized follow-up report. J Clin Periodontol 2005;32:480–487.

25. Schropp L, Kostopoulos L, Wenzel A. Bone healing following immediate versus delayed placement of titanium implants into extraction sockets: A prospective clinical study. Int J Oral Maxillofac Implants 2003;18:189–199.

26. Schropp L, Wenzel A, Kostopoulos L, Karring T. Bone healing and soft tissue contour changes following single-tooth extraction: A clinical and radiographic 12-month prospective study. Int J Periodontics Restorative Dent 2003;23:313–323.

27. Botticelli D, Berglundh T, Lindhe J. Hard-tissue alterations following immediate implant placement in extraction sites. J Clin Periodontol 2004;31:820–828.

28. Araújo MG, Sukekava F, Wennström JL, Lindhe J. Ridge alterations following implant placement in fresh extraction sockets: An experimental study in the dog. J Clin Periodontol 2005;32:645–652.

29. Araújo MG, Sukekava F, Wennström JL, Lindhe J. Tissue modeling following implant placement in fresh extraction sockets. Clin Oral Implants Res 2006;17:615–624.

30. Mankoo T. Contemporary implant concepts in esthetic dentistry—Part 2: Immediate single-tooth implants. Pract Proced Aesthet Dent 2004;16:61–68.

31. Araújo M, Linder E, Wennström J, Lindhe J. The influence of Bio-Oss Collagen on healing of an extraction socket: An experimental study in the dog. Int J Periodontics Restorative Dent 2008;28:123–135.

32. Cornelini R, Cangini F, Martuscelli G, Wennström J. Deproteinized bovine bone and biodegradable barrier membranes to support healing following immediate placement of transmucosal implants: A short-term controlled clinical trial. Int J Periodontics Restorative Dent 2004;24:555–563.

33. Nevins M, Camelo M, De Paoli S, et al. A study of the fate of the buccal wall of extraction sockets of teeth with prominent roots. Int J Periodontics Restorative Dent 2006;26(1):19–29.

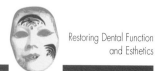

Restoring Dental Function and Esthetics

34. Mankoo T. Restoration of failing single teeth in compromised anterior sites with immediate or delayed implant placement combined with socket preservation—A report of two cases. Eur J Esthet Dent 2007;2:352–368.

35. Mankoo T. Contemporary implant concepts in aesthetic dentistry—Part 3: Adjacent immediate implants in the aesthetic zone. Pract Proced Aesthet Dent 2004;16:327–334.

36. Mankoo T. Maintenance of interdental papillae in the aesthetic zone using multiple immediate adjacent implants to restore failing teeth—A report of ten cases at 2–7 year follow up. Eur J Esthet Dent 2008;3:304–322.

37. Salama H, Salama MA, Garber D, Adar P. The interproximal height of bone: A guidepost to predictable aesthetic strategies and soft tissue contours in anterior tooth replacement. Pract Periodontics Aesthet Dent 1998;10:1131–1141.

38. Tarnow D, Elian N, Fletcher P, et al. Vertical distance from the crest of bone to the height of the interproximal papilla between adjacent implants. J Periodontol 2003;74:1785–1788.

39. Buser D, Martin W, Belser UC. Optimizing esthetics for implant restorations in the anterior maxilla: Anatomic and surgical considerations. Int J Oral Maxillofac Implants 2004;19(suppl):43–61.

40. Buser D, Chen ST, Weber HP, Belser UC. Early implant placement following single-tooth extraction in the esthetic zone: Biologic rationale and surgical procedures. Int J Periodontics Restorative Dent 2008;28:441–451.

41. Kan JY, Rungcharassaeng K, Sclar A, Lozada JL. Effects of the facial osseous defect morphology on gingival dynamics after immediate tooth replacement and guided bone regeneration: 1-year results. J Oral Maxillofac Surg 2007;65(suppl 1):13–19.

42. Mankoo T. Single tooth implant restorations in the aesthetic zone—Contemporary concepts for optimization and maintenance of soft tissue esthetics in replacement of failing teeth in compromised sites. Eur J Esthet Dent 2007;2:274–295.

43. Jemt T, Lekholm U. Measurements of buccal tissue volumes at single-implant restorations after local bone grafting in maxillas: A 3-year clinical prospective study case series. Clin Implant Dent Relat Res 2003;5(2):63–70.

44. Jemt T, Lekholm U. Single implants and buccal bone grafts in the anterior maxilla: Measurements of buccal crestal contours in a 6-year prospective clinical study. Clin Implant Dent Relat Res 2005;7(3):127–135.

45. Becker W, Hujoel P, Becker BE. Effect of barrier membranes and autologous bone grafts on ridge width preservation around implants. Clin Implant Dent Relat Res 2002;4(3):143–149.

46. Araújo MG, Sonohara M, Hayacibara R, Cardaropoli G, Lindhe J. Lateral ridge augmentation by the use of grafts comprised of autologous bone or a biomaterial. An experiment in the dog. J Clin Periodontol 2002;29:1122–1131.

47. Berglundh T, Lindhe J. Healing around implants placed in bone defects treated with Bio-Oss. An experimental study in the dog. Clin Oral Implants Res 1997;8:117–124.

48. Norton MR, Odell EW, Thompson ID, Cook RJ. Efficacy of bovine bone mineral for alveolar augmentation: A human histologic study. Clin Oral Implants Res 2003;14:775–783.

49. Esposito M, Grusovin MG, Coulthard P, Worthington HV. The efficacy of various bone augmentation procedures for dental implants: A Cochrane systematic review of randomized controlled clinical trials. Int J Oral Maxillofac Implants 2006;21:696–710.

50. Jensen SS, Aaboe M, Pinholt EM, Hjørting-Hansen E, Melsen F, Ruyter IE. Tissue reaction and material characteristics of four bone substitutes. Int J Oral Maxillofac Implants 1996;11:55–66.

51. Hämmerle CH, Lang NP. Single stage surgery combining transmucosal implant placement with guided bone regeneration and bioresorbable materials. Clin Oral Implants Res 2001;12:9–18.

52. Choquet V, Hermans M, Adriaenssens P, Daelemans P, Tarnow DP, Malevez C. Clinical and radiographic evaluation of the papilla level adjacent to single-tooth dental implants. A retrospective study in the maxillary anterior region. J Periodontol 2001;72:1364–1371.

Restoring Dental Function and Esthetics

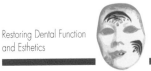

53. Jemt T. Regeneration of gingival papillae after single-implant treatment. Int J Periodontics Restorative Dent 1997;17:326–333.
54. Small PN, Tarnow DP. Gingival recession around implants: A 1-year longitudinal prospective study. Int J Oral Maxillofac Implants 2000;15:527–532.
55. Cardaropoli G, Lekholm U, Wennström JL. Tissue alterations at implant-supported single-tooth replacements: A 1-year prospective clinical study. Clin Oral Implants Res 2006;17:165–171.
56. Funato A, Salama MA, Ishikawa T, Garber DA, Salama H. Timing, positioning, and sequential staging in esthetic implant therapy: A four-dimensional perspective. Int J Periodontics Restorative Dent 2007;27:313–323.
57. Jung RE, Sailer I, Hämmerle CHF, Attin T, Schmidlin P. In vitro color changes of soft tissues caused by restorative materials. Int J Periodontics Restorative Dent 2007;27:251–257.
58. Sclar AG. Guidelines for flapless surgery. J Oral Maxillofac Surg 2007;65(suppl 1):20–32.
59. Fickl S, Zuhr O, Wachtel H, Bolz W, Huerzeler M. Tissue alterations after tooth extraction with and without surgical trauma: A volumetric study in the beagle dog. J Clin Periodontol 2008;35:356–363.
60. Fickl S, Zuhr O, Wachtel H, Bolz W, Huerzeler MB. Hard tissue alterations after socket preservation: An experimental study in the beagle dog. Clin Oral Implants Res 2008;19:1111–1118.
61. Fickl S, Zuhr O, Wachtel H, Stappert CF, Stein JM, Hürzeler MB. Dimensional changes of the alveolar ridge contour after different socket preservation techniques. J Clin Periodontol 2008;35:906–913.

Scientific Advances in Tooth-Whitening Processes

7

Wyman Chan, BDS, LDS, RCS, IADFE

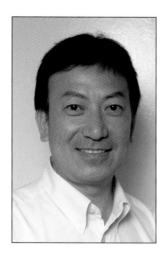

Wyman Chan, BDS, LDS, RCS, IADFE

Wyman Chan qualified at Guy's Hospital Dental School, London, UK. He is a dedicated teeth whitening dentist and founder of smilestudio London and the International Tooth-whitening Academy. He has trained more than 1,500 dentists, dental hygienists, dental therapists, dental surgery assistants, and other dental team members over the past 5 years.

Dr Chan has worked with all major home and power whitening systems. His innovative research in the field of teeth whitening has led to five UK patents and several more pending patents. Dr Chan won the prestigious Procter and Gamble Investigator Award at the 2008 International Association for Dental Research meeting in Toronto, Canada. He is a part-time PhD research student at the Centre for Materials Research and Innovation, University of Bolton, UK. Through his research and experience of treating thousands of patients, Dr Chan has discovered some important phenomena in the texture of teeth and has used them to establish some important protocols and metrics that have contributed to the understanding and improvement of the safety and efficacy of teeth whitening processes. He lectures internationally, has published many articles in dental journals, and is regarded as an expert in this field.

Email: smilestudiouk@aol.com

A whiter smile has become an essential part of an attractive, successful image as well as a sign of good health. Currently, the demand for tooth-whitening treatment is at an all-time high. In a 2004 survey of 3,215 subjects in the United Kingdom, 50% perceived that they had some class of tooth discoloration,[1] while a 2000 study of an adult population in the United States discovered that 34% of participants were dissatisfied with the current color of their teeth.[2] Since tooth-whitening procedures have become such a lucrative sphere of cosmetic dentistry, the market has responded with an ever-expanding range of commercially available tooth-whitening products, leaving dental practitioners exposed to aggressive marketing and the often-exaggerated claims of manufacturers. In the end, the clinician needs to have a thorough understanding of how the whitening process works and how various whitening agents may affect patients' teeth, and should use this knowledge to choose the safest and most efficient product and technique for each case.

Stains are dark discolorations in the teeth caused either by the deposition of pigmented organic and inorganic molecules within the crystalline structure of enamel and dentin or by the ingestion of chromogenic agents such as tetracycline. They are commonly bleached via an oxidative process initiated by the primary generation of hydroxyl radical ($^{\bullet}$OH) from hydrogen peroxide (H_2O_2), which is present as a bleaching agent in various professional tooth-whitening products. The acceleration of this oxidative process effectively enhances the bleaching potential of a tooth-whitening agent. A number of techniques have been developed to assist the conversion of hydrogen peroxide to hydroxyl radical, including exposure to heat, ultraviolet light or alternative light sources of specific wavelengths, a variety of coapplied chemical accelerators and, more recently, lasers. In general, as with many other (nonenzymatic) physiologically relevant chemical reactions performed in the laboratory, for every 10°C the temperature rises, the bleaching effect of hydrogen peroxide is doubled.

With so many options available, the choice of the safest and most effective bleaching product and technique has never been a bigger challenge. In addition, the degree of shade improvement achieved by any bleaching agent at the termination of a standard treatment time may vary greatly. The result depends on a combination of factors in each clinical case, particularly the initial tooth shade, nature of the stain, and sites of the discoloration within the tooth structure. The unique physiologic characteristics of patients' teeth—such as enamel porosity, which determines the permeability of the enamel—and agents present in the saliva that may promote tooth discoloration (eg, dietary-derived reducing sugars and aldehydes) also are of critical importance. Full comprehension of how these etiologic and physiologic factors can affect the tooth-whitening process will help alleviate the inconsistent results experienced by clinicians who offer chairside/power bleaching systems in their practices.

Restoring Dental Function
and Esthetics

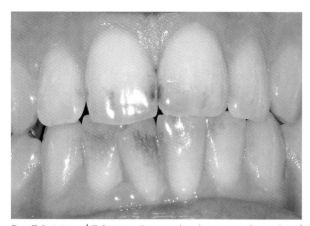 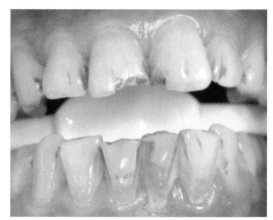

Figs 7-1 (left) and 7-2 (right) Extrinsic discoloration on the teeth surfaces.

Etiology of Tooth Stains

The color of teeth is influenced by a very wide range of physical factors that originate in the patient as well as the immediate environment. These include *(1)* the relative translucency, opacity, and color of enamel; *(2)* the thickness and color of underlying dentin; and *(3)* the nature and quality of incident light and other optical and visual effects. For example, the yellow or brown coloration of dentin is superimposed by the green, pink, and blue hues of enamel, which results in a wide range of hues and values even within a single tooth. Tooth color is therefore a consequence of all factors affecting both enamel and dentin.

The discolorations of human teeth can be classified as arising from an extrinsic, internalized, or intrinsic source.

Oral bacteria and mycotic organisms are often involved in extrinsic discoloration. Other extrinsic sources of stains include beverages, food, tobacco smoke, mouthrinses, medications, and industrial agents (Figs 7-1 and 7-2). This type of stain is lodged in the pellicle layers of the teeth and can be removed effectively by good tooth brushing with an appropriate dentifrice, combined with scaling and polishing procedures, which can be performed by the clinician or a dental hygienist.

The internalized form of staining is caused by penetration of the extrinsic stains into the enamel and dentin substructures, and the scaling and polishing mentioned above will not be able to remove this class of stain at these sites (Fig 7-3).

The third type of stain, intrinsic discoloration, can arise from a variety of systemic and pulpal factors operating during odontogenesis, such as fluorosis, enamel hypoplasia, pulp trauma, tetracycline therapy, hemolytic disease, amelogenesis, and dentinogenesis imperfecta.

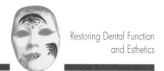

Restoring Dental Function
and Esthetics

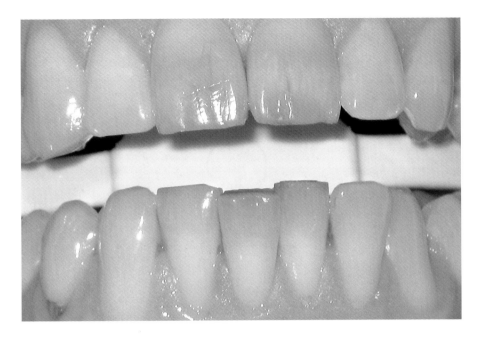

Fig 7-3 Internalized discoloration on the maxillary central incisors and the mandibular right central incisor and first premolars.

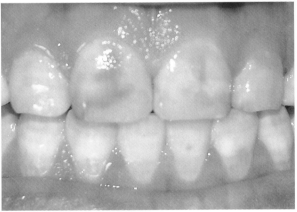

Fig 7-4 Fluorosis-stained teeth with stains ranging from light to dark brown.

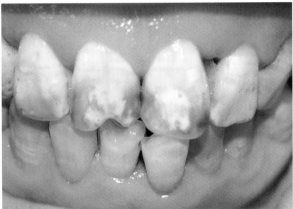

Fig 7-5 White patches and enamel pitting in a patient with fluorosis.

Fluorosis

Fluorosis is a type of intrinsic stain that can arise from the ingestion of fluoride (F^-) at a concentration of greater than 1 ppm in drinking water. This excess fluoride causes metabolic modifications in ameloblasts during amelogenesis, which leads to a defective matrix and calcification. Fluorosis can be a form of hypoplasia and can affect a child's dentition from the second trimester in utero until 8 or 9 years of age.[3,4] The affected teeth may be pitted, and they often display dark brown stains that cover part of the enamel (Figs 7-4 and 7-5). Any pigmentation of stain is usually confined to the outer third of the enamel, which can appear chalky.[5,6]

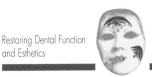

Restoring Dental Function and Esthetics

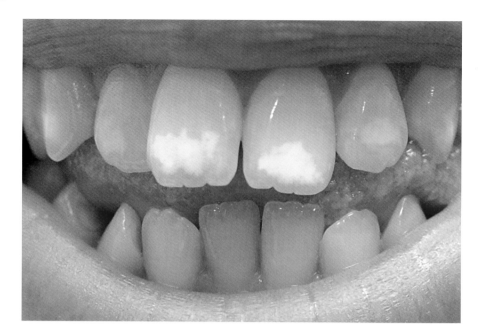

Fig 7-6 White patches in this patient with enamel hypoplasia are especially prominent in the maxillary teeth.

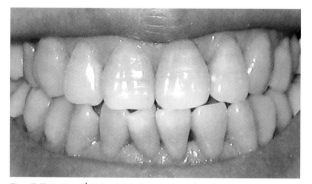 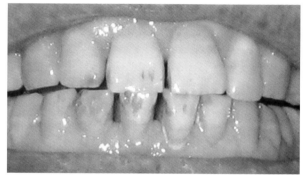

Figs 7-7 (left) and 7-8 (right) Tetracycline discoloration is prominent at the cervical third of the teeth because the stains show through thin enamel in this area.

Enamel hypoplasia

Enamel hypoplasia is responsible for a defective matrix and calcification of enamel, and is clinically observed as white patches on the enamel surfaces. The teeth can appear chalky white when dry, and the condition sometimes affects the entire enamel surface (Fig 7-6). This differs from fluorosis in that the enamel, which is more hypocalcified than that affected by fluorosis, does not display brown stains or pitting.

Age-induced stains

The dentin becomes darker as we age as a result of the formation of the more discolored secondary and tertiary dentin. At the same time, the enamel may become thinner due to erosion from acidic food and drinks in the diet and wear from excessive tooth brushing and the use of abrasive dentifrice. The stains in the dentin travel outward to the enamel

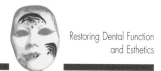

Restoring Dental Function and Esthetics

(a hypothesis of the author), which contribute to the discoloration, and become more visible in the thinner layer of enamel. Other factors contributing to age-induced stains are internalized discoloration and inflammation and necrosis of the pulpal tissues. The latter may explain why the discoloration in a single traumatized tooth (see Fig 7-19) may take months and sometimes years to manifest and be visible in the enamel.

Tetracycline-induced stains

The nature and extent of tetracycline-induced stains depend on the specific class of drug administered,[7,8] the dosage,[8] and the duration of administration.[9] This antibiotic agent forms a complex with Ca^{2+} and becomes incorporated into hydroxyapatite at the mineralizing front of enamel and dentin.[10] The staining is attributable to a photo-oxidative process that yields a red/purple product, 4,12 anhydro-4-oxo dedimethylaminotetracycline[11,12] (AODTC). The coloration observed depends on the particular molecular form of this adduct (Figs 7-7 and 7-8). Oxytetracycline and chlorotetracycline have been shown to cause only minimal discoloration in both in vitro and enamel-based investigations.[13,14]

Tetracycline is detectable in both enamel and dentin,[15–17] but much higher levels are present in the latter. Tetracycline crosses the placenta and is incorporated into developing enamel and dentin; hence, a neonate will develop staining if the mother receives this agent during pregnancy.[6]

Background of Tooth-Whitening Processes

Tooth whitening is a bleaching process that removes stains in the enamel and dentin of teeth. The diffusion of bleaching agents into the teeth substructures is critical to remove staining chromophores, a process that effectively improves the color shade of teeth. The bleaching agents used by the dental profession today are hydrogen peroxide (H_2O_2) and carbamide peroxide ($CH_4N_2O.H_2O_2$), or CP, an equimolar addition complex of urea with hydrogen peroxide.

According to Zaragoza,[18] the first technique for tooth bleaching was published in 1877 by Chapple, who used oxalic acid as a bleaching agent. Hydrochloric acid was subsequently tested and clinically employed by Kane in 1916[19] as an alternative bleaching agent. Because of the significant risk of enamel demineralization by high levels of acid, Ames chose to use hydrogen peroxide to bleach mottled teeth and reported his findings in 1937.[20]

The use of CP in tooth-whitening trays warrants historical consideration because it is the first bleaching agent that was discovered accidentally. In 1968, Dr William Klusmier, an American orthodontist, attempted to treat gingival inflammation in his patients. He first used

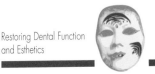

Gly-Oxide (GlaxoSmithKline), a 10% (by weight) CP oral antiseptic solution, and later moved on to Proxigel (Reed and Carnrick Pharmaceuticals), a 10% CP oral antiseptic gel placed in patients' nightguard retainers.[21] The side effect of each treatment was whiter teeth. Since the first scientific report of nightguard/tray bleaching published in 1989, hydrogen peroxide has been introduced as an alternative to CP.[22] In the early preparations of both CP and hydrogen peroxide products, clear and single-barrelled syringes were used in the manufacturing processes. The pH of CP ranges from 6.2 to 7.0, which is safe for enamel because the enamel matrix only starts to dissolve at pH values of less than 5.0. However, hydrogen peroxide is only stable in acidic formulations.

Compared with CP, hydrogen peroxide is a more convenient and practical agent for bleaching teeth since it requires a shorter contact time with the teeth surfaces, and patients can have their teeth bleached while awake, rather than using it overnight. If a double-barrelled syringe is used, the hydrogen peroxide can be prepared in a gel form and stabilized at low pH in one of the barrels. The other barrel can house an alkaline activator to raise the pH to a safe level (usually above 7.0 and preferably above 10.0) and hence enhance the bleaching effect by *(1)* generating the perhydroxyl anion (HO_2^-), and *(2)* catalyzing its conversion to the hydroxyl radical ($^{\bullet}OH$) so that the entire bleaching process can proceed at a clinically rapid rate (30 minutes). A patented tray system invented by the author for in-office delivery of bleaching agents includes internal seals that prevent escape of the bleaching agent to the exposed dentin and soft tissue; therefore, it is safe to use even with higher concentrations of hydrogen peroxide that may otherwise damage surrounding vital tissues.[23,24]

Bleaching Mechanisms of Tooth-Whitening Agents

The low molecular mass of hydrogen peroxide and its ability to denature proteins allow it to move more freely than CP within the tooth.[25] Because of the variable inherent porosity and selective permeability of enamel and dentin, hydrogen peroxide is able to penetrate their structures and therefore remove not only superficial stains on the surface of the teeth but also those present within enamel and dentin.[3,26,27]

Since hydrogen peroxide loses its efficacy upon exposure to air and chromophores, this bleaching agent is dispensed in small quantities: 0.25 mL (0.30 mg) is sufficient for each home whitening application on both arches. A higher dose (3.0 mg) is required for each chairside procedure for both arches.

It is generally accepted that the whitening effect can be attributed to the degradation (by the hydroxyl radical) of the high-molecular-mass complex organic chromophores, which are responsible for the color of the stain. These chromophores reflect a specific wavelength of light in

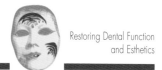

the visible region of the electromagnetic spectrum. Flaitz and Hicks postulated that the chromophores degrade to products of lower molecular mass that reflect more light and result in a reduction or elimination of tooth discoloration.[28]

The bleaching process is generally safer with the double-barrelled technique described above, since the contact time of the bleaching agent with the teeth is much shorter, sometimes by as much as 80%, compared with the single-barrelled bleaching technique. This procedure achieves similar or better results than those of methods that do not use an effective activator/initiator. A study presented in 2006 at the International Association for Dental Research (IADR) conference in Brisbane, Australia, showed that an amino-alcohol activator enhanced the bleaching effect of hydrogen peroxide by 300%.[29]

Hypotheses for Effective Treatment

Extensive clinical experience and careful observation of all patients often provide the main tools for a clinician to fully understand the effects of bleaching agents and techniques on various patients' teeth. Because no two patients are entirely alike, consistent and effective results may be achieved by assessing the porosity and, subsequently, the translucency of the enamel before beginning treatment.[30] Methods to assess the porosity have been proposed, and the influence of dentin color on effective bleaching of more translucent enamel is currently under examination. Typically, enamel consists of 80% to 90% inorganic hydroxyapatite mineral and 10% to 20% (by volume) interprism pores, the latter filled with fluid and organic matter. Nonetheless, enamel can be either highly porous (consisting of more than 20% pores) or highly dense (with less than 10% pores).

The author advanced a hypothesis[30] that the differing textures of enamel are based on the rate and extent of enamel dehydration under standard clinical tooth-whitening conditions. Indeed, this hypothesis postulates that the greater the dehydration rate of the enamel, the more porous it is. Enamel is porous and loses moisture through the enamel pores when left to dry; it is translucent when wet in the normal oral cavity, and white and opaque when dry. This difference can be measured by comparing the baseline shade (A) of the enamel before dehydration against its dehydrated shade (B) after drying in a standardized manner, a process that prevents saliva from hydrating this matrix via the blockage of entry into this biofilm for a preselected period of time. The greater the difference between A and B, the more porous is the enamel. A further hypothesis of the author is that the more porous the enamel, the greater diffusion rate through more porous enamel and less dilution of the bleaching solution, since its pores are empty subsequent to dehydration.

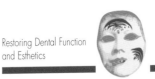

Restoring Dental Function
and Esthetics

The first hypothesis, which focuses on enamel porosity, would explain why some teeth respond better than others to a standardized bleaching protocol. Clinical experience has demonstrated that porous teeth whiten better than dense teeth. This may be due to quicker diffusion of the bleaching agent within the enamel, allowing a brighter overall effect in a similar period.

Another hypothesis, centered around enamel translucency, postulates that porous enamel is usually translucent whereas dense enamel is usually opaque. The more porous the enamel, the more translucent it is. If the enamel is very translucent, the underlying color of the dentin shows through the enamel. Therefore, the dentin would need to be whitened as well to effectively change the color of the overall tooth. This makes very translucent enamel difficult to bleach because the underlying dentin needs to be bleached so that the lightened effect can be transmitted through the very translucent enamel. The "rebound" effect on this type of enamel is also greater because in most chairside bleaching, the bleaching agent does not travel to the dentin. The immediate whiter result is due to dehydration of the enamel, which appears whiter, and the teeth revert back to their baseline shade a few days later after the enamel is rehydrated by the saliva in the oral cavity. On the other hand, if the enamel is less translucent and more opaque and the underlying color of the dentin does not show through, then only changes to the color of the enamel are necessary to change the color of the tooth. Comprehension of these optical properties of the enamel is fundamental to help the clinician determine which sites of the discoloration need to be bleached, and at what concentration or length of time. The second hypothesis also would explain the rebound effect in chairside/power whitening, in which the teeth darken after bleaching and may require a second or further treatment, as the dentin in these translucent-enamel teeth may not have been properly lightened.

Tooth-Whitening Procedures

Types of systems

Three types of professional tooth-whitening systems are commonly used today:

1. Home whitening systems that use customized trays
2. "Jump-start" systems that use the same home whitening trays before home treatment begins
3. Chairside/power whitening, an in-office bleaching procedure that employs a high-concentration bleaching agent (15% to 38% hydrogen peroxide)

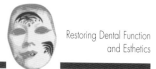

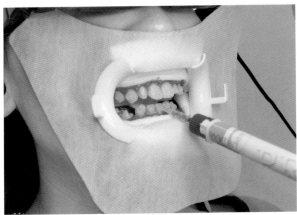 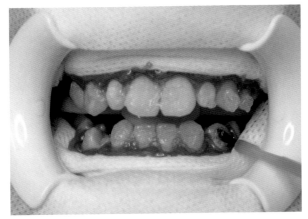

Figs 7-9 *(left)* and **7-10** *(right)* Exposed dentin and soft tissues are protected by paint-on dam.

The first article on nightguard vital bleaching was published in 1989 by Haywood and Heymann and recommended a 10% CP solution in an overnight bleaching protocol.[22] Many clinicians still prescribe 10% CP to their patients for home whitening procedures; this is a weak bleaching agent that takes many weeks of use to whiten teeth to a desired shade.

Jump-start systems became popular in the early 1990s and employ a more concentrated bleaching agent (usually 35% to 45% CP gel) that is administered at the dental practice. Patients normally sit in the waiting room for this procedure, usually for 30 to 60 minutes, without further clinician supervision. This process provides an initial portion of the overall bleaching necessary for the desired shade to increase the efficacy of subsequent home whitening.

The chairside/power or in-office systems were first used in the 1970s with an aqueous solution of 35% hydrogen peroxide, combined with rubber dam (Figs 7-9 and 7-10) to protect the soft tissues from the potentially harmful effects of this agent that are present at this concentration. A specific type of heat lamp is employed to heat the hydrogen peroxide and accelerate the bleaching process. Available materials (eg, paint-on dam) can protect the soft tissues and exposed dentin effectively against hydrogen peroxide–induced side effects, and hydrogen peroxide can be stabilized and prepared into a paste form so that it is able to remain on the tooth surfaces without escaping to the surrounding soft tissues (which causes severe discomfort in patients). Because of these advances, the chairside systems can be very safe and effective if conducted professionally and if the clinician understands and respects the science underlying tooth-whitening processes.

Conscious bleaching

It is recommended that, within reason, hydrogen peroxide be used when home whitening is chosen. Although unconscious bleaching (ie, in which patients wear trays while asleep) has been considered relatively safe in the past due to the reduced flow of saliva and jaw motion during sleep, there is still a significant risk that patients may inadvertently swallow the bleaching gel. Therefore, in light of other methods available, unconscious bleaching may be outdated and unnecessary. The author has designed customized trays that allow conscious bleaching for a period of 30 minutes twice a day, which is recommended to reduce the risk of sensitivity to the teeth and the soft tissues because the bleaching agent is sealed inside these particular trays[23,25] (Fig 7-11). This technique is described in more detail below. It is of paramount importance that the bleaching trays remain firmly seated over the tooth surfaces to prevent movement of the trays and any subsequent leakage of the bleaching agent. To ensure that the trays remain still, the patient must be awake while undergoing the home whitening procedure.

Additional methods of conscious home and chairside bleaching procedures are currently being researched. The hope is that techniques will be discovered that prevent the bleaching agent from coming into contact with the oral environment. Soft tissues and exposed dentin contain nerve endings that cause severe discomfort to the patient when contacted by a bleaching agent, so less exposure results in more satisfactory treatment. Moreover, improved techniques would minimize contact with saliva, which contains many hydrogen peroxide–scavenging biomolecules.

The wy10 technique

The wy10 tooth-whitening technique combines all three classes of professional tooth-whitening systems mentioned above. It consists of 30 minutes of jump-start bleaching using customized trays, followed by one week of home whitening and then a final chairside procedure.

The patented wy10 Perfect Trays (Wyten Technology) used in this technique are fabricated with internal seals to prevent the escape of the bleaching agent to the exposed dentin and gingival tissues. Location marks in these trays direct the patient to place them at the exact locations with a specific amount of bleaching agent. As Fig 7-12 shows, the tray has no reservoirs and is non-scalloped. The tray extends 2 to 3 mm above the gingival margin to prevent the saliva from entering, which can dilute and metabolize the bleaching agent rapidly (saliva metabolizes 29 mg of naturally produced hydrogen peroxide per minute). The bleaching agent is placed over these location marks, which have small dimples to house the agent. While the internal seals (see Fig 7-12) prevent leakage of the bleaching agent, they also serve to push the hydroxyl radical back inside the enamel pores, thereby enhancing the bleaching effect.

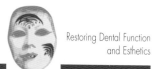

Restoring Dental Function
and Esthetics

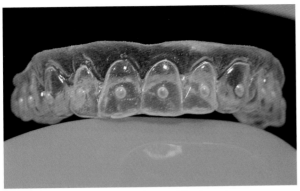

Fig 7-11 Home whitening tray designed by the author.

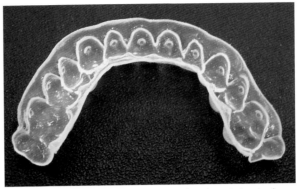

Fig 7-12 View of the tray showing internal seals and dimples for placement of bleaching agent.

The procedure for this technique is as follows:

1. Impressions of the teeth are taken so that the customized wy10 bleaching trays can be fabricated.
2. Photographs are taken, and the baseline/initial shades are recorded for the six maxillary anterior teeth. Based on the value (lightness) of the teeth, the Vita Classical shade guide (Vident) can be rearranged (Fig 7-13).
3. A small amount of the bleaching agent (wy10, 25% hydrogen peroxide) is loaded onto the dimples (Figs 7-14 and 7-15).
4. The tray is seated over the teeth to be bleached (Fig 7-16), and jump-start bleaching occurs for 30 minutes, usually while the patient sits in the waiting room.
5. The patient completes 7 days of at-home conscious bleaching, using 6% hydrogen peroxide (wy10, 6% hydrogen peroxide) for 30 minutes twice a day.
6. After the 7 days, chairside/power whitening is performed with the paint-on dam procedure that uses a high-concentration bleaching agent (wy10, 25% hydrogen peroxide) and a thermal diffuser with variable power output to control the temperature (Figs 7-17 and 7-18). At this stage of the process, the clinician can vary the contact time (normally 3 × 10 minutes) of the bleaching agent on the teeth surfaces to whiten the patient's teeth to the desired final shade.
7. Photographs are taken and posttreatment shades are recorded for the same six anterior teeth.

This technique is very simple, and the teeth usually end at six to ten shades lighter than their initial value according to the Vita Classical shade guide. The final result depends on the porosity of the teeth and the nature and sites of the original stains. This protocol provides more effective and comfortable treatment for patients since clinicians are not under

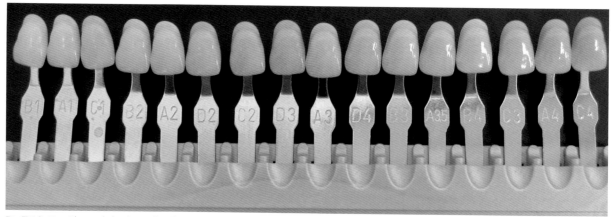

Fig 7-13 Vita Classical shade guide. This arrangement demonstrates shades in order of increasing darkness. From left to right, the shades are identified as B1 (lightest), A1, C1, B2, A2, D2, C2, D3, A3, D4, B3, A3.5, B4, C3, A4, and C4 (darkest).

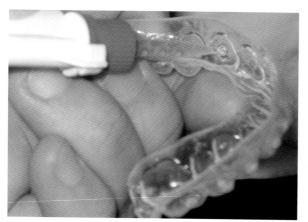

Fig 7-14 Loading the bleaching agent.

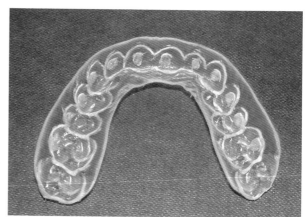

Fig 7-15 Fully loaded bleaching tray.

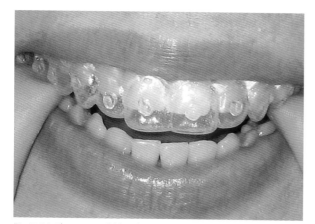

Fig 7-16 Placement of bleaching tray in patient.

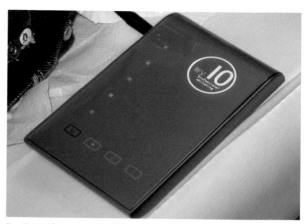

Fig 7-17 The wy10 TD (Wyten Technology) can vary its power to warm up the bleaching agent on the teeth surfaces by 5°C to 10°C.

Restoring Dental Function
and Esthetics

pressure to produce a six- to ten-shade change at the initial jump-start session. The jump-start and 7-day conscious bleaching stages contribute up to 50% of the bleaching result, and the final chairside/power whitening session accomplishes the other 50%.

Figures 7-19 and 7-20 represent two cases before and after whitening with the wy10 technique.

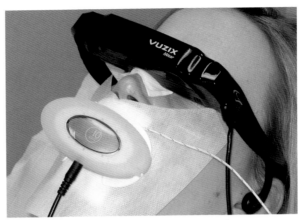

Fig 7-18 View of the wy10 TD over a retractor in the patient.

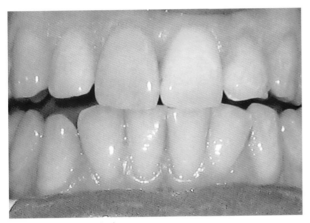

Fig 7-19a A patient before treatment.

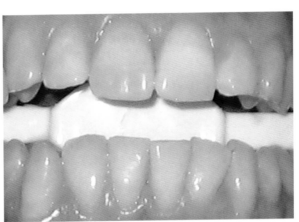

Fig 7-19b Improved esthetics after treatment using the wy10 technique.

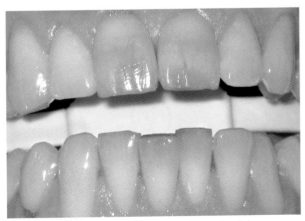

Fig 7-20a Before treatment, this patient presented with brown internalized stains on the maxillary central incisors.

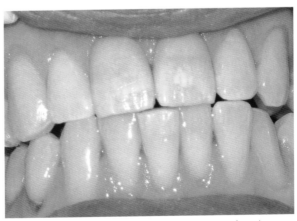

Fig 7-20b After treatment, the brown stains are gone from the central incisors.

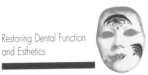

Restoring Dental Function and Esthetics

Prevention of Side Effects Involving Oral Soft Tissues and Exposed Dentin

Most of the literature that reports on side effects of various tooth-whitening procedures focuses on treatment of the side effects after the patient has already experienced them. However, by better understanding the main symptoms and causes of these side effects in patients, the clinician may be able to prevent them altogether.

Symptoms

The side effects of tooth whitening can be classified into three categories: *(1)* soft tissue irritation, *(2)* dentin hypersensitivity, and *(3)* pulpal inflammation. These side effects can be very painful, and clinical studies on home whitening have reported sensitivity in as many as 80% of the subjects tested.[31–33] In 2003, the Clinical Research Associates (CRA) tested eight chairside systems and found that all of them caused tooth sensitivity during and/or after the treatment.[34] Symptoms of soft tissue irritation include stinging and/or tingling sensations and tissue blanching. The symptoms of dentin hypersensitivity or pulpal inflammation usually involve dull to sharp/acute toothache. Severe discomfort of the oral tissues often is a central reason that patients do not continue with bleaching.[35] Most of the symptoms subside within 24 to 48 hours; however, no reports are available on permanent damage to pulpal tissue.

Causes

The main cause of soft tissue irritation is a bleaching agent that inadvertently comes into contact with the oral soft tissue. If the exposed dentin is not fully protected against bleaching agents, dentin hypersensitivity occurs, likely as a result of the fluid displacement in the dentinal tubules by these bleaching agents.[36] Dentin hypersensitivity can be increased when the affected teeth are stimulated by other factors such as hot or cold temperatures or the acidity of citrus fruit.[29–31] The bleaching agent can reach the pulp of the teeth within 15 to 30 minutes of bleaching, a process that can cause pulpal inflammation and give rise to acute pain.[37,38]

Prevention

The science of tooth-whitening techniques should involve a method to prevent contact of bleaching agents with exposed dentin and soft tissues in the oral cavity. As mentioned earlier, both these sites have nerve endings and can cause severe pain and discomfort to patients. In humans, enamel is the only nonvital erupted tissue in the oral cavity, so for safety reasons, it is essential to target the placement of bleaching agents on

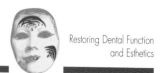

Restoring Dental Function and Esthetics

enamel surfaces only, with no contact with local vital tissues. Such a procedure diminishes the risk of discomfort and pain in patients. Conscious bleaching in home whitening procedures plays an important role in preventing the bleaching agent from inadvertent contact with dentin and soft tissue. The short bleaching time (30 minutes) in conscious bleaching also decreases the risk that the bleaching agent will travel to the pulp and cause severe discomfort in the patient.

Conclusion

As tooth-whitening procedures continue to increase in popularity, additional techniques and products will doubtless be developed to provide consistently effective and comfortable results for all patients. The clinician can benefit from the recommendations in this chapter to further study the individual characteristics of patients' teeth, the etiology of tooth stains, and the prevention of side effects before any treatment is begun. Proper use of the methods and agents described, combined with an understanding of their influence on the final tooth appearance, is essential for consistent results.

References

1. Alkhatib MN, Holt R, Bedi R. Age and perception of dental appearance and tooth colour. Gerodontology 2005;22:32–36.
2. Odioso LL, Gibb RD, Gerlach RW. Impact of demographic, behavioral, and dental care utilization parameters on tooth color and personal satisfaction. Compend Contin Educ Dent 2000;21(suppl):35S–41S.
3. McInnes J. Removing brown stain from teeth. Ariz Dent J 1966;12(4):13–15.
4. Eisenberg E. Anomalies of the teeth with stains and discolorations. J Prev Dent 1975;2(1):7–14,16–20.
5. McEvoy SA. Chemical agents for removing intrinsic stains from vital teeth. II. Current techniques and their clinical application. Quintessence Int 1989;20:379–384.
6. Bailey RW, Christen AG. Bleaching of vital teeth stained with endemic dental fluorosis. Oral Surg Oral Med Oral Pathol 1968;26:871–878.
7. Feinman RA, Goldstein RE, Garber DA. Bleaching Teeth. Chicago: Quintessence, 1987.
8. Weyman J. The clinical appearances of tetracycline staining of the teeth. Br Dent J 1965;118:289–291.
9. Bevelander G, Nakahara H. The effects of diverse amounts of tetracycline on fluorescence and coloration of teeth. J Pediatr 1966;68(1):114–120.
10. Swallow JN. Discoloration of primary dentition after maternal tetracycline ingestion in pregnancy. Lancet 1964;2(7360):611–612.
11. Cooley R. Dilemma of the discolored teeth due to tetracycline staining. Current Dent 1974;5:587–592.
12. Davies AK, Cundall RB, Dandiker Y, Slifkin MA. Photo-oxidation of tetracycline adsorbed on hydroxyapatite in relation to the light-induced staining of teeth. J Dent Res 1985;64:936–939.

13. Davies AK, McKellar JF, Phillips GO, Reid AG. Photochemical oxidation of tetracycline in aqueous solution. J Chem Soc, Perkins Trans II 1979:369–375.

14. Ibsen KH, Urist MR, Sognnaes RF. Differences among tetracyclines with respect to the staining of teeth. J Pediatr 1965;67:459–462.

15. Walton RE, O'Dell NL, Myers DL, Lake FT, Shimp RG. External bleaching of tetracycline stained teeth in dogs. J Endod 1982;8:536–542.

16. Hoerman KC. Spectral characteristics of tetracycline-induced luminescence in rat teeth and bones. J Dent Res 1975;54(special issue B):B131–B136.

17. Bevelander G, Rolle GK, Cohlan SQ. The effect of the administration of tetracycline on the development of teeth. J Dent Res 1961;40:1020–1024.

18. Zaragoza VMT. Bleaching of vital teeth technique. Estomodeo 1984;9:7–30.

19. McCloskey RJ. A technique for removal of fluorosis stains. J Am Dent Assoc 1984;109:63–64.

20. Ames JW. Removing stains from mottled enamel. J Am Dent Assoc 1937; 24:1674–1677.

21. Albers HF. Tooth-Colored Restoratives: A Syllabus for Selection, Placement and Finishing, ed 6. Cotati, CA: Alto, 1984.

22. Haywood VS, Heymann HO. Nightguard vital bleaching. Quintessesnce Int 1989;20:173–176.

23. Chan W [inventor]. Tray for dental use. UK patent GB2416310. 4 Jun 2008.

24. Chan W [inventor]. Tray for dental use. UK patent GB2445298. 27 Aug 2008.

25. Cox CS. Roles of Maillard Reactions in Diseases. London: HMSO, 1991.

26. Stewart DJ. Tetracyclines: Their prevalence in children's teeth. Br Dent J 1968;124:318–320.

27. Griffin RE Jr, Grower MF, Ayer WA. Effects of solutions used to treat dental fluorosis on permeability of teeth. J Endod 1977;3(4):139–143.

28. Flaitz CM, Hicks MJ. Effects of carbamide peroxide whitening agents on enamel surfaces and caries-like lesion formation: An SEM and polarized light microscopic in vitro study. ASDC J Dent Child 1996;63(4):249–256.

29. Blackburn J, Grootveld M, Silwood C, Lynch E. Bleaching of tooth discolouration compounds by a novel chairside gel. Presented at the 84th IADR General Session and Exhibition, Brisbane, 28 June 2006.

30. Chan W [inventor]. Teeth whitening. UK Patent GB2416309. 16 Jul 2008.

31. Haywood VB, Leonard RH, Nelson CF, Brunson WD. Effectiveness, side effects and long-term status of nightguard vital bleaching. J Am Dent Assoc 1994;125:1219–1226.

32. Gerlach RW, Jeffers MJ, Pernik PS, Sagel PA, Zhou X. Impact of prior tooth brushing on whitening strip clinical response. Presented at the 30th Annual Meeting of the AADR, 7–10 Mar 2001.

33. Browning WD, Blalock JS, Frazier KB, Downey MC, Myers ML. Duration and timing of sensitivity related to bleaching. J Esthet Restor Dent 2007;19:256–264.

34. New Generation in-office vital tooth bleaching. Part 1 and Part 2. CRA Newsletter. Nov 2002, Mar 2003.

35. Chan W. Home whitening without the sensitivity. Private Dentistry Dec 2006-Jan 2007;11(10):80–82.

36. Brookfield S, Addy M, Alexander D, Benhamou V, Dolman B, Gagnon V. Consensus-based recommendations for the management of dentin hypersensitivity. J Can Dent Assoc 2003;69:221–226.

37. Cooper JS, Bokmeyer TJ, Bowles WH. Penetration of the pulp chamber by carbamide peroxide bleaching agents. J Endod 1992;18(7):315–317.

38. Joiner A, Thakker G. In vitro evaluation of a novel 6% hydrogen peroxide tooth whitening product. J Dent 2004;32(suppl 1):19–25.

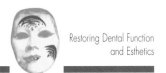

Restoring Dental Function
and Esthetics

Parameters for Integrating Esthetics with Function

8

Sergio Rubinstein, DDS

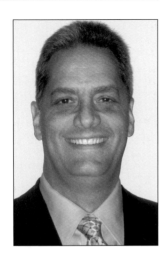

Sergio Rubinstein, DDS

Sergio Rubinstein received his dental degree in 1980 from the Universidad Tecnologica de Mexico. From 1980 to 1982 he completed his specialty training in periodontal prosthesis at the University of Illinois at Chicago, where he was an assistant professor until 1992. Dr Rubinstein is the coinventor of a custom abutment to prosthetically correct misaligned implants. He has lectured nationally and internationally, given hands-on courses in adhesive dentistry, and published several articles in adhesive dentistry and implant prosthodontics.

Email: oralrehab1@gmail.com

In 1974, Amsterdam stated that "there may be different ways of treating a disease, but there can be but one correct diagnosis."[1] This is still true today: Regardless of the scientific and technological advances dentistry has undergone, treatment is still based upon accurate identification of the underlying problem.

A treatment plan is created when a knowledgeable diagnosis of a clinical problem is used to form a practical series of procedures that effectively resolve it. Once the diagnosis is made and the different treatment options have been evaluated, the best option is that which usually provides the best result with the least overall compromise. The rationale for such a decision is to offer the patient a solution that is, if possible, more conservative and long lasting than other available options. The cases presented in this chapter demonstrate examples of how proper treatment planning can provide the patient with a satisfactory solution from biologic, esthetic, and functional perspectives. A conservative approach is always recommended in cases where tooth structure is to be preserved, especially in the young patient, because some treatment modalities could involve irreversible procedures.

Diagnosis and Problem Analysis

The diagnosis dictates creation of a sequence that results in an ideal treatment based on the final expectations of the clinician and patient. Basic aspects of any successful treatment plan depend on *(1)* an accurate diagnosis, *(2)* evaluation of the risk involved with the chosen treatment, *(3)* prognosis of each therapeutic option based on relative risk, *(4)* consultation with other healthcare professionals as appropriate, and *(5)* proper execution of each step of the procedure. A correct diagnosis usually leads to a specific treatment option or range of options that are appropriate for the patient. *Prognosis* refers to the probable or expected result of the course of therapy. This is dependent upon the risk involved, however, which requires the clinician to fully comprehend the complexity of any given case so as to define the predictability of the selected treatment. When choices are made that increase risk, it is important that the patient, restorative dentist, and treating specialists understand how the prognosis may be subsequently affected. Consultation with other dental clinicians or specialists is frequently necessary to ensure that the original diagnosis is warranted. Recommended treatment should be directly related to the diagnosis and presented as a series of options.

An incorrect diagnosis usually results in improper treatment that needs to be redone or is altogether unnecessary. In Figs 8-1 and 8-2, three different oral surgeons diagnosed a localized cyst in a patient. Treatment recommendations included extraction and bone grafting, possible osteodistraction, implants, and/or implant-supported crowns.

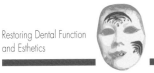

Fig 8-1 *(left)* Radiograph of patient scheduled for extraction of mandibular right canine and premolar.

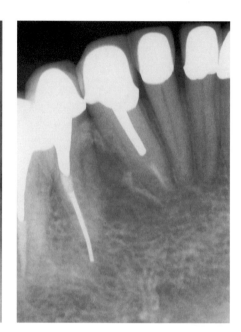

Fig 8-2 *(right)* Root canal treatment results in retention of the natural teeth and confirms that the original diagnosis and proposed treatment plan were incorrect. (Treatment by Paul Bery, DDS, Evanston, IL.)

Even with contemporary treatment modalities, procedures such as extraction of the canine and premolar, cleaning the surgically curetted area, and placement of a bone graft(s), combined with additional techniques such as osteodistraction, could have led to a permanent defect due to the size of the involved area. Furthermore, the adjacent teeth could face a guarded prognosis even with the most well-executed treatment. Reexamination of the problem led to the correct diagnosis and successful treatment.

It is essential to break down the specific problem in terms of its etiology and location and to visualize the desired result before any procedure is initiated. Detailed knowledge of the problem's origin and the treatment goal helps the clinician determine the appropriate course of treatment and thus should lead to a favorable prognosis. Box 8-1 outlines parameters to be closely evaluated in every patient to create the best possible treatment plan. Although clinical experience can lead to good decision making, the most successful treatment plans are created when a practitioner is able to, as Gladwell notes, "analyze a complex problem and reduce it to its simplest elements by recognizing an identifiable underlying pattern."[2]

Treatment Guidelines

It is simpler to establish an appropriate course and sequence of action after the problem has been identified and a diagnosis made. If a question exists regarding treatment sequence, it is important to know

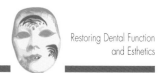

Restoring Dental Function and Esthetics

whether reversible options are available, and at what point in the sequence those exist, so as to maintain a predictable outcome. If proper healing time after the selected procedure is allowed and the patient is monitored closely for signs of potential problems, the outcome is more likely to be predictable and successful as well.

When the initial objective changes in the middle of treatment or other problems are encountered, the clinician should set new goals and be prepared to make the necessary adjustments to meet them. The original plan should be discussed with and accepted by the patient before procedures are begun, and any deviation from this plan should be explained before it is undertaken. Skillful execution based on scientific information and knowledge, combined with thorough communication with both the patient and the laboratory throughout the treatment process, leads to the best possible results.

Case Studies

The following four cases demonstrate the treatment-planning concepts outlined above. As each patient's chief complaint is examined to discover the source of the problem, the clinician is challenged to provide a solution that integrates acceptable esthetics and proper function, while keeping in mind the parameters listed in Box 8-1.

Case 1: Replacement of a maxillary crown

A 21-year-old woman presented with a complaint that she was unhappy with the surrounding periodontal tissue and color of the maxillary left central incisor crown, which was completed following an accident less than a year earlier. Medical history was noncontributory. Upon clinical examination, the color of the crown was found to be unsatisfactory. The gingiva was irritated and displayed subgingival recession that was 2 mm deeper than that of the adjacent natural central incisor (Fig 8-3a). Marginal fit of the restoration was slightly overcontoured and bulky. It was unclear whether the gingival recession, which was the main clinical problem, was the result of the incorrect fit of the crown, the original trauma to the tooth, or a combination of both.

After the crown was removed and the prepared tooth could be directly evaluated, it was determined that the restoration was slightly underprepared, with an unacceptable shape and marginal definition (Figs 8-3b and 8-3c). The tooth was re-prepared, and a provisional crown was fabricated. Placement of the provisional crown allowed a new evaluation of the tissue response, which was the most important factor in this case. Tooth contours and color were also assessed to determine the ideal course of action (Figs 8-3d and 8-3e).

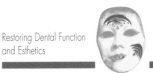

Box 8-1 Parameters to consider in treatment planning

- **Tooth**
  - Anatomic/structural/biomechanical factors
    - i. Weakened by caries lesions
    - ii. Endodontic treatment
    - iii. Previous restorative treatment
    - iv. Position
  - Periodontal factors
    - i. Tooth mobility
    - ii. Edentulous area
- **Bone**
  - Quantity
  - Quality/density
  - Width
  - Height
- **Soft tissues**
  - Biotype
  - Location
  - Quantity
- **Systemic and physiologic factors**
  - Occlusion
  - Growth and development
  - Parafunctional activity
  - Temporomandibular joint conditions
- **Intrinsic/extrinsic factors**
  - Pathology
  - Iatrogenic conditions

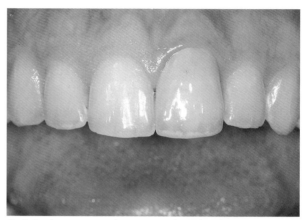

Fig 8-3a Anterior view of crown completed less than 1 year prior to current presentation.

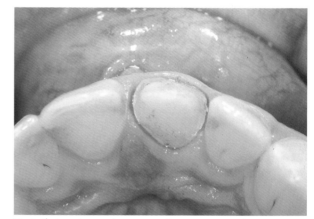

Fig 8-3b Incisal view showing rough preparation with poor marginal definition.

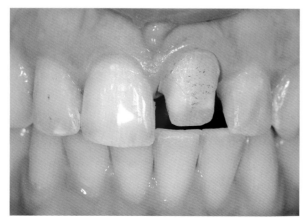

Fig 8-3c Anterior view with crown removed.

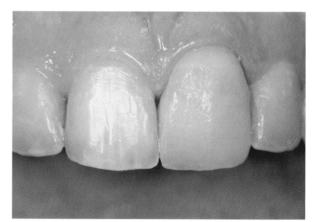

Fig 8-3d Anterior view of patient 1 week postoperatively with acrylic resin provisional restoration.

Restoring Dental Function and Esthetics

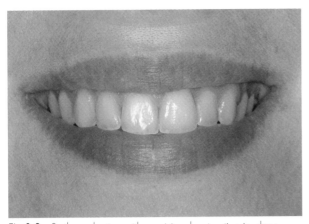

Fig 8-3e Smile evaluation with provisional restoration in place.

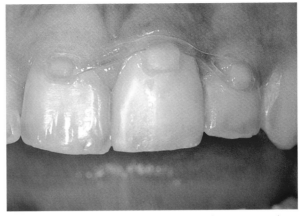

Fig 8-3f Simple short-term orthodontics are used to supraerupt the maxillary left central incisor and maintain esthetics. An Essix retainer (Dentsply Raintree Essix) is worn at night to prevent any undesirable movement of the abutment teeth.

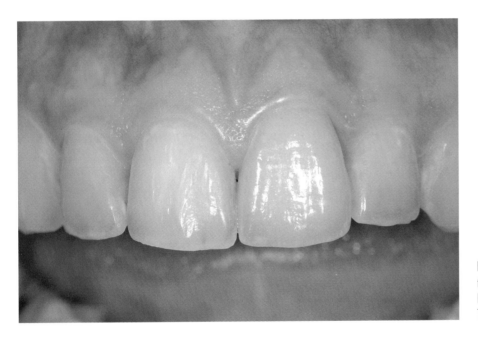

Fig 8-3g Anterior view of definitive Procera crown (Nobel Biocare). (Laboratory work by Toshi Fujiki, RDT, Skokie, IL.)

Simple short-term orthodontics was considered essential to obtain the best possible result, and the patient consented to this treatment plan (Fig 8-3f). The goal was to improve the ratio of crown length to width in the provisional and future crown restorations through supraeruption of the tooth, which would alter gingival levels by bringing down the bone and periodontal tissue.[3–5] The lingual surface and incisal edge of the provisional restoration were reduced to allow the supraeruption to occur without secondary occlusal trauma (Fig 8-3g).

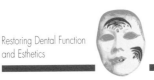

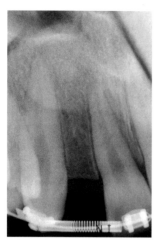

Fig 8-4a Periapical radiograph showing unfinished orthodontic treatment with inadequate room for implant placement.

Case 2: Replacement of a congenitally missing tooth

A 17-year-old girl in the midst of orthodontic treatment arrived for a consultation, requesting permanent replacement of a congenitally missing maxillary right lateral incisor (Fig 8-4a). She did not wish to have a removable prosthesis, but her parents asked for the most conservative treatment available. Medical history was noncontributory.

It is not possible to have two objects in the same place at the same time. If a tooth or teeth are in the incorrect position, orthodontic treatment is a top consideration if the desired results are to be achieved without compromise. Quite often, roots are in an undesirable position, and the practitioner will prepare teeth to accommodate esthetic restorations even though the teeth remain crowded. In a situation with such proximity, if an interdental periodontal problem develops, it could be quite complicated to correct and to obtain long-term healthy and predictable results. When the treatment plan involves implants, as seen in this case, it is even more important to respect the required distance between teeth, teeth and implants,[6-11] or adjacent roots. Orthodontics can prevent the problems caused by hasty or improper treatment that can lead to compromised long-term peri-implant periodontal health, or a problem as straightforward as the loss of papillae.[12]

Smile evaluation and soft tissue display in an individual play very important roles in the effect that implant depth and soft tissue manipulation have on the overall expected esthetic outcome (Figs 8-4b and 8-4c). If the surgeon is not the restorative dentist, a model-based or computer-based surgical guide is essential to assist in proper implant placement, especially for anterior tooth replacement (Fig 8-4d). The more anterior the restoration, the more critical the patient will be of the final result.[11]

Communication with the laboratory technician is essential if optimal esthetics is to be achieved. A black-and-white photograph should be provided so that the value of the referenced adjacent teeth can be assessed, which is the first and most important step of the shade selection. Teeth can present with different colors; but even when the shade selection is slightly incorrect, if the correct value is chosen, the restoration will still blend in with the adjacent dentition.[11]

The next step is to select the required hue and chroma to reproduce the tooth's color, which is generally easier for clinicians to communicate to a technician compared with the concepts of *value* or *depth*. It is critical that the teeth are moist and not dehydrated when a shade is selected.[13] Although more resin composites and porcelains are under development to give laboratory technicians better options to accurately re-create value and depth, this is an area that will evolve for years to come. In addition to the previously described esthetic concepts, a detailed anatomical assessment of the tooth or teeth textures to be repli-

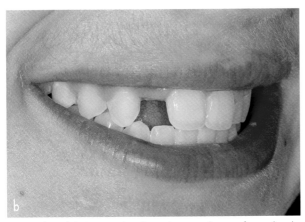

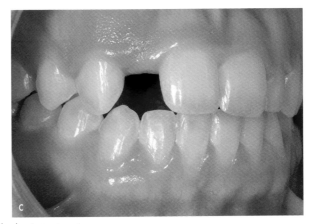

Figs 8-4b and 8-4c Lateral smile and retracted view of completed orthodontic treatment.

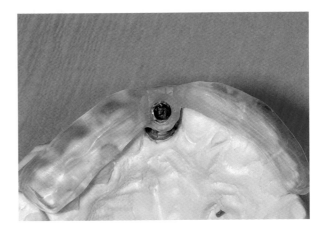

Fig 8-4d Model-based surgical guide in place with metal sleeve to guide surgeon for ideal implant position.

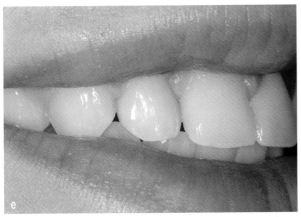

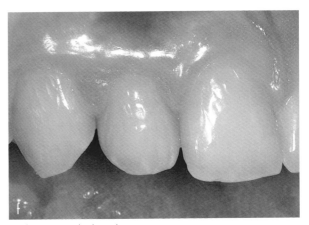

Figs 8-4e and 8-4f Lateral smile and retracted view of the implant-supported crown on the lateral incisor.

cated allows the technician to create the desired illusion by deflecting the light in different directions (Figs 8-4e and 8-4f). Creation of a natural-looking restoration is as significant to the final result as is the soft tissue management during all phases of implant placement.[14]

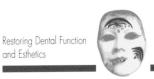

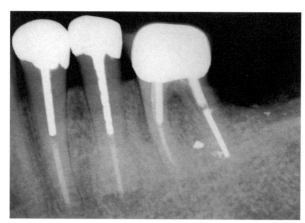

Fig 8-5a Mandibular left first molar with root fracture and hopeless prognosis.

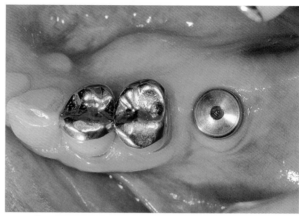

Fig 8-5b Occlusal view of implant with healing abutment.

Case 3: Esthetic solutions for posterior teeth

The patient, a 62-year-old woman, reported pain upon chewing on the mandibular left first molar. Medical history was noncontributory. A radiograph of the tooth in question revealed a vertical fracture (Fig 8-5a). After the tooth was extracted and the area was bone grafted, the patient requested replacement of the missing tooth with a single implant-supported crown instead of a removable prosthesis.

Molars with fractures or localized periodontal problems have historically been treated with root amputations or hemisections, which proved an excellent alternative to extraction of the affected tooth and allowed patients to keep these teeth for several years with very good results.[15,16] Nevertheless, the inception of the osseointegrated implant[17] and the evolution of its design over the last two decades have allowed for better bone preservation in cases where careful extraction is exercised and a bone graft placed, if necessary, followed by implant placement. Single- or two-stage surgery is effective, as is either delayed or immediate placement.

The implant was placed at the correct buccolingual orientation relative to the available bone, adjacent teeth, and opposing teeth (Fig 8-5b). When the implant is oriented accurately, the abutment crown demonstrates optimal contours and function along the axis of the implant, thus preventing undesirable lateral forces.[18–21]

A three-dimensional visualization of the clinical case, proper treatment planning, and proper orientation of the implant placement simplifies achievement of the prosthetic goals. Implant placement at an adequate depth is extremely helpful to create space for an abutment with subgingival margins and a proper emergence profile of the crown (Fig 8-5c).

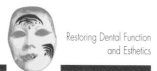

Restoring Dental Function and Esthetics

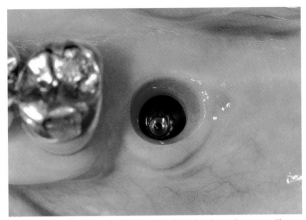

Fig 8-5c Occlusal view of implant without healing abutment. The excellent implant position in relation to the adjacent tooth and the healthy peri-implant soft tissue allow a clean impression to be taken.

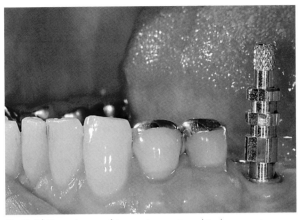

Fig 8-5d Buccal view of impression post used in the open tray technique.

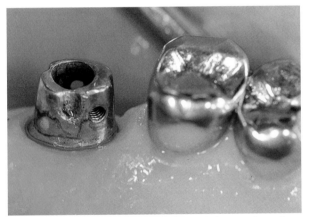

Fig 8-5e A custom abutment is tapped through the mesiolingual line angle to allow for a screw-retained crown and permit the creation of a crown with ideal occlusal anatomy.

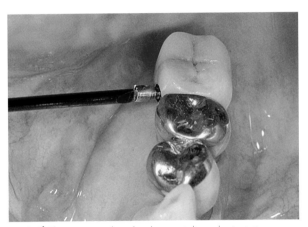

Fig 8-5f The screw is placed with a mesiolingual orientation.

When impressions of implants are taken, an open or closed tray can be used. The open tray impression technique is preferred for its greater accuracy, especially in cases with multiple implants. Proper placement in a mesiodistal and buccolingual orientation (Fig 8-5d) allows the abutment to have optimal design, regardless of whether the crown is cemented or screw retained (Figs 8-5e to 8-5g).

Although the majority of clinicians prefer to cement the implant-supported crowns (either with temporary or permanent cement), the advantages of using a screw-retained crown are numerous, beginning with the ease of retrieval.[11] When the crown is cemented, it is impossible to ascertain whether the cement has been removed in its entirety

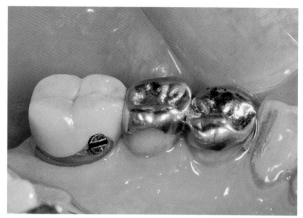

Fig 8-5g Sharp edge of the screw is filed down with a no. 4 round carbide bur and brownie rubber point.

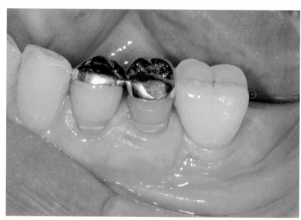

Fig 8-5h Definitive crown in place. Note the excellent anatomic contours. (Laboratory work by Toshi Fujiki, RDT, Skokie, IL.)

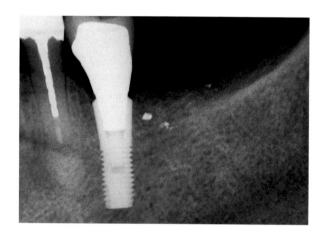

Fig 8-5i Postoperative radiograph showing implant and crown. (Implant placement by Kenneth H. Peskin, DDS, Skokie, IL.)

unless the crown has supragingival margins. As seen in Figs 8-5h and 8-5i, however, excellent gingival tissue response is routinely seen when a screw-retained abutment is used.

Case 4: Replacement of a fixed partial denture with implant

A 46-year-old man with a mandibular left fixed partial denture (FPD) and recurrent caries under the premolar asked for a restorative solution that would allow him to have separate teeth. Medical history was noncontributory. A 20-year-old FPD served as a replacement for the missing first molar. The patient reported pain upon chewing and felt that the FPD was loose around the premolar abutment (Fig 8-6a).

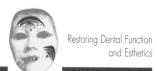

Restoring Dental Function
and Esthetics

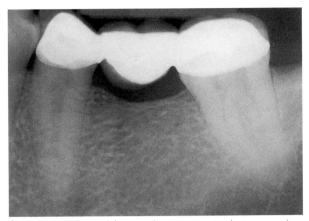

Fig 8-6a Mandibular left FPD with recurrent caries lesion around the premolar.

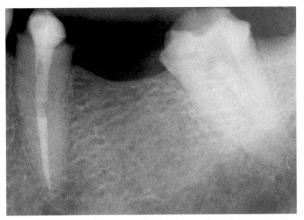

Fig 8-6b The premolar is treated endodontically and restored with a Peerless Post (SybronEndo).

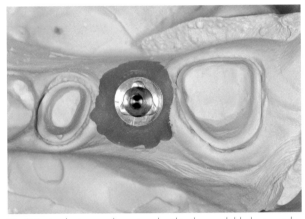

Fig 8-6c Implant properly centered within the available bone and adjacent teeth. One of the tri-lobes has a lingual rather than buccal position.

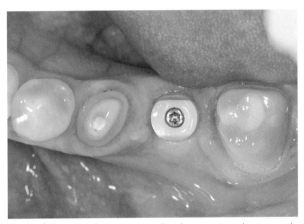

Fig 8-6d Zirconia abutment inserted at the correct angle. A smooth tooth preparation is critical for accurate impression reproduction.

Radiographs revealed that the premolar was in need of endodontic treatment. After the initial complaint of pain had been addressed and root canal therapy completed, the tooth was rebuilt in a conservative manner (Fig 8-6b). Cast posts have been the norm for restoring endodontically treated teeth for the past century.[22–26] Prefabricated posts also can be used because they closely resemble the flexural strength of dentin and can strengthen the root, thus reducing the risk of root fracture.[27–33]

When teeth were extracted in the past, very little emphasis was placed on preservation of the ridge and buccal plate. However, close attention must be paid to (1) preparation of the extraction site, (2) execution of the chosen technique, and (3) soft tissue manipulation if an implant is to help preserve the bone and function properly with the final restoration.

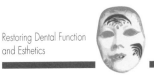

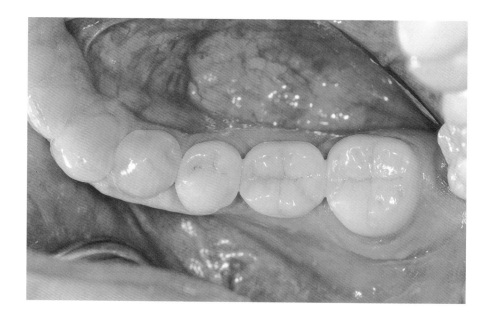

Fig 8-6e Occlusal view of definitive crowns.

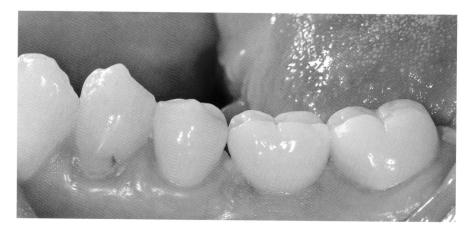

Fig 8-6f Buccal view of definitive Procera crowns. (Laboratory work by Toshi Fujiki, RDT, Skokie, IL.)

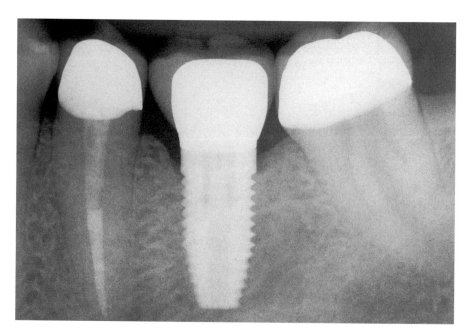

Fig 8-6g Final radiograph showing individual restorations. (Implant placement by Robert Bressman, DDS, Skokie, IL.)

Restoring Dental Function and Esthetics

Even when a single implant will be placed and stock or customized components are to be used (Figs 8-6c and 8-6d), the path of insertion of the abutment and definitive restoration is very important. Creation of the proper contours in these components not only enhances esthetics but also contributes to ideal periodontal and peri-implant health (Figs 8-6e and 8-6f).

If natural teeth are included as abutments for the definitive restoration, a well-defined preparation and margin must be established. An electric handpiece is a beneficial tool to achieve this goal because the operator can control torque and speed. The final impression must be accurate and dimensionally stable to duplicate the prepared teeth and the implant position. Modern techniques and materials allow the clinician to create computer-based copings and porcelains that can closely mimic the natural dentition. To deliver the highest possible quality of dental care, communication between the patient and clinician and between the clinician and laboratory technician is as essential as the integration of the clinicians' and laboratory technicians' knowledge and talent. In this case, correct diagnosis, astute planning, and meticulous execution led to the desired results (Fig 8-6g).

References

1. Amsterdam M. Periodontal prosthesis: Twenty-five years in retrospect. Alpha Omegan 1974;67(3):8–52.
2. Gladwell M. Blink. New York: Little, Brown and Co, 2005.
3. Salama H, Salama M. The role of orthodontic extrusive remodeling in the enhancement of soft and hard tissue profiles prior to implant placement: A systematic approach to the management of extraction site defects. Int J Periodontics Restorative Dent 1993;13:312–333.
4. Kois JC. Altering gingival levels: The restorative connection. Part I: Biologic variables. J Esthet Dent 1994;6:3–9.
5. Salama H, Salama M, Garber D, Adar P. Developing optimal peri-implant papillae within the esthetic zone: Guided soft tissue augmentation. J Esthet Dent 1995;7(3):125–129.
6. Tarnow DP, Magner AW, Fletcher P. The effect of distance from the contact point to the crest of bone on the presence or absence of the interproximal dental papilla. J Periodontol 1992;63:995–996.
7. Salama H, Salama MA, Garber D, Adar P. The interproximal height of bone: A guidepost to predictable aesthetic strategies and soft tissue contours in anterior tooth replacement. Pract Periodontics Aesthet Dent 1998;10(9):1131–1141.
8. Tarnow DP, Cho SC, Wallace SS. The effect of inter-implant distance on the height of inter-implant bone crest. J Periodontol 2000;71:546–549.
9. Kois JC, Kan JY. Predictable peri-implant gingival aesthetics: Surgical and prosthodontic rationales. Pract Proced Aesthet Dent 2001;13:691–698.
10. Kois J. Predictable single-tooth peri-implant esthetics: Five diagnostic keys. Compend Contin Educ Dent 2004;25:895–905.
11. Rubinstein S, Nidetz A, Heffez LB, Fujiki T. Prosthetic management of implants with different osseous levels. Quintessence Dent Technol 2006;29:147–156.
12. Arnoux JP, Weisgold AS, Lu J. Single-tooth anterior implant: A word of caution. Part I. J Esthet Dent 1997;9(6):225–233.

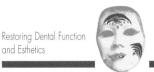

13. Sensi LG, Marson FC, Roesner TH, Baratieri LN, Junior SL. Fluorescence of composite resins: Clinical considerations. Quintessence of Dent Technology 2006;29:43–53.
14. Garber DA, Salama MA. The aesthetic smile: Diagnosis and treatment. Periodontol 2000 1996;11:18–28.
15. Staffileno HJ. Surgical management of the furca invasion. Dent Clin North Am 1969;13(1):103–119.
16. Rubinstein S. Restoration of hemisected teeth [thesis, in Spanish]. Mexico City: Universidad Tecnologica of Mexico, 1982.
17. Brånemark P-I, Zarb GA, Albrektsson T. Tissue-Integrated Prostheses: Osseointegration in Clinical Dentistry. Chicago, IL: Quintessence, 1985.
18. Stanford CM. Biomechanical and functional behavior of implants. Adv Dent Res 1999;13:88–92.
19. Stanford CM, Brand RA. Toward an understanding of implant occlusion and strain adaptive bone modeling and remodeling. J Prosthet Dent 1999;81:553–561.
20. Gapski R, Wang HL, Mascarenhas P, Lang N. Critical review of immediate implant loading. Clin Oral Implants Res 2003;14:515–527.
21. Stanford CM. Application of oral implants to the general dental practice. J Am Dent Assoc 2005;136:1092–1100 [erratum 2005;136(10):1372].
22. Frank, AL. Protective coronal coverage of the pulpless tooth. J Am Dent Assoc 1959;59:895–900.
23. Rosen H. Operative procedures on mutilated endodontically treated teeth. J Prosthet Dent 1961;11:972–986.
24. Silverstein WH. The reinforcement of weakened pulpless teeth. J Prosthet Dent 1964;14:372–381.
25. Ingle JI. Endodontics. Philadelphia: Lea & Febiger, 1965.
26. Federick DR, Serene TP. Secondary intention dowel and core. J Prosthet Dent 1975;34(1):41–47.
27. Fredriksson M, Astbäck J, Pamenius M, Arvidson K. A retrospective study of 236 patients with teeth restored by carbon fiber-reinforced epoxy resin posts. J Prosthet Dent 1998;80(2):151–157.
28. Mannocci F, Ferrari M, Watson TF. Intermittent loading of teeth restored using quartz fiber, carbon-quartz fiber and zirconium dioxide ceramic root canal posts. J Adhes Dent 1999;1(2):153–158.
29. Glazer B. Restoration of endodontically treated teeth with carbon fibre posts: A prospective study. J Can Dent Assoc 2000;66(11):613–618.
30. Ferrari M, Vichi A, Garcia-Godoy F. Clinical evaluation of fiber-reinforced epoxy resin posts and cast post and cores. Am J Dent 2000;13(special issue):15B–18B.
31. Ferrari M, Vichi A, Mannocci F, Mason PN. Retrospective study of the clinical performance of fiber posts. Am J Dent 2000;13(special issue):9B–13B.
32. Kogan E, Kuttler S. Integrating fundamental restorative and endodontic concepts: A new post system. Dent Today 2006;25(2):66–67 [erratum 2006;24(4):8].
33. Rubinstein S, Bery P. Endodontic-restorative symbioses: Diagnosis and treatment. Endo Tribune 2007;2(5):1,8–10,12.

Soft and Hard Tissue Augmentation in the Posterior Mandible

9

Cobi J. Landsberg, DMD

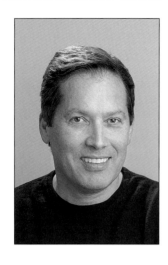

Cobi J. Landsberg, DMD

Cobi Landsberg graduated from Hebrew University Hadassah School of Dental Medicine, Jerusalem, in 1977. In 1984 he graduated from specialized study in periodontics at Boston University, and he is a diplomate of the American Board of Periodontology (1992).

Dr Landsberg is a past chairman of the Israel Periodontal Society and was formerly an instructor in periodontics at the specialized study program at the Department of Periodontology, Faculty of Dental Medicine, Hebrew University Hadassah School of Dental Medicine. Dr Landsberg has published numerous scientific and clinical articles on periodontology and implant dentistry in the international dental literature and has lectured extensively in Israel and abroad. He is currently a member of the editorial board of *Practical Procedures & Aesthetic Dentistry*.

Dr Landsberg maintains a private practice limited to periodontics and implant and regenerative surgery in Tel Aviv, Israel.

Email: Cobi@Landsberg.co.il

The introduction of osseointegration and evolution of related biomaterials and surgical techniques have contributed to an increased application of dental implants in the restoration of partially and completely edentulous patients.

An examination of these patients often reveals soft and hard tissue defects resulting from various causes such as infection, trauma, or tooth loss. These defects are often responsible for an anatomic foundation that is less than favorable for ideal implant placement.

In prosthetic-driven dental implant placement, reconstruction of the alveolar bone through a variety of regenerative surgical procedures has become an option with a predictable outcome. To guarantee a good long-term prognosis for a restoration, hard tissue augmentation may be necessary either prior to implant placement or at the time of implant surgery. Hard and soft tissues with adequate volume and quality are required if the functional and esthetic goals of implant dentistry are to be fulfilled.

The predictability of the corrective, reconstructive procedures is influenced by the anatomy of the edentulous ridge at the operative site in addition to the quality of the remaining soft and hard tissues. A stable outcome also depends significantly on the technique and biomaterials chosen and the experience, knowledge, and clinical skills of the surgeon.

Through a series of clinical cases centered around patients with inadequate hard or soft tissues, this chapter aims to demonstrate the implementation of contemporary tissue augmentation techniques in the posterior region of the mandible. Proper analysis, thorough treatment planning, and knowledge of suitable materials in each case lead to predictable results that effectively address each patient's chief complaint.

Case 1: Guided Bone Regeneration

Overview

A 45-year-old woman was referred to the clinic for implant therapy on the posterior right mandible. The main problem was identified as inadequate conditions for implant placement due to horizontal ridge resorption. Guided bone regeneration (GBR) was the treatment of choice.

To date, there are insufficiently well-controlled evidence-based studies to substantiate a clear clinical advantage of one bone regeneration technique over another. The clinician's preference for using a specific technique is based mainly on personal experience. In any case, the decision as to which technique to implement must be preceded by a thorough study of the clinical and radiographic findings of the case.

In this patient, the highly positioned inferior alveolar nerve at both the donor and the recipient sites obviated the safe execution of other

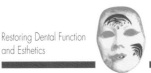

surgical techniques such as ridge splitting or onlay bone grafting. In contrast, although it is an extremely technique-sensitive procedure, GBR seldom jeopardizes the inferior alveolar nerve. Furthermore, in the author's clinical experience, grafting particulated autogenous cortical and cancellous bone under a stabilized titanium-reinforced expanded poytetrafluoroethylene (e-PTFE) membrane usually results in regenerated bone tissue that exhibits superior clinical properties. The ability to augment the ridge simultaneously with implant placement might be considered an advantage over other bone regenerative techniques, such as onlay bone grafts in which implant placement is delayed for about 5 months following bone grafting.

Procedure

Clinical examination of the patient revealed a severely horizontally resorbed edentulous alveolar ridge that extended mesially to the mandibular right first premolar. As is typical in this kind of situation, the quantity of remaining keratinized tissue at the crest of the ridge was minimal.

A computed tomography (CT) scan confirmed the significant resorption and revealed an inferior alveolar nerve canal in a high position. Consequently, ridge splitting or ramus onlay graft harvesting procedures were considered hazardous to the nerve, and a GBR procedure was determined adequate to augment the ridge (Figs 9-1a and 9-1b). A total of 6 mL of 2% lidocaine with 1:100,000 epinephrine was used in buccal and lingual infiltration for analgesia and hemostasis.

The plan for the flap design took the following factors into consideration:

- To accurately approximate flaps at the suturing stage, it is advantageous to have keratinized tissue on both buccal and lingual aspects. Accordingly, a midcrestal incision was performed, starting mesially at the distal aspect of the premolar and extending distally to the retromolar area.
- To provide optimal access and visibility, proper membrane placement, and coronal flap extension, the midcrestal incision was extended to the buccal and lingual sulci of the mandibular right canine and first premolar. Releasing incisions for the buccal flap were added vertically at the mesial line angle of the canine and in a lateral-posterior direction in the retromolar area (Fig 9-1c).
- To prevent lingual nerve or blood vessel damage, no vertical releasing incision was made on the lingual side.

The area intended for ridge augmentation was prepared with cortical penetrations to recruit bone-forming cells to the wound. Three implants

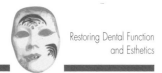

Restoring Dental Function
and Esthetics

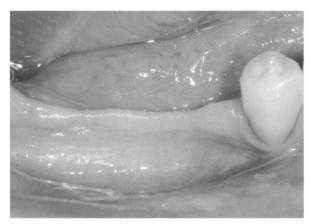

Fig 9-1a Clinical view of the edentulous mandibular region demonstrates extensive horizontal resorption.

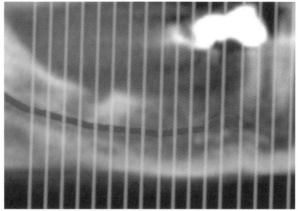

Fig 9-1b CT scan reveals that the inferior alveolar nerve was located high enough to present a considerable risk.

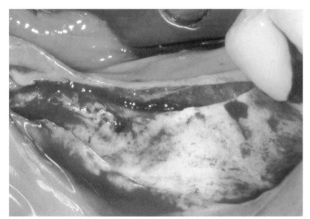

Fig 9-1c Midcrestal incision with releasing incisions allows optimal flap manipulation.

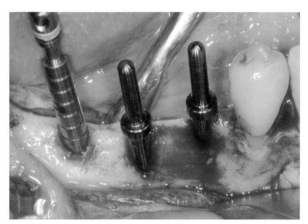

Fig 9-1d Three guide pins are inserted to ensure correct implant positioning.

were placed, with various amounts of their buccal and interproximal surfaces exposed. A space of 3 to 4 mm between the implants was ensured in order to maintain inter-implant bone (Figs 9-1d and 9-1e).

A titanium-reinforced e-PTFE membrane was then prepared. To do this, the membrane was first trimmed and adapted to the ridge and relieved in the area of the mental foramen to prevent any stress on the mental branches. A buccal extension was prepared on the mesial portion to minimize invasion of the connective tissue cells. The membrane was attached buccal-

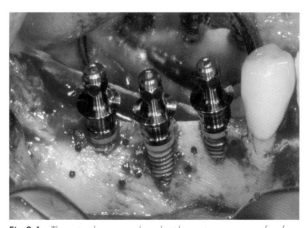

Fig 9-1e Three implants are placed with varying amounts of surfaces remaining exposed.

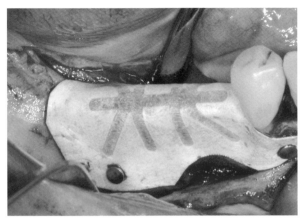

Fig 9-1f The e-PTFE membrane is placed and attached with two tacks.

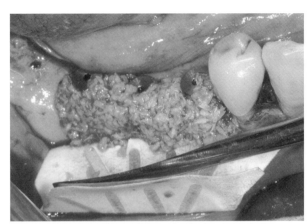

Fig 9-1g Autogenous bone chips are grafted underneath the membrane.

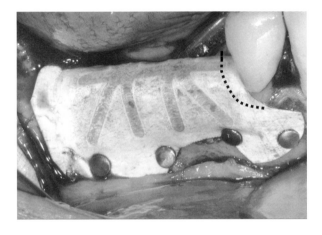

Fig 9-1h The membrane is reattached with two more tacks to hold the bone graft. The part of the membrane in contact with the root surface is removed with sharp scissors (dotted line) to facilitate connective tissue reattachment and to prevent bacterial invasion.

ly at the inferior border by two tacks, that provided sufficient initial stability yet allowed adequate flexibility for accurate placement of the bone graft to follow.

Autogenous bone chips were harvested from the posterior mandible and packed at the recipient site to cover the exposed surfaces of the implants. Care was taken to isolate the wound from any salivary contamination emanating from the floor of the mouth or the buccal vestibule. The membrane was repositioned, and two tacks were added in the center of the inferior border to ensure optimal isolation of the grafted bone. The part of the membrane in contact with the root surface was removed with sharp scissors to facilitate connective tissue reattachment and to prevent bacterial infection (Figs 9-1f to 9-1h).

An additional tack was placed on the lingual aspect to prevent membrane dislodgement, and excess membrane material was removed with a surgical blade. To release muscle tension and to facilitate coronal flap extension, the periosteum on both buccal and lingual flaps was dissected anteroposteriorly to a minimum depth by the tip of a no. 15 scalpel blade.

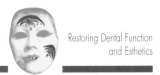

Restoring Dental Function and Esthetics

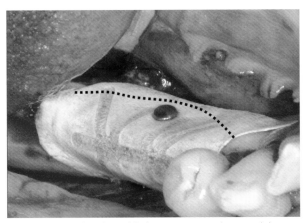

Fig 9-1i A lingual tack is added to improve membrane stabilization. Extra membrane on the lingual side *(dotted line)* is removed with scissors and a surgical blade.

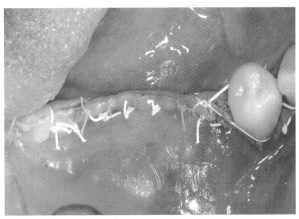

Fig 9-1j Flaps are sutured.

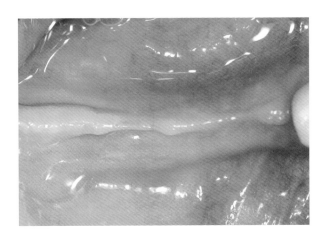

Fig 9-1k Healing after 6 months. Complete membrane isolation has been successfully maintained.

Flaps were sutured as follows:

1. Horizontal mattress 5-0 e-PTFE sutures were used for flap eversion and approximation to facilitate immediate broad contact between the flaps.
2. Simple interrupted 5-0 vicryl sutures were added between the horizontal mattress sutures to ensure tight flap adaptation.
3. An anchoring sling 5-0 e-PTFE suture was wrapped closely around the premolar to ensure intimate contact between the flaps and the tooth. This would help prevent bacterial plaque contamination of the underlying membrane.

During the 6-month healing period, the membrane remained completely covered by the soft tissues, and there were no signs or symptoms of infection. At the end of this period, a visible gain in ridge width had been achieved (Figs 9-1i to 9-1k).

A second surgical procedure removed the membrane and exposed the implants. A thin layer of fibrous tissue is normally interposed between the membrane and the underlying bone. Following removal of the membrane and the fibrous layer, the previously exposed implant surfaces were found to be fully embedded in newly regenerated bone. The healing abutments were connected, and the flaps were reapproximated using 6-0 monofilament polyamide sutures (Figs 9-1l to 9-1n).

After a 6-week healing period, the peri-abutment tissue was confirmed as mature, and the patient was referred for the restorative phase. The definitive restoration consisted of a cement-retained metal-ceramic fixed partial denture (FPD). Despite the thin band of peri-implant keratinized mucosa, soft tissue health had been maintained. Periodic follow-ups in cases like this are essential to assess the need for future soft tissue augmentation (Figs 9-1o to 9-1q).

Case 2: Ramus Onlay Bone Graft

Overview

A 51-year-old woman was referred to the clinic for implant therapy on the posterior right mandible. She presented with inadequate conditions for implant placement due to horizontal ridge resorption. As mentioned earlier, the clinician's preference for a specific technique is based mainly on personal experience. After careful evaluation of the clinical and radiographic situation, a ramus onlay bone graft was chosen.

In this patient, unlike in Case 1, the lower position of the inferior alveolar nerve and the adequate dimensions of the ascending ramus allowed for safe implementation of an onlay bone augmentation procedure, in which the ascending ramus is the donor site.

Because a potentially infection-provoking tooth (mandibular right canine) remained at the border of the ridge defect, there was a clear advantage in using the onlay graft procedure versus GBR (which is much more sensitive to infection). When rigid fixation of the grafted onlay bone to the recipient site must be achieved, the author's preference is to maintain adequate space between the donor and the recipient bone. This provides adequate interpositioning of particulated bone material and encourages increased bone outgrowth from the recipient site. Thus, the ridge may recapture the preferred anatomic and physiologic qualities (namely, cancellous-type bone interpositioned between two cortical plates) for implant placement.

Procedure

Clinical examination revealed a severely horizontally resorbed edentulous alveolar ridge that extended mesially to the mandibular right canine. A moderate amount of keratinized tissue remained at the crest of the

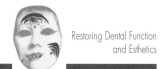

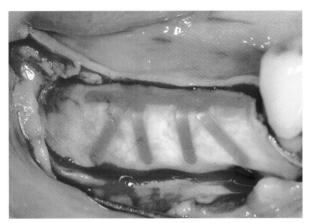

Fig 9-1l Uncovering of the grafting site. A thin layer of fibrous tissue is normally interposed between the membrane and the underlying bone.

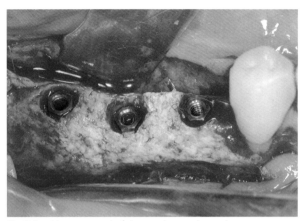

Fig 9-1m Upon removal of the membrane, the implants are seen embedded in the new bone tissue.

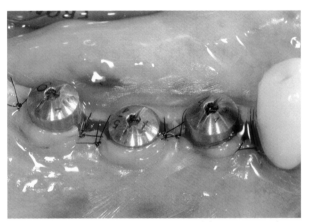

Fig 9-1n Healing abutments are placed, and flaps are sutured.

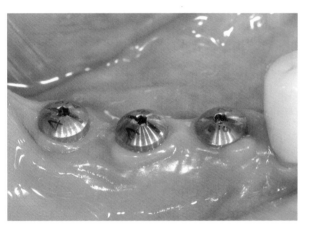

Fig 9-1o After an additional 6 weeks, the soft tissue surrounding the healing abutments is ready for the next phase.

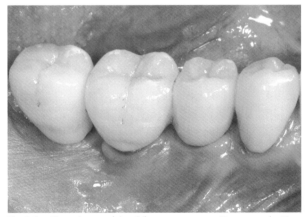

Fig 9-1p Clinical view of the definitive restoration. (Restoration by Dr Joseph Azuelos, Tel-Aviv, Israel, and Mr Alex Copitt, Tel-Aviv, Israel.)

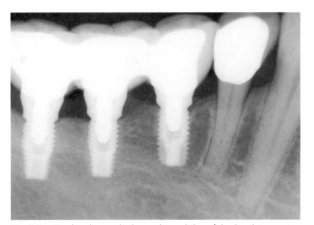

Fig 9-1q Final radiograph shows the stability of the hard tissues in the peri-implant region.

Restoring Dental Function
and Esthetics

ridge. Due to the significant resorption of the ridge, a regenerative procedure was necessary before implant placement could be considered (Fig 9-2a).

CT scans demonstrated that the inferior alveolar nerve canal in the region of the posterior oblique ridge and the ascending ramus was located more than 10 mm inferiorly to the mandibular crest, and the width of the mandibular body in that area exceeded 10 mm (Fig 9-2b). In consideration of these dimensions, it was assumed that a ramus block harvesting procedure could be safely performed, and the placement of four or five implants was determined as adequate to restore posterior occlusal relationships.

A total of 7 mL of 2% lidocaine with 1:100,000 epinephrine was used for an inferior alveolar neurovascular block and as an analgesic and a hemostatic agent in buccal and lingual infiltration. A no. 15 scalpel blade was used to make a midcrestal incision through the right retromolar pad that extended approximately 1 cm posteriorly and obliquely into the buccinator muscle. The incision continued anteriorly around the intrasulcular area of the canine and lateral incisor, with a further oblique releasing incision into the buccal vestibule at the mesial line angle of the lateral incisor.

The full-thickness buccal and lingual flaps were then elevated to expose the entire ridge defect, the mental neurovascular bundle and foramen, and the angle of the mandible down to the inferior border. A large round bur and straight fissure burs were used to outline the recipient site for the monocortical block graft. The outline began distal to the canine and continued posteriorly for approximately 18 mm. The vertical extent of the decortication inferiorly from the crest of the ridge measured approximately 13 mm. A 0.8-mm round bur was used to penetrate the cortical plate for the recruitment of bone-forming cells (Fig 9-2c)

Harvesting of the bone block had begun at this point. With the aid of a 702L bur, a superior osteotomy was performed approximately 4 mm medial to the lateral surface of the body of the mandible, beginning opposite the area of the first and second molars and continuing posteriorly for a length of approximately 22 mm. Next, the vertical osteotomies were completed at the anterior and posterior extent of the previous osteotomy to a length of approximately 12 mm.

A no. 8 round bur was used to make the inferior score to connect the inferior aspect of both previous vertical osteotomies. A series of two bone spreaders was used to remove the block graft. The sharp edges of the donor site were smoothed with a large round bur, and a collagen-based hemostatic agent was used as a pack in the donor site area.

The edges of the block graft were contoured with a large bur, and the graft was secured in the recipient site with two titanium alloy screws 1.5 mm in diameter and 12-mm long. At this point, no attempt was made to fully adapt the bone graft to the recipient site (Figs 9-2d to 9-2f).

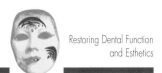

Restoring Dental Function and Esthetics

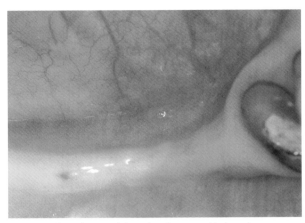

Fig 9-2a Clinical view of the edentulous mandibular ridge.

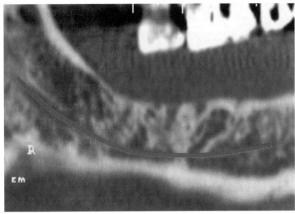

Fig 9-2b CT scan verifies that the location of the inferior alveolar nerve and the mandibular dimensions make the ramus a good donor site for a graft procedure.

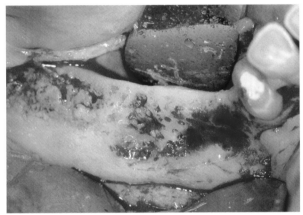

Fig 9-2c Flaps are elevated to expose the ridge, and the recipient site is decorticated.

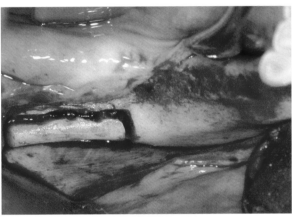

Fig 9-2d The donor bone is prepared using a series of bone burs and spreaders.

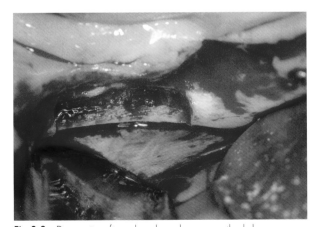

Fig 9-2e Donor site after edges have been smoothed down.

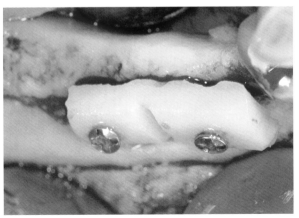

Fig 9-2f Block graft secured at the recipient site with titanium alloy screws. No attempt is made to achieve full adaptation.

Autogenous cortical bone shavings were collected by a bone scraper and placed in the spaces left between the block and recipient site (Fig 9-2g). The periosteum was scored inferiorly with a no. 15 scalpel blade to appropriately release a buccal mucoperiosteal flap, and a curved hemostat was used for muscle spreading. Then the periosteum was carefully scored with the tip of a sharp periosteal elevator to release the lingual flap. Primary closure of the recipient site was achieved with 5-0 e-PTFE horizontal mattress sutures, combined with 5-0 vicryl simple sutures in the posterior region (Fig 9-2h).

After a healing period of 5 months, the mucosa covering the bone graft appeared intact and free of any signs of inflammation. The little bump visible through the thin mucosa suggested that minor horizontal resorption around the fixation screw head had occurred (Fig 9-2i). A midcrestal incision that left 2 to 3 mm of keratinized mucosa in each flap was performed over the grafted area. To fully visualize the grafted area and the mental foramen, the midcrestal incision continued with a sulcular incision around the right lateral incisor and canine, ending with a vertical releasing incision on the mesial line angle of the incisor. The occlusal view demonstrated continuous bony texture of the healed ridge that suggested an organic union between the graft and the recipient bone. Slight horizontal resorption (0.5 mm) was evident around the screw heads (Fig 9-2j).

The following surgical steps were undertaken to prevent possible dislodgment of the graft during the preparation of the osteotomies:

- The process adhered to a strict sequential transition. A narrower drill was initially used, and the operator progressed to increasingly larger drills.
- The osteotomies at the premolar and first molar sites were carefully prepared slightly larger than necessary.
- To ensure smooth implant insertion, pretapping was used in all three osteotomies.

Finally, direction indicators were inserted to check for appropriate three-dimensional implant positioning, and the three implants were placed with their heads located approximately 0.5 mm supracrestally. The healing caps were immediately connected, and the buccal and lingual flaps were replaced and sutured (Figs 9-2k to 9-2m).

Two months later, the peri-implant mucosa had healed nicely. The canine, however, exhibited periodontal deterioration and hence was extracted and immediately replaced with an additional implant. A flapless approach was used for this final implant placement (Figs 9-2n and 9-2o).

Recall sessions to supplement meticulous home oral hygiene were scheduled every 2 to 3 weeks for hygiene that included bacterial plaque

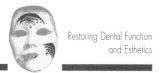

Restoring Dental Function
and Esthetics

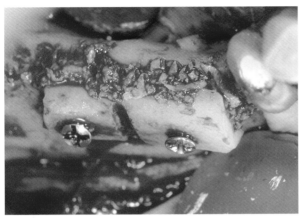

Fig 9-2g Autogenous bone shavings in place.

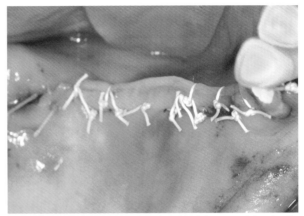

Fig 9-2h The flaps are sutured in place, and the site is left to heal.

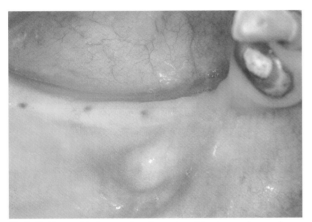

Fig 9-2i The visible bump after 5 months of healing indicates that some resorption has taken place around one of the screw heads.

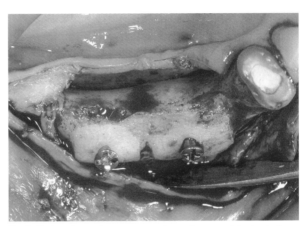

Fig 9-2j A midcrestal incision is performed to reveal the healed graft and minor resorption.

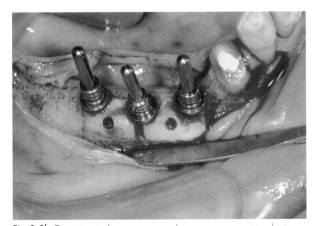

Fig 9-2k Direction indicators are used to ensure correct implant positioning.

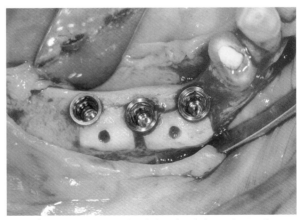

Fig 9-2l Implants are placed with their heads located partially above crest level.

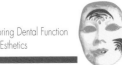

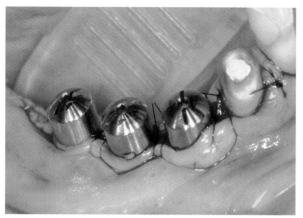

Fig 9-2m Healing abutments in place with sutured flaps.

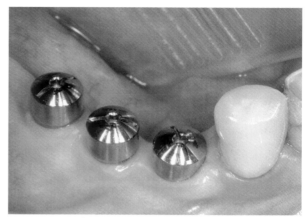

Fig 9-2n View of the healed site 2 months later.

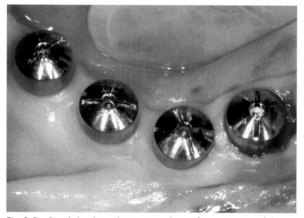

Fig 9-2o Fourth healing abutment in place after extraction of the canine and immediate placement of another implant.

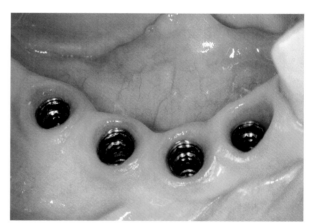

Fig 9-2p The peri-abutment soft tissues are kept clean and healthy.

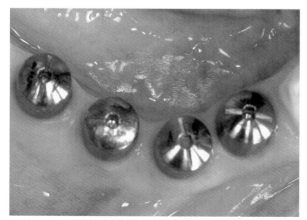

Fig 9-2q View of the healed site 2 months after implant placement at the site of the canine.

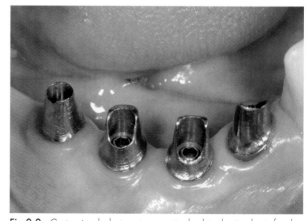

Fig 9-2r Customized abutments are attached to the implants for the definitive restoration.

Restoring Dental Function
and Esthetics

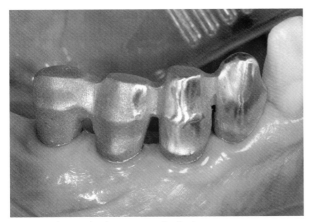

Fig 9-2s The metal substructure is checked.

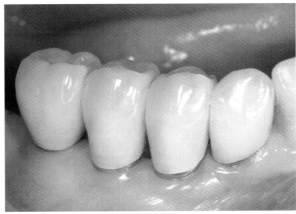

Fig 9-2t Definitive metal-ceramic restoration in place.

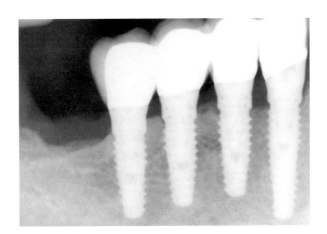

Fig 9-2u The final radiograph shows solid, well-preserved bony profiles.

and calculus removal. Occasionally, the healing caps were removed and the implants and peri-implant mucosa dipped in a disinfecting solution such as povidone iodine or chlorhexidine gluconate.

Two months after the implant for the mandibular right canine was placed, all implant sites demonstrated healthy peri-implant mucosa and adequate bony profiles. Customized anatomic titanium abutments were connected to the implants (Figs 9-2p to 9-2r), and a metal-ceramic FPD was cemented. All implants displayed solid and well-preserved bony profiles (Figs 9-2s to 9-2u).

After the patient was provided with the final fixed prosthesis, she requested an additional implant at the mandibular right second molar site to improve masticatory function. A full-thickness mucoperiosteal flap was elevated to allow adequate access for implant placement and to

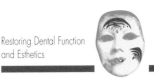

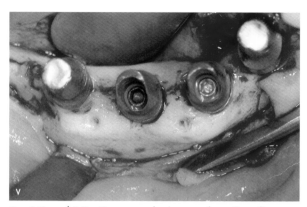

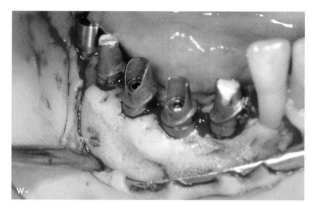

Figs 9-2v and 9-2w Two years after bone grafting. Open-flap procedure to place an implant in the second molar site.

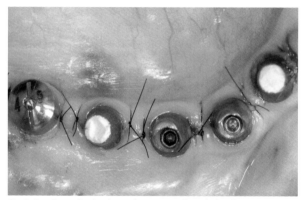

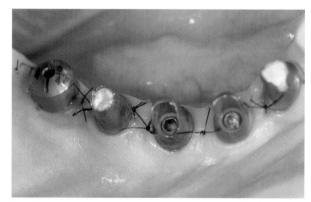

Fig 9-2x Once the healing abutment is placed, the flaps are secured around the abutments with polyamide sutures.

Fig 9-2y One week postoperatively, the tissues have healed, and the sutures can be removed.

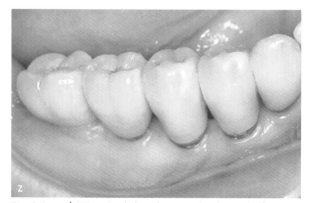

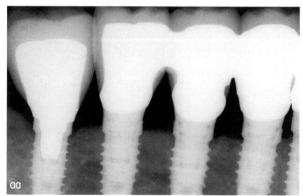

Figs 9-2z and 9-2aa Final clinical view and radiograph of restorations showing good esthetics and support. (Restoration by Dr Elie Sawdayee, Tel Aviv, Israel, and Mr Yossi Pinto, Jerusalem, Israel.)

visualize and assess the bone block graft, which at this point had been performed a full 2 years earlier. It was evident that the bone graft had undergone slight remodeling, although no major volumetric changes had occurred except for minimal peri-implant crestal resorption, as is usually expected.

Once the healing abutment was connected to the mandibular second molar implant, the flaps were repositioned and adapted to all abutments by simple interrupted 6-0 monofilament sutures (Figs 9-2v to 9-2x).

The peri-abutment tissues had healed nicely 1 week postoperatively, and the sutures were removed. Treatment concluded with an additional screw-retained restoration to replace the second molar. Final clinical photographs and radiographs demonstrated healthy peri-implant tissues (Figs 9-2y to 9-2aa).

Case 3: Hard and Soft Tissue Augmentation

Overview

A 43-year-old woman presented with an ill-fitting FPD in the right posterior mandible. A large pontic of a ridge lap design had prevented adequate plaque control and had resulted in thin and inflamed soft tissue at the alveolar ridge (Figs 9-3a and 9-3b). To replace the ill-designed pontic, an implant restoration in the mandibular right first molar site was planned. Due to ridge deficiency at this site, guided bone regeneration with simultaneous implant placement was implemented. It was noted that due to the poor quality of the lining mucosa, membrane coverage by the flaps was inadequate, and indeed, early membrane exposure had occurred. Although bone regeneration around the implant appeared to be successful, a complete loss of keratinized tissue at the buccal aspect of the implant had resulted. Lack of keratinized tissue around an implant restoration may lead to reduced plaque control, decreased resistance to infection, a tendency toward soft tissue recession, and peri-implant bone resorption.

An epithelialized free graft harvested from the palatal masticatory mucosa is relatively easily manipulated and may predictably increase the width of keratinized tissue at the recipient site. Its survival and satisfactory acceptance by the surrounding tissues depends significantly on the presence of a periosteum that is truly vascularized and attached to the bone. In the author's clinical experience, the reconstitution of such a periosteum may take 6 to 9 months post-initiation of the GBR procedure.

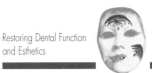

Restoring Dental Function
and Esthetics

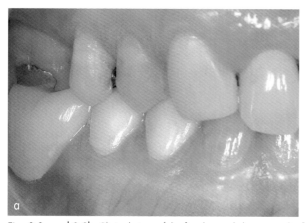 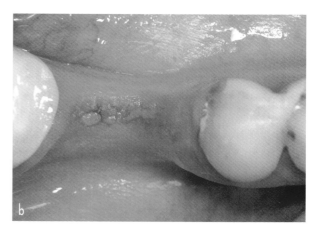

Figs 9-3a and 9-3b Clinical view of the fixed partial denture and inflamed tissue at the alveolar ridge.

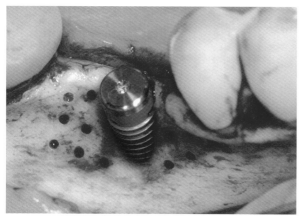 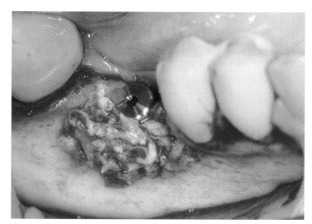

Fig 9-3c Full-thickness flap elevation reveals the exposed buccal side of the implant.

Fig 9-3d Autogenous bone chips are placed over the exposed implant surfaces.

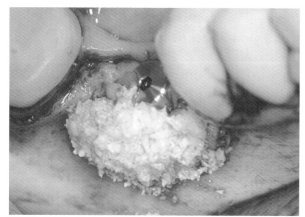 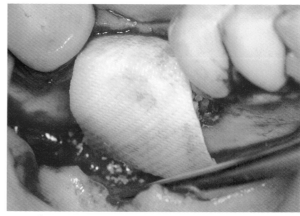

Fig 9-3e Particles of deproteinized bovine bone are added as a second layer.

Fig 9-3f A slowly resorbable xenogeneic membrane is trimmed and placed over the layers of grafted bone.

Procedure

A midcrestal incision with a continuous sulcular incision and vertical releasing incision at the mesiobuccal line angle of the mandibular right first premolar facilitated the elevation of full-thickness flaps. This enabled an adequate inspection of the mental foramen so that the full extent of the residual defect could be discovered. Following transcortical penetration and osteotomy preparation, the implant was positioned according to prosthetic standards; however, almost its entire buccal surface remained exposed (Fig 9-3c).

Hard tissue augmentation was performed using the sandwich bone augmentation technique, as follows:

1. Autogenous bone chips, which potentially contained live bone cells, were harvested from the posterior mandible and placed as a first layer adjacent to the implant surface.
2. A second layer, composed of bovine bone mineral, was added to maintain ideal space for the regenerating bone.
3. A xenogeneic, slowly resorbable membrane was layered on top of the bone graft materials to isolate them from soft tissue elements. This particular membrane was preferred in this case because of its ability to resist infection even if exposed prematurely to the oral environment (Figs 9-3d to 9-3f).

Indeed, the poor quality of the covering mucosa dictated a complicated flap management procedure and suturing (Fig 9-3g) and, as expected, 1 week later some tissue sloughing occurred, resulting in minor membrane exposure. A meticulous maintenance program served as a safeguard to prevent contamination of the membrane, although part of the membrane over the cover screw had evidently been prematurely lost, leaving the cover screw completely exposed. This resulted in a very narrow band of keratinized mucosa on the buccal aspect of the implant (Figs 9-3h and 9-3i).

In an attempt to increase the width of keratinized mucosa, a free gingival graft procedure was performed 8 months after the augmentation procedure. Along with a horizontal incision placed immediately buccal to the cover screw, two vertical releasing incisions enabled a split-thickness miniflap elevation that left the periosteum attached to the regenerated bone. (A properly organized periosteum is necessary for soft tissue graft suturing and its initial revascularization. The periosteum is likely to be well reestablished and attached to highly vascularized bone that was regenerated via a GBR procedure. This is contrary to poorly vascularized grafted bone blocks on which periosteal-like tissue reformation is not predictable, even a few years postoperatively). The graft was accurately positioned and held in place by four simple sutures, and a

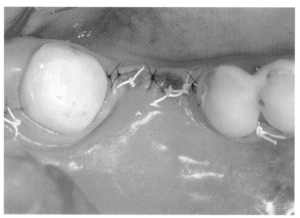

Fig 9-3g Flaps are sutured closed over the bone graft materials.

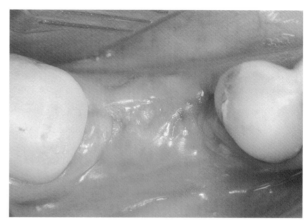

Fig 9-3h One week later, some tissue sloughing is evident.

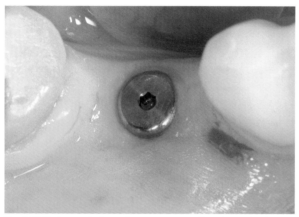

Fig 9-3i Eight months later, the coverscrew is found completely exposed with an inadequate narrow band of keratinized mucosa at the buccal aspect.

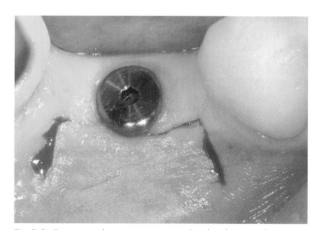

Fig 9-3j Two vertical incisions connected with a horizontal incision are made.

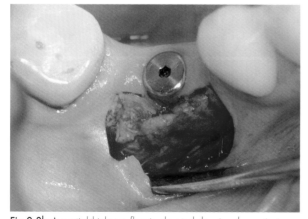

Fig 9-3k A partial-thickness flap is elevated, leaving the periosteum over the newly regenerated bone.

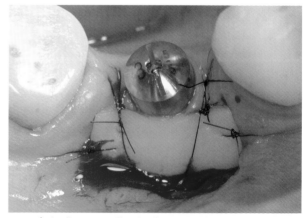

Fig 9-3l The flap is cut off and a free gingival graft adapted to the recipient site with sutures.

Restoring Dental Function
and Esthetics

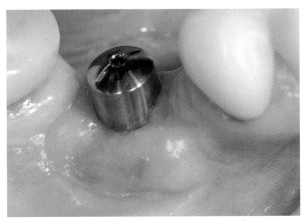

Fig 9-3m Clinical view of graft 4 weeks postoperatively.

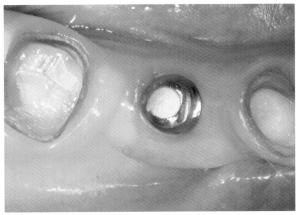

Fig 9-3n After 3 months of healing, the prosthetic abutment is placed.

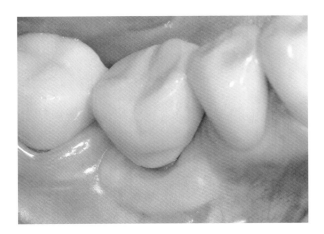

Fig 9-3o An acrylic provisional crown is cemented. A slight exposure of the implant head is noted.

circumferential periosteal suture was added to enhance the stabilization and adaptation of the graft (Figs 9-3j to 9-3l).

Four weeks later, the graft was almost completely keratinized (Fig 9-3m). After increased maturation and keratinization was observed 3 months post–graft placement, a titanium abutment with a provisional crown was connected to the implant. Minor recession of the soft tissue was noted. The minimal exposure of the implant head that resulted had negligible functional or esthetic implications (Figs 9-3n and 9-3o). Approximately 9 months after grafting of the soft tissue, no further significant radiographic or clinical changes had occurred, and a metal-ceramic crown was cemented (Figs 9-3p and 9-3q).

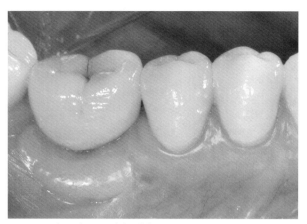

Fig 9-3p Clinical view of the definitive restoration. (Restoration by Dr Joseph Azuelos, Tel-Aviv, Israel, and Mr Alex Copitt, Tel-Aviv., Israel.)

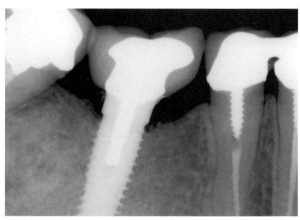

Fig 9-3q Radiographic appearance of the implant and surrounding bone.

Case 4: Split-Thickness Free Gingival Graft

Overview

A 61-year-old man presented to the office with a request to restore the right mandibular area with an implant-supported restoration. The central challenge here was the lack of adequate width of keratinized tissue presenting at the crest of the ridge, which could lead to implant restorations surrounded by nonkeratinized soft tissue. As noted in Case 3, a lack of keratinized tissue around an implant restoration may lead to reduced plaque control, decreased resistance to infection, a tendency toward soft tissue recession, and peri-implant bone resorption.

Keratinized tissue width can be relatively easily gained with an epithelialized mucosal graft, which should be performed prior to dental implant placement. This may allow the preservation of an adequate band of keratinized tissue in both buccal and lingual flaps during the implant surgery.

(A significant point to consider: Contrary to the present case, in bone augmentation procedures, the inclusion of previously grafted, thick, scar-like, keratinized tissue in the flaps may eventually lead to failure of the approximated flaps to fully unite. This may result from the decreased vascularized surfaces of the abutting flap margins. In such cases it might prove advantageous to maintain only a thin band of keratinized tissue in the flaps and perform the soft tissue grafting after the bone regeneration process has been completed.)

Procedure

The alveolar ridge at the site where the implants were to be placed was slightly horizontally resorbed but maintained sufficient width to allow

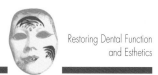

Restoring Dental Function and Esthetics

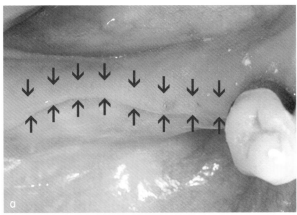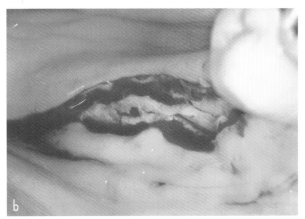

Figs 9-4a and 9-4b *(a)* Arrows indicate the keratinized band borders on the slightly resorbed alveolar crest. *(b)* A split-thickness flap is elevated in anticipation of the graft.

regular platform implant placement. However, only a narrow band (2 to 3 mm) of keratinized mucosa had remained at the ridge crest. It was predicted that during flap manipulation at implant surgery, additional loss of keratinized tissue would occur, leaving thin or no attached keratinized peri-implant mucosa. This could compromise plaque control, lead to peri-implant bone loss, and negatively affect the esthetic appearance. It was therefore decided to augment the attached tissue first.

Initial steps were taken to prepare the recipient site. Starting distal to the mandibular right first premolar and progressing about 2 cm distally, a horizontal incision was made that followed the buccal border of the keratinized tissue. Short vertical incisions were added at the distal line angle of the premolar and at the distal end of the horizontal incision. A buccal split-thickness flap was elevated to a depth of 8 to 10 mm (Figs 9-4a and 9-4b).

A split-thickness free gingival graft was harvested from the palate. It was initially anchored to the attached mucosa by simple 6-0 polyamide sutures, then firmly adapted to the periosteum by the addition of two periosteal sutures (Fig 9-4c). To retard muscle creeping and "swallowing" of the graft, the free vestibular muscular margins were cut off, and a periodontal dressing that extended the entire depth of the vestibular pouch was placed on the grafted tissue.

A hemostatic agent was placed on the exposed palatal connective tissue, and a 5-0 e-PTFE sutured mesh was prepared to help retain the hemostatic agent and maintain the periodontal pack, which was adapted to the mesh and teeth (Fig 9-4d).

Eight weeks later, the grafted tissue appeared to be fully keratinized and ready for implant surgery (Fig 9-4e). A midcrestal incision was used to divide the tissue covering the ridge into buccal and lingual well-keratinized flaps. Three implants were placed, and the flaps were

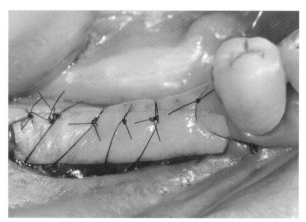

Fig 9-4c A split-thickness graft is harvested from the palate and sutured into place.

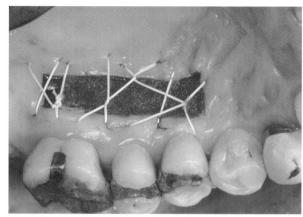

Fig 9-4d The donor site is packed with a hemostatic agent and sutured.

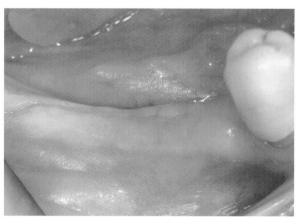

Fig 9-4e View of the recipient site 8 weeks later.

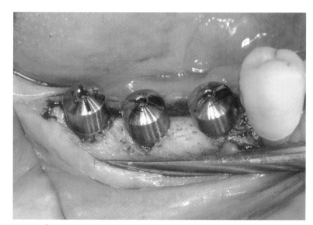

Fig 9-4f Implants are placed.

readapted to the bone and healing abutments with 6–0 polyamide simple interrupted sutures. The peri-implant mucosa matured over a 4-week healing period, at which point the patient was referred for the restorative phase (Figs 9-4f to 9-4h).

The implants were restored by a cemented metal-ceramic FPD, which contributed to a pleasing presentation of adequately keratinized pericrown mucosa. The postoperative radiographic image demonstrated intimate bone-to-implant contact with an appearance of solid crestal profiles (Figs 9-4i and 9-4j).

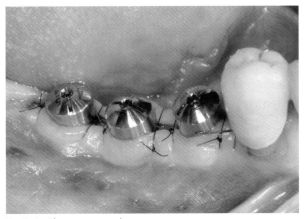

Fig 9-4g Flaps are sutured.

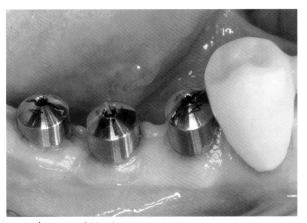

Fig 9-4h Uneventful healing.

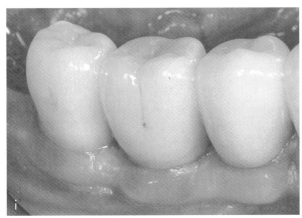

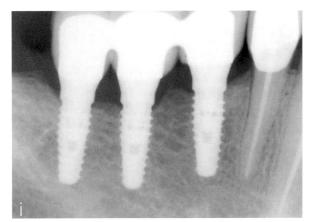

Figs 9-4i and 9-4j Final clinical and radiographic appearance of the definitive restoration shows adequate hard and soft tissues. (Restoration by Dr Yossi Pinkas, Ramat Gan, Israel, and Mr Shmulik Pertman, Petah-Tikva, Israel.)

Acknowledgments

The author would like to thank Ms Julie Elisha, Tel-Aviv, Israel, and Dr Harry Cshweidan, Raanana, Israel for their editorial assistance.

Bibliography

Becker W, Hujoel P, Becker BE. Effect of barrier membranes and autologous bone grafts on ridge width preservation around implants. Clin Implant Dent Relat Res 2002;4(3):143–149.

Bouri A Jr, Bissada N, Al–Zahrani MS, Faddoul F, Nouneh I. Width of keratinized gingiva and the health status of the supporting tissues around dental implants. Int J Oral Maxillofac Implants 2008;23(2):323–326.

Chiapasco M, Zaniboni M, Boisco M. Augmentation procedures for the rehabilitation of deficient edentulous ridges with oral implants. Clin Oral Implants Res 2006;17(suppl 2):136–159.

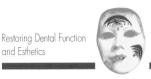

Restoring Dental Function and Esthetics

Chung DM, Oh TJ, Shotwell JL, Misch CE, Wang HL. Significance of keratinized mucosa in maintenance of dental implants with different surfaces. J Periodontol 2006;77(8):1410–1420.

Hämmerle CH, Jung RE, Yaman D, Lang NP. Ridge augmentation by applying bioresorbable membranes and deproteinized bovine bone mineral: A report of twelve consecutive cases. Clin Oral Implants Res 2008;19(1):19–25.

Landsberg CJ, Grosskopf A, Weinreb M. Clinical and biologic observation of demineralized freeze-dried bone allografts in augmentation procedures around dental implants. Int J Oral Maxillofac Implants 1994;9:586–592.

Landsberg CJ. Complete flap coverage in augmentation procedures around dental implants using the everted crestal flap. Pract Periodontics Aesthet Dent 1995;7(2):13–22.

Mankoo T. Functional, biologic, and esthetic considerations in the contemporary management of posterior edentulous areas in extensive rehabilitation. J Esthet Dent 1997;9(3):137–145.

Misch CM. Use of the mandibular ramus as a donor site for onlay bone grafting. J Oral Implantol 2006;26(1):42–49.

Park SH, Lee KW, Oh TJ, Misch CE, Shotwell J, Wang HL. Effect of absorbable membranes on sandwich bone augmentation. Clin Oral Implants Res 2008;19(1):32–41.

Pikos MA. Mandibular block autografts for alveolar ridge augmentation. Atlas Oral Maxillofac Surg Clin North Am 2005;13(2):91–107.

Schwartz-Arad D, Levin L, Sigal L. Surgical success of intraoral autogenous block onlay bone grafting for alveolar ridge augmentation. Implant Dent 2005;14(2):131–138.

Simion M, Fontana F, Rasperini G, Maiorana C. Vertical ridge augmentation by expanded-polytetrafluoroethylene membrane and a combination of intraoral autogenous bone graft and deproteinized anorganic bovine bone (Bio Oss). Clin Oral Implants Res 2007;18(5):620–629.

Simion M, Jovanovic SA, Trisi P, Scarano A, Piattelli A. Vertical ridge augmentation around dental implants using a membrane technique and autogenous bone or allografts in humans. Int J Periodontics Restorative Dent 1998;18(1):8–23.

Smukler H, Chaibi MS. Ridge augmentation in preparation for conventional and implant-supported restorations. Compend Suppl 1994;(18):706S–710S.

Strub JR, Gaberthüel TW, Grunder U. The role of attached gingiva in the health of peri-implant tissue in dogs. 1. Clinical findings. Int J Periodontics Restorative Dent 1991;11(4):317–333.

Tal H, Kozlovsky A, Artzi Z, Nemcovsky CE, Moses O. Long-term bio-degradation of cross-linked and non-cross-linked collagen barriers in human guided bone regeneration. Clin Oral Implants Res 2008;19(3):295–302.

Tinti C, Parma-Benfenati S. Vertical ridge augmentation: Surgical protocol and retrospective evaluation of 48 consecutively inserted implants. Int J Periodontics Restorative Dent 1998;18(5):434–443.

von Arx T, Cochran DL, Hermann JS, Schenk RK, Buser D. Lateral ridge augmentation using different bone fillers and barrier membrane application. A histologic and histomorphometric pilot study in the canine mandible. Clin Oral Implants Res 2001;12(3):260–269.

Zigdon H, Machtei EE. The dimensions of keratinized mucosa around implants affect clinical and immunological parameters. Clin Oral Implants Res 2008;19(4):387–392.

Zubery Y, Goldlust A, Alves A, Nir E. Ossification of a novel cross-linked porcine collagen barrier in guided bone regeneration in dogs. J Periodontol 2007;78(1):112–121.

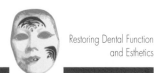

Restoring Dental Function
and Esthetics

Porcelain Laminate Veneers: Predictable Tooth Preparation for Complex Cases

10

Galip Gürel, MSc

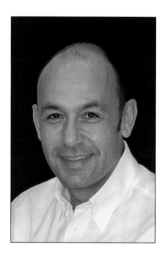

Galip Gürel, MSc

Galip Gürel graduated from the Istanbul University School of Dentistry and continued his education at the University of Kentucky in the Department of Prosthodontics. He is the founder and president of EDAD (the Turkish Academy of Esthetic Dentistry). Dr Gürel is editor-in-chief of the *Quintessence Magazine* in Turkey and serves on the editorial boards of the *Journal of Cosmetic Dentistry* and *Spectrum*. One of the true pioneers in esthetic dentistry, he lectures extensively all over the world and is a visiting lecturer at the Center for Continuing Education at New York University College of Dentistry, lecturing on the latest advances in this field. He is a diplomate of the American Board of Aesthetic Dentistry. Dr Gürel maintains a private practice in Istanbul, Turkey, where he specializes in esthetic dentistry.

Email: info@galipgurel.com
        dentis@superonline.com

Porcelain laminate veneers (PLVs) have proved to be one of the most conservative esthetic techniques available over the past two decades. Patients and doctors prefer this technique to the conventional fixed partial denture restoration because it is generally more esthetic and does not require risky or extensive invasive procedures. Careless planning and insufficient or improper tooth preparation, however, can quickly lead to failed PLV restorations and disappointed patients. This chapter uses two case studies to review the step-by-step procedures for obtaining PLV restorations that may not be "ideal" in every way but still successfully address patients' concerns in various situations. Helpful tips offered throughout the described procedures should allow the clinician to execute treatments that are predictable and long lasting.

PLVs in Acceptably Aligned Teeth

Patient 1 presented with a moderate central diastema. This is a very common situation where PLVs can be used to close the space without movement of the teeth or any additional procedures (Figs 10-1a to 10-1c). In such cases, when teeth are properly aligned in the dental arch, the diagnosis and treatment plan look simple. Yet because it is not recommend-

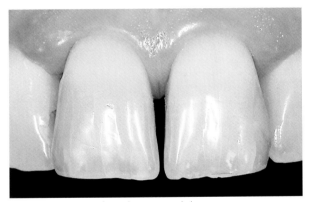

Fig 10-1a Patient with moderate central diastema.

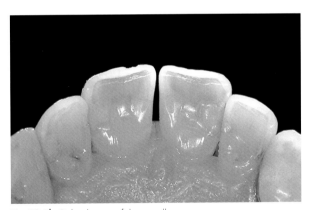

Fig 10-1b Palatal view of the maxilla.

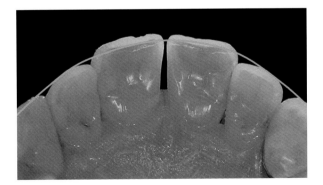

Fig 10-1c An arc sketched from canine to canine shows that the maxillary teeth are properly aligned in the dental arch.

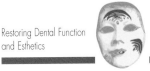

Restoring Dental Function and Esthetics

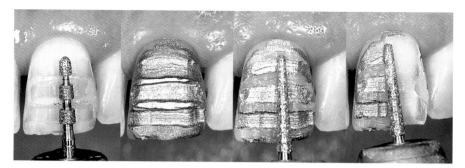

Fig 10-1d Depth cutters of different sizes (measured in millimeters) enable creation of the necessary depth all over the tooth enamel.

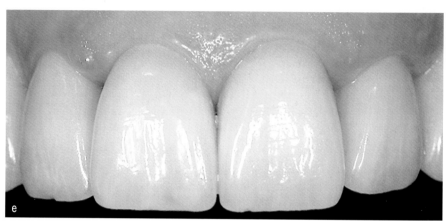

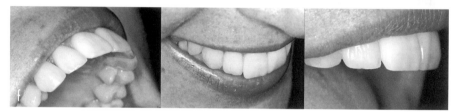

Figs 10-1e and 10-1f Anterior and smile views of the final result. Note the harmony of the PLVs with the adjacent teeth and the beautiful color matching.

ed to move the facial aspect of the teeth more buccally, it is important to ensure that enough of the original tooth is retained to keep the integrity of the arch.

A standard tooth preparation technique for PLVs is recommended in such cases. Depth cutters of 0.3 mm, 0.5 mm, or 0.7 mm were used to begin the preparation and create the necessary depth all over the tooth enamel. Then, the tooth surface was painted for precise depth preparation. Long round-ended cylindrical diamond burs were used to prepare the surface of the tooth. Depending on the initial color of the tooth and the type of porcelain to be used, a preparation can be deepened by as much as 0.4 to 0.8 mm (Fig 10-1d).

Once the PLVs are placed, the final result should look very natural and elegant from every angle (Figs 10-1e and 10-1f). The patient was pleased with the esthetic outcome of this conservative treatment. Results like this are easily attained when the standard preparation technique is used to limit and control the tooth structure removal.

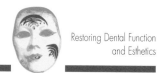

Restoring Dental Function
and Esthetics

PLVs on Malaligned Teeth

The standard technique is excellent when the teeth are aligned properly in the dental arch, but the situation changes if those teeth are not properly aligned. Malalignment can take the form of teeth that overlap or are in an undesirable position in the dental arch (ie, anteroposterior and/or mesiodistal displacement). It is always best to return those teeth to their ideal locations in the arches and then restore them with PLVs. However, if the patient refuses orthodontic treatment and the teeth need to be restored with PLVs, the preparation suddenly presents a significant challenge.

How can these teeth be prepared precisely, predictably, and more importantly, with a minimally invasive technique? This situation requires a well-planned treatment approach, for which the clinician must take precise steps in a synchronized manner from beginning to end.

Patient 2 lost his maxillary right central incisor when he was 12 years old. During smile, a distinct midline shift toward his right side was visible (Figs 10-2a and 10-2b). Modern orthodontics could be used to reopen the space for the missing tooth by shifting the left and right quadrants with orthodontic mini-implants for absolute anchorage, and the space could be restored with an implant. The patient declined this treatment plan, however.

Kokich Jr et al have questioned and examined whether it is necessary to correct minimal discrepancies[1,2] (eg, midline shift, uneven tooth size, or bite plane canting). Most mild asymmetries are not noticed by laypeople, and occasionally, dental clinicians and specialists such as orthodontists might not notice them either. The key factors to an esthetic outcome are *(1)* maintenance of the harmony between teeth, gums, and face, and *(2)* preservation of a midline that is perpendicular to the eyeline. In this way, midline shifts of as much as 3 to 4 mm can be esthetically acceptable. In many cases, the focus on these key factors enables the clinician to offer a much more conservative treatment, with minimally invasive procedures, in much less time compared with an "ultimate" treatment plan that would restore the perfect midline. Diagnostics and treatment planning are the most essential steps in such cases.

Case analysis

In Patient 2, it was decided to attempt restoration of the anterior region with PLVs. The smile first should be analyzed carefully and systematically, as described in recent literature.[3–5] When the smile was analyzed from an oblique angle (which is one of the three important views of the smile according to Sarver[6]), the maxillary right premolars and the maxillary left lateral incisor seemed to have negative torque (too palatal), and the maxillary left canine was too buccal (Figs 10-2c and 10-2d). The debate was whether to bulk the teeth to the bigger perimeter—that is, to add

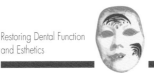

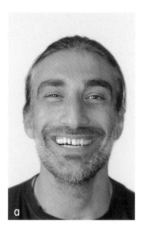

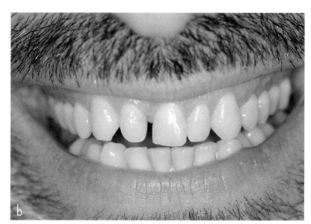

Figs 10-2a and 10-2b Anterior view of the face and smile of Patient 2, showing the unesthetic appearance due to early loss of the maxillary right central incisor and a distinct midline shift.

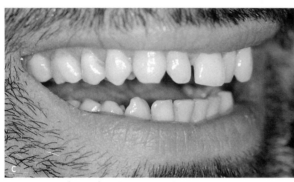

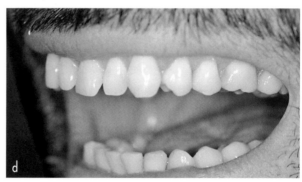

Figs 10-2c and 10-2d Oblique view of the patient during smile. Note the crowded positions of the maxillary left central incisor, lateral incisor, and canine.

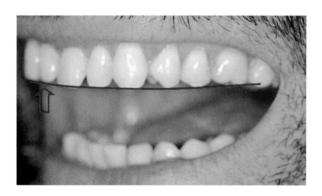

Fig 10-2e Lateral view of the patient during smile. Note the unesthetic plane of occlusion.

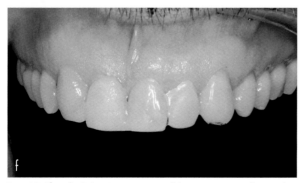

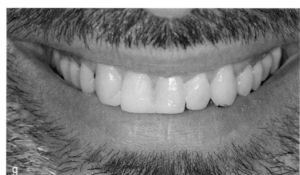

Figs 10-2f and 10-2g Anterior view of the patient's maxillary esthetic zone with resin composite buildup to mimic the shape of the future restorations. Note the parallelism between the new shape of the teeth and the lower lip line.

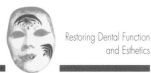

Restoring Dental Function and Esthetics

volume to the palatally placed teeth—or to aggressively grind the canine in an attempt to establish a more continuous arch. The patient's occlusal plane also needed some correction due to its flatness and unattractive smile arc. The anterior teeth were significantly shorter than required to create a parabolic type of smile line.

Wax-up procedure

Although the initial complaint of the patient was the unesthetic appearance around the missing tooth, after a full analysis it was concluded that the entire esthetic zone needed modification so that the pleasant smile could be synchronized with the lower lip line (Fig 10-2e). To define the treatment goals and to communicate better with the patient, the first step in this type of situation is to create a mock-up in the mouth with resin composite.[7] Although the experienced clinician may have executed thousands of veneers over time, this stage should never be skipped. When any type of resin composite is used, the smile can be built up and pictures taken from different angles so as to examine not only the shape of each tooth but also its harmony with supporting structures such as the gingiva and the lips.

Because the patient had a retruded upper lip and retroclined teeth, it was decided to add resin composite to the teeth rather than grind down the maxillary left canine (Fig 10-2f). Although a midline shift of about 4 to 5 mm still existed after this adjustment, the smile was acceptable to the clinic staff and the patient (Fig 10-2g).

The next steps in this type of procedure occur in the laboratory, where the predicted outcome could be better evaluated because of the opportunity to slice the teeth slightly to shift the midline at least 1 mm to the left side. Again, the clinician should keep in mind that any changes to the tooth dimensions should preserve tooth proportion, preferably within the golden proportion rule of a 1:1.6 ratio between the length and the width of each tooth. The support of the soft tissue and the interdental papillae should be considered as well.[8,9]

For better proportions, a rough wax-up copy was created to indicate whether the mock-up guide worked well proportionally and functionally in the patient's mouth (Figs 10-2h and 10-2i). This can be checked with the help of an articulator. This laboratory procedure is a marvelous educational tool for both the technician and the clinician: It can help to determine how much buildup material (resin composite or porcelain) should be layered or how much reduction should be performed to achieve the best tooth proportions. Later, this information can be transferred to the preparation of the actual teeth.

Once the wax-up was completed, an impression was taken and a template made of polyvinyl siloxane (PVS) that could be filled later by the clinician with a flowable resin composite in the patient's mouth. It is

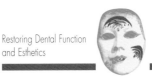

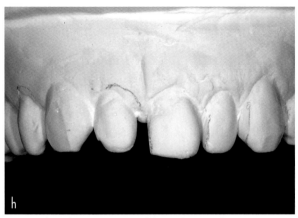
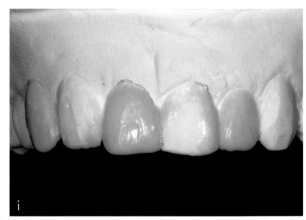

Figs 10-2h and 10-2i Wax-up of the teeth. Note the recontouring of the right lateral incisor to the shape of a central incisor while the right canine is modified to the shape of a lateral incisor.

essential to understand that at this stage, this is still a diagnostic procedure; no tooth has been prepared yet. The provisional was placed in the patient's mouth before any tooth was prepared or the patient anesthetized. These trial provisionals, called *esthetic pre-evaluative temporaries*,[10] provide an excellent opportunity to see not only the likely esthetic outcome of the restoration but also its effect on the teeth's support of the lips, the appearance of the smile line, and the phonetics of the patient (Figs 10-2j to 10-2n). The need for this extra diagnostic tool arose from the silicone index's inability to help the clinician define the amount by which tooth material should be reduced and determine the best preparation method to use. As shown in Figs 10-2o to 10-2q, a difference exists between the amount of material that needs to be removed from the teeth and the actual gap left between the silicone index and the outer enamel.

The method most clinicians have been accustomed to was the use of the silicone index as the only guideline to prepare the teeth for PLV restorations.[11] In this trial-and-error method, clinicians needed to come back to the patient repeatedly during the preparation and check the silicone index against the teeth to see how the preparation was progressing. Once the index was removed to prepare the teeth, there was no reference for how much had already been trimmed or how much reduction was still required. In cases where it was realized too late that too much tooth material had been removed, there was no way to rebuild that natural structure.

Since the esthetic pre-evaluative temporaries were already prepared and exactly mimicked the contours of the definitive veneers, it was suddenly realized they could help in the diagnostic phase or for provisionalization as well as in the preparation process itself. It was decided to leave the esthetic pre-evaluative temporaries on the teeth and just prepare through them[12–14] (Figs 10-2r to 10-2t).

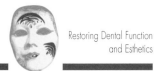

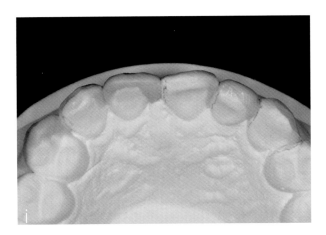

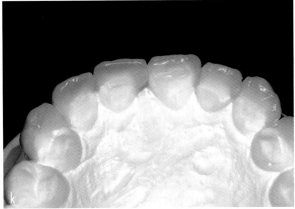

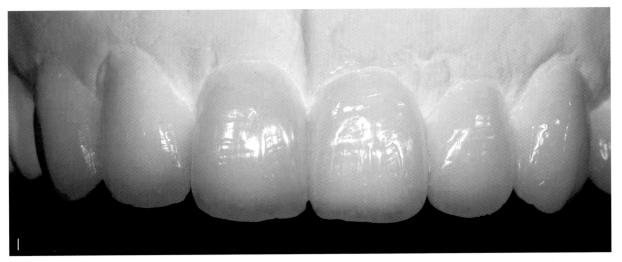

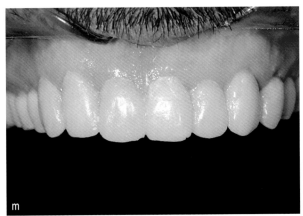

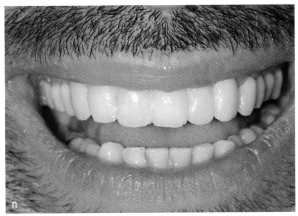

Figs 10-2j to 10-2n Wax-up preparation transferred from model to the patient's mouth. Note how well this provisional restoration (*esthetic pre-evaluative temporary*) integrates with all the supporting structures (lips, gums, and smile). Although the midline is still shifted, the smile is well accepted by both patient and clinician.

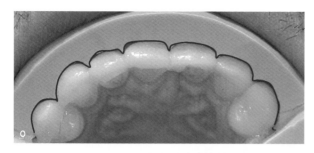
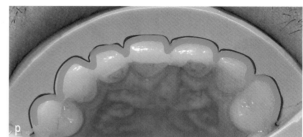
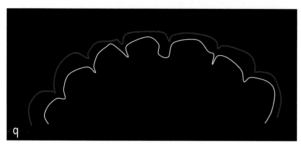

Figs 10-2o to 10-2q The blue line (o) indicates the silicone index. The green zone (p) indicates the amount of tooth structure that should be removed so that the porcelain will be layered equally on every tooth. The white line (q) describes the way the teeth are aligned (or, in this case, malaligned) and their unequal distance from the silicone index.

Once an esthetic pre-evaluative temporary is placed, the case can be treated like a very simple case with well-aligned teeth. If some teeth are lingually or otherwise malpositioned, such as the maxillary left lateral incisor in Patient 2, the tooth structure may not be visible at all during preparation.

Preparation of teeth and soft tissue

After the facial tooth reduction was finished, the silicone index was checked to ensure ideal preparation depth for all PLV restorations (Fig 10-2u). The amount of incisal reduction was much more than expected in this technique. For improved esthetics, a space had to be created 1.5 to 2.0 mm incisally, and a butt joint was formed. The esthetic pre-evaluative temporaries are a precise tool that allows more tooth structure to be preserved. Once the initial preparation was finished (Fig 10-2v), the esthetic pre-evaluative temporaries were removed. In all the areas that were untouched, such as the maxillary left lateral incisor (Fig 10-2w), the prismatic layer of the enamel was removed for better etchability and better bonding.[15,16]

At this stage, the soft tissues were recontoured as had been planned at the laboratory stage. Since the anterior diastema was to be closed by enlarging the right lateral incisor, the gingival structure in that area needed modification. The plan was to squeeze and reshape the papilla slightly downward to close the black triangle and attain a better emergence profile for the veneer (see Figs 10-2w and 10-2x). It was also important to prepare the teeth on either side of the diastema.

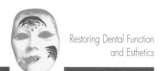
Restoring Dental Function
and Esthetics

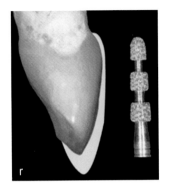
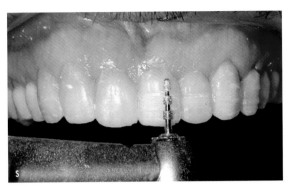

Figs 10-2r and 10-2s Preparation of teeth for PLV restoration through the esthetic pre-evaluative temporary placed on the buccal surface.

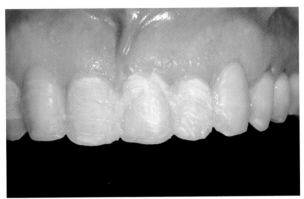

Fig 10-2t Facial view of the anterior teeth after preparation has taken place through the esthetic pre-evaluative temporary: Note that the maxillary left lateral incisor that was retroclined still has remnants of the esthetic pre-evaluative temporary on the buccal surface.

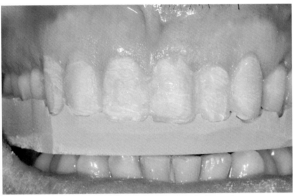

Fig 10-2u Facial view of the preparation with the esthetic pre-evaluative temporary and incisal silicone index.

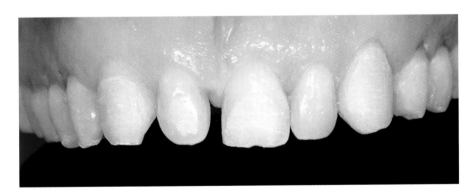

Fig 10-2v Facial view of the teeth after preparation was finalized. Note that some teeth, such as the maxillary left lateral incisor, have not been touched.

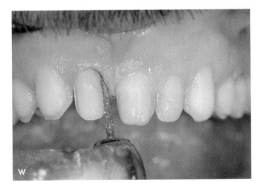
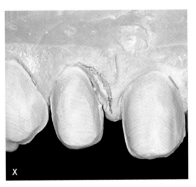

Figs 10-2w and 10-2x Preparation of the soft tissue at the mesial of the maxillary right lateral incisor according to the laboratory plan. Note the subgingival preparation so that the veneer will push the papilla slightly downward to enable a crisp triangular shape.

Restoring Dental Function and Esthetics

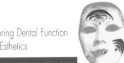

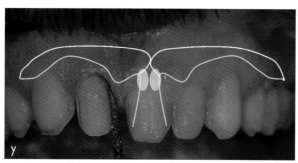
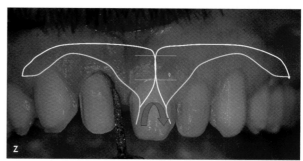

Figs 10-2y and 10-2z Preparation of the teeth close to the diastema to be closed with PLV restoration should extend interproximally to avoid the black appearance and food impaction (as shown in Fig 10-2z).

A standard preparation could lead to two problems. First, the contact area between the veneers would be so thin that the darkness of the mouth's interior would show through the veneers and result in a darker appearance of that veneer. Second, the sharp angulations in the area where the PLVs would connect to the teeth could result in food impaction. Therefore, it was decided to extend the preparation line interproximally slightly toward the palate on both sides to allow for a thicker connection to be attained between the veneers. This would block out any dark discoloration and enable better oral hygiene (Figs 10-2y and 10-2z).

Fabrication of the veneers

Once the teeth and soft tissues are prepared, the rest is up to the ceramist, who fabricates the veneers to be placed in the patient's mouth. In accordance with the treatment goals, the technician also *(1)* lengthened the teeth for better crown exposure during rest position and at smile; *(2)* shifted the midline very slightly to the patient's left side; *(3)* converted the maxillary right lateral incisor to a central incisor; *(4)* converted the canine to a lateral incisor; and *(5)* converted the maxillary right premolar to a canine.

Although the final result still displayed a midline shift and a missing maxillary central incisor (Figs 10-2aa to 10-2ee), the harmony and the integration with the supporting elements—lips, gums, and face—was most satisfactory, both to the clinician and to the patient.

Conclusion

Whether a patient presents with a simple or complex situation to be restored with PLVs, treatment that requires some compromise in ideal esthetics can still provide functional results with an acceptable appearance. This chapter provides some diagnostic tools that can be used to analyze and treat complex cases when applied within the following guidelines:

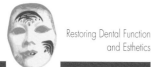

Restoring Dental Function
and Esthetics

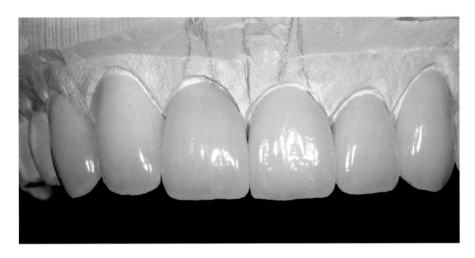

Fig 10-2aa Final PLV restoration placed on the working model.

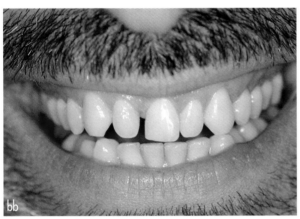

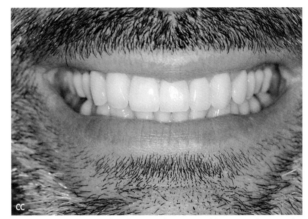

Figs 10-2bb and 10-2cc Final restoration as viewed from close-up anterior view (*cc*) compared to the initial situation (*bb*). Note that maxillary midline shift and missing tooth are no longer easily recognized.

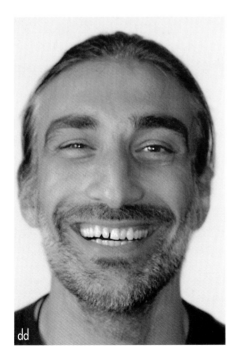

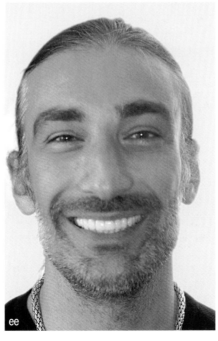

Figs 10-2dd and 10-2ee Anterior view of the patient's face during smile before and after treatment. Note the improvement in smile arc and the total esthetic improvement.

Restoring Dental Function and Esthetics

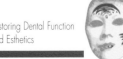

1. Start with a mock-up, and analyze the smile from every aspect possible.
2. Transfer all the anatomic and clinical information to the laboratory so the technician can create an effective wax-up, and then apply the outcome to a provisional restoration to be tried in the patient's mouth.
3. Check the esthetic outcome before anything is irreversibly prepared! If the wax-up doesn't match the expectations of the patient because the patient was allowed to expect the impossible, the situation can be a very good moment to discontinue treatment. If the patient is told what to expect early, a lot of unhappiness and disappointment can be prevented.
4. Once the esthetic pre-evaluative temporary is in the mouth, it is possible to prepare the teeth through the restoration, which allows the exact depth that is needed for the veneers to be created. This minimizes structural loss.
5. Pay attention to the width of the final restoration, especially in areas where spaces need to be closed.
6. Creation of self-cleaning areas in the interproximal areas can prevent food impaction.

References

1. Kokich VO Jr, Kokich VG, Kiyak HA. Perceptions of dental professionals and laypersons to altered dental esthetics: Asymmetric and symmetric situations. Am J Orthod Dentofacial Orthop 2006;130:141–151.
2. Kokich VO Jr, Kiyak HA, Shapiro PA. Comparing the perception of dentists and lay people to altered dental esthetics. J Esthet Dent 1999;11(6):311–324.
3. Ker AJ, Chan R, Fields HW, Beck M, Rosenstiel S. Esthetics and smile characteristics from the layperson's perspective: A computer-based survey study. J Am Dent Assoc 2008;139(10):1318–1327.
4. Krishnan V, Daniel ST, Lazar D, Asok A. Characterization of posed smile by using visual analog scale, smile arc, buccal corridor measures, and modified smile index. Am J Orthod Dentofacial Orthop 2008;133(4):515–523.
5. Gill DS, Naini FB, Tredwin CJ. Smile aesthetics. Dent Update 2007;34(3):152–154, 157–158.
6. Sarver DM. The importance of incisor positioning in the esthetic smile: The smile arc. Am J Orthod Dentofacial Orthop 2001;120(2):98–111.
7. Gürel G (ed). The Science and Art of Porcelain Laminate Veneers. Hanover Park, IL: Quintessence, 2003.
8. Bukhary SM, Gill DS, Tredwin CJ, Moles DR. The influence of varying maxillary lateral incisor dimensions on perceived smile aesthetics. Br Dent J 2007;20(12)3:687–693.
9. Ward DH. A study of dentists' preferred maxillary anterior tooth width proportions: Comparing the recurring esthetic dental proportion to other mathematical and naturally occurring proportions. J Esthet Restor Dent 2007;19(6):324–337.
10. Gürel G. Permanent diagnostic provisionals: Predictable outcomes using porcelain laminate veneers. Quint Dent Technol 2007;30:43–55.
11. Gürel G. Predictable tooth preparation for porcelain laminate veneers in complicated cases. Quintessence Dent Technol 2003;26:99–111.

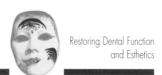

Restoring Dental Function and Esthetics

12. Magne P. Perspectives in esthetic dentistry. Quintessence Dent Technol 2000;23:86–89.
13. Gürel G. Predictable, precise and repeatable tooth preparation for porcelain laminate veneers. Pract Proced Aesthet Dent 2003;15(1):17–24.
14. Gürel G. Permanent diagnostic provisional restorations for predictable results when redesigning the smile. Pract Proced Aesthet Dent 2006;18(5):281–286.
15. Shimada Y, Tagami J. Effects of regional enamel and prism orientation on resin bonding. Oper Dent 2003;28(1):20–27.
16. Chaiyabutr Y, McGowan S, Phillips KM, Kois JC, Giordano RA. The effect of hydrofluoric acid surface treatment and bond strength of a zirconia veneering ceramic. J Prosthet Dent 2008;100(3):194–202.

Innovative Concepts in Orthodontic Therapy

III

Carlos F. Navarro

Jorge A. Villanueva

Marco A. Navarro

Silvia Geron

P. Emile Rossouw

Georges L. S. Skinazi

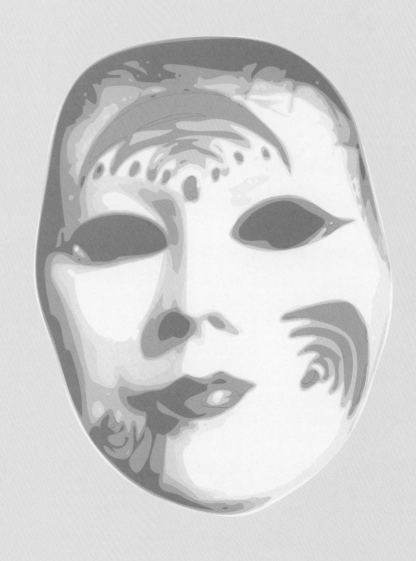

The Proportions of Facial Balance: An Esthetic Appraisal

11

Carlos F. Navarro, DDS,
  MSD
Jorge A. Villanueva, DDS

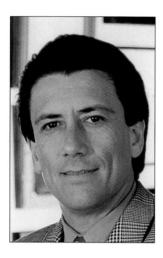

Carlos F. Navarro, DDS, MSD

Carlos Navarro received his CD from Coahuila State University in 1976. He completed his preceptorship in orthodontics at the Mexican Center of Orthodontics and Maxillofacial Orthopedics in 1979 and his fellowship in surgical orthodontics at the University of Texas, Dallas in 1981. Dr Navarro received his certificate of specialty in orthodontics, his DDS, and his MS from Baylor Dental School in 1981, 1984, and 1985, respectively. He is a diplomate of the American Board of Orthodontics. He has also lectured internationally and is a member of the Roth-Williams International Society of Orthodontics. Dr Navarro maintains a private practice limited to orthodontics in Dallas, Texas.

Email: drcarlosnavarro@mac.com

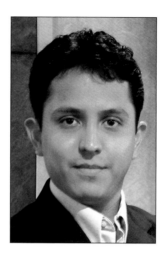

Jorge A. Villanueva, DDS

Jorge A. Villanueva received his DDS from the Universidad Autonoma de Nueva Leon in 2001 and has since lectured there and at the Universidad Autonoma de Coahuila. In 2009, he completed the Roth-Williams Course, and he is currently serving an internship in orthodontics at the University of Southern Nevada. He has been collaborating with Dr Navarro since 2005.

Email: jorgevillanueva@orthos.com.mx

Innovative Concepts in
Orthodontic Therapy

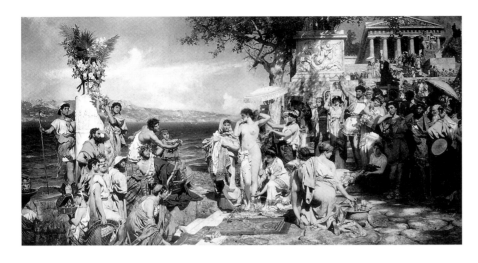

Fig 11-1a Henryk Siemiradzki. *Phryne at the Festival of Poseidon in Eleusin,* 1889.

Factors in the Discussion of Beauty

"Beauty is in the eye of the beholder."
Margaret Wolfe Hungerford, 1878

Throughout time, civilizations around the world have shared a sense of what beauty is regardless of the subject's race, ethnic background, or age (Fig 11-1). Cultures have been able to apply labels of *beautiful* to experiences such as watching a sunset or to objects such as the teeth that clinicians see in everyday practice. How is it possible to define all of the numerous variables that create beauty?

Beauty is a trait of a person, object, place, or idea that provides a perceptual experience of pleasure, affirmation, meaning, or goodness. The subjective experience of beauty often involves the interpretation of some entity as being in balance and harmony with nature. This leads to

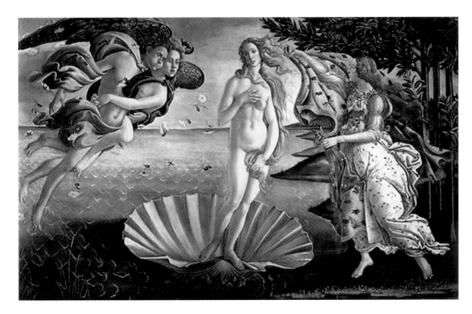

Fig 11-1b Sandro Botticelli. *The Birth of Venus,* 1486.

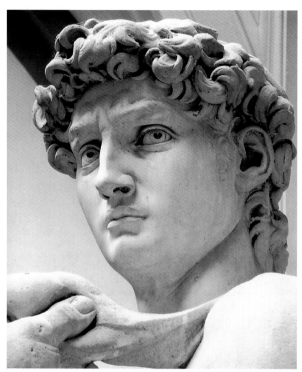

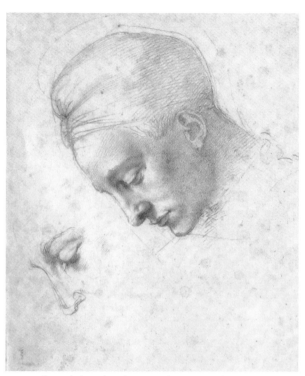

Fig 11-2a Michelangelo's *David*, one of the most beautiful sculptures in the world, shows a soft tissue structure indicative of a Class II, division 2 malocclusion.

Fig 11-2b Michelangelo's drawings demonstrate that appreciation of ideal facial proportions was emphasized even during the Renaissance.

feelings of attraction and emotional well-being. In terms of human perception, facial beauty is associated with success and social power, and it has an affirmative influence on well-being and confidence.

One common idea suggests that the appraisal of beauty is related to the appearance of people and things that are "good." For example, a good apple will be perceived as more beautiful than a bruised one. In terms of human form, recognition of something as good or beautiful is more subjective and influenced by cultural preference. A perfectly proportioned face may display myriad variations in coloring and in shapes of the individual facial features (eyes, eyebrows, lips, nose, etc) that give rise to the distinctive appearance of each race and provide for endless variations in beauty. Although norms may change with time and evolution, we could say that Michelangelo's *David* is beautiful despite a skeletal Class II, division 2 malocclusion (Fig 11-2a).

In discussions of beauty, terms such as *symmetry*, *balance*, and *harmony* have been used repeatedly without much attention to their definitions. *Symmetry* can be defined as mirror imaging about an axis. *Balance* is equality of magnitudes on either side of a division. *Harmony* is the presence of recurring themes within an entity. From these definitions, it is possible to see that absolute symmetry would have balance, but balance may not necessarily have symmetry.[1]

Innovative Concepts in
Orthodontic Therapy

The golden ratio

Throughout history, human beings have been aware of beauty and facial esthetics in terms of harmony and quality of parts (Fig 11-2b). The golden ratio of the Greeks, known during the Renaissance as the *divine proportion, golden mean,* or *golden section,* is a number (approximately 1:1.618) often encountered in recorded ratios of distances within simple geometric figures such as the pentagon, decagon, and dodecahedron. Leonardo de Pisa (c1180 to c1250), better known as Fibonacci, described a mathematical sequence that is closely connected to the golden ratio. This sequence appears consistently in natural settings such as the branches of trees, pineapples, the curves of a nautilus, and the scales of pinecones. It is connected to a perception of beauty; as a result, objects with these proportions tend to elicit a positive emotional response.[2–7]

The human face communicates an incredible array of emotions that are an integral element of total beauty. The lines and angles of a smiling face conform most closely to the golden proportion, and a person is also generally perceived as more beautiful when smiling. During the Renaissance, esthetic studies became the domain of painters, sculptors, and philosophers. Artists and architects since that time have fashioned works influenced by the golden rectangle, in which the ratio of the longer side to the shorter side matches the golden ratio, in the belief that this proportion is esthetically pleasing. Leonardo da Vinci applied the golden ratio to the human face in an illustration from *De Divina Proportione* (Fig 11-3), and it is thought that he incorporated the golden ratio into his own paintings as well. Some suggest that his *Mona Lisa,* for example, employs the golden ratio in its geometric equivalents.[8–10]

Applications to dentistry

Researchers in many fields of dentistry such as orthodontics, maxillofacial surgery, and plastic surgery have conducted studies of the human face and profile that have contributed to esthetic awareness. These have been used to establish guidelines that enable the clinician to make an appropriate treatment plan, select proper treatment mechanics, and move the teeth to produce facial changes that are esthetically and functionally favorable.[11]

An orthodontic diagnosis, for example, involves clinical and cephalometric assessments. These assessments involve all of the procedures essential to describe, analyze, measure, and predict results for the dentofacial structures.[12]

A stable maxillofacial relationship that exhibits the correct balance between centric occlusion (CO) and centric relation (CR) is key to the success of any orthodontic treatment. Poor maxillomandibular function

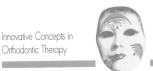

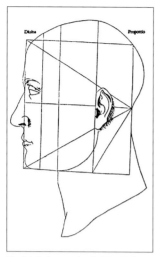

Fig 11-3 Leonardo da Vinci's illustration from *De Divina Proportione* applies the golden ratio to the human face. Leonardo's thoughts on bodily proportions and the golden ratio have led a number of scholars to speculate that he incorporated the golden ratio into his own paintings.

produces attrition, abrasion, abfraction, and erosion, which result in tooth surface loss and reduced esthetics.[13] All elements of the dentofacial complex interact harmoniously with each other to play a part in a comfortable, pleasing, and physiologic whole that includes *(1)* an occluded dentition; *(2)* the correct vertical dimension of occlusion; *(3)* the right degree of overbite and overjet; *(4)* condyles in their most superior position, in intimate contact with discs against the distal surface of the articular eminences; and *(5)* the CR position during maximum intercuspation.

The appraisal of facial proportions presented in this chapter is an objective evaluation triggered by visual stimulus. The process is explained through simple methods that match soft and hard tissue landmarks and connect esthetics to physiology to achieve the best clinical outcome. The authors' intention is to present an individualized method of analysis that can be performed during the evaluation of different facial structures. A systematic initial examination with this element of consistency maximizes the objectivity of the evaluation of the areas in question and minimizes the risk that other discrepancies will be overlooked. Several general facial parameters on both anterior and profile views are considered and then reviewed in more detail.

The full visual examination consists of a facial examination and a buccodental examination; this chapter focuses on the facial examination, which evaluates the esthetics of the face and the relationship between dentoalveolar abnormalities, esthetics, and any dysfunction.

Natural Head Position

For years orthodontists have studied the soft tissue contour of facial profiles to understand how movement of teeth and supporting bone affects the arrangement of facial soft tissue. In the past, facial profile esthetics was described subjectively. More recently, various objective methods of soft tissue assessment have been developed.[14–18]

Natural head position (NHP) has been defined by Cole as "the relationship of the head to the true vertical," while natural head posture was defined as "the relationship of the head to the cervical column."[19] As a reproducible factor, NHP is useful for comparison of different treatment stages in the same patient or for cephalometric comparisons between patients. NHP is established early in life and is influenced by balance (the vestibular canals of the middle ear), vision (the need to maintain a horizontal visual axis), and proprioception from joints and muscles in the erect posture. NHP is less variable than other intracranial reference lines. Profile assessment on a lateral cephalogram can be a highly accurate process if the head is held in its natural position and sufficient soft tissue data are collected.

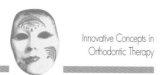

Innovative Concepts in
Orthodontic Therapy

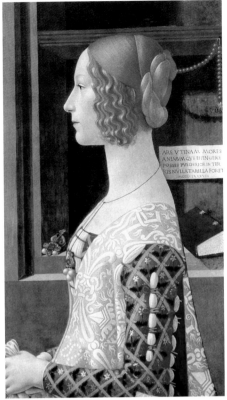

Fig 11-4 Domenico Ghirlandaio. *Portrait of Giovanna Tornabuoni.* 1488. Museo Thyssen-Bornemisza, Madrid, Spain. Renaissance artists used gravity lines to position the head for profile paintings. The profile view was their first choice because it did not show the damaged smiles or missing teeth common in those times.

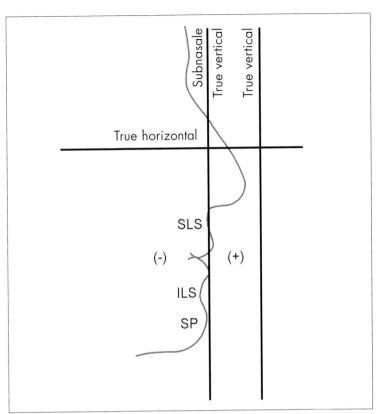

Fig 11-5 Profile assessment on a lateral cephalogram can be a highly accurate process if the head is held in its natural position and sufficient soft tissue data are collected. The subnasale vertical has become the most statistically reproducible landmark, evidence of Jacobs' foresight more than 30 years ago. (SLS, superior labial sulcus; ILS, inferior labial sulcus; SP, soft tissue pogonion.)

The greatest facial diagnostic innovation occurred in 1978 when Jacobs modified the González-Ulloa analysis to employ a true vertical reference plane through the subnasale (Sn). This measurement is obtained by dropping a weighted line that hangs freely from the ceiling.[20,21] Italian Renaissance artists used similar gravity lines to position the head for profile paintings (Fig 11-4). Jacobs' method has proven the most statistically reproducible position of the head, facial lateral view components, and profile landmarks (Fig 11-5).

At about the same time as Jacobs' development, Burstone, James, and Legan used similar methodology to create the glabella's (gb) true vertical analysis.[22] In the authors' opinion, however, this is statistically unreliable due to variations in the location of the pneumatic cavity of the frontal sinus and in forehead dimensions in diverse ethnic groups.

In 1979, Jacobson used an extracranial true vertical reference plane, obtained from NHP, and proposed this as the most accurate method for profile assessment from a lateral cephalogram.[14] However, this study mainly looked at sagittal jaw discrepancies and not linear or angular soft tissue relationships to the true vertical.

The authors use the NHP as the reference tool to appraise facial proportions through clinical photographs and for cephalometric radiographs and analysis. To record NHP, the patient sits in front of a mirror and stares straight ahead with the head vertical, feet slightly spread, and arms hanging. The lips and all muscles of the jaw and neck should be relaxed (Fig 11-6).

Clinical Evaluation of the Face and Oral Components

To perform a full clinical evaluation, the face is recorded in several views: full face anterior, full smile anterior, right profile, and at a 45-degree profile angle (left and right). The last view is recorded to obtain a more natural image, since this is the maximum angle in which patients can see themselves (Fig 11-7).[23]

Anterior view evaluation
Facial type

Three distinct facial patterns describe the biometric scale of the face as discussed by Ricketts: mesofacial, brachyfacial, and dolichofacial (Fig 11-8).[16] Individuals with a mesofacial pattern show proportionally equivalent horizontal and vertical dimensions. The brachyfacial pattern is characterized by a low facial height with a wide transverse face. The dolichofacial pattern exhibits increased facial height and a narrow face. Muscle patterns also differ due to the different vectors seen in these facial types. Brachyfacial-type individuals have strong facial muscles, but the muscles of dolichofacial types are weak. In profile, the bone structure of the dolichofacial type is convex, whereas that of the brachyfacial type is straighter or even concave. The distance between nasion (N) and menton (Me) is proportionally greater in dolichofacial-type individuals.[24]

Facial balance

All human beings have a slight asymmetry between their left and right sides that is within normal tolerance. Nevertheless, orthodontic treatment can influence some asymmetries, such as those within the lower facial third from below the nose (Sn) to the chin (Me), a very important area in orthodontics and maxillofacial surgery. Facial asymmetry is closely related to temporomandibular joint (TMJ) status, occlusal function, tooth alignment, and esthetics (Fig 11-9).[25]

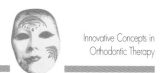

Innovative Concepts in
Orthodontic Therapy

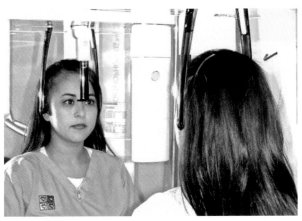

Fig 11-6 To record NHP, the patient sits in front of a mirror staring straight ahead with head vertical, feet slightly spread, and arms hanging. The lips and all muscles of the jaw and neck should be relaxed.

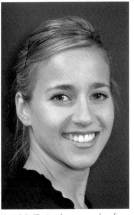

Fig 11-7 A photograph of the 45-degree profile is obtained in addition to the lateral and anterior views.

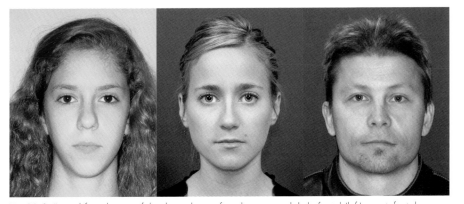

Fig 11-8 Frontal facial view of the three distinct facial patterns: dolichofacial (left), mesiofacial (center), and brachyfacial (right).

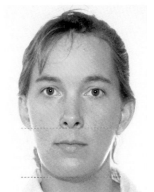

Fig 11-9 Photograph of a young patient shows a deviation of her chin to the right due to a TMJ disturbance.

Asymmetry can be functional or skeletal. Functional asymmetry is defined as an inadequate mandibular position due to lateral displacement by premature occlusal contact, unilateral posterior crossbite, or TM joint or muscle problems.[26] Skeletal asymmetry involves displacement of the teeth toward the right or left side due to a shorter condyle or ramus on that side, which also causes the chin to deviate in that direction. When the chin is the only deviated structure of the face, the patient has mandibular asymmetry. Skeletal asymmetry cannot be repaired with orthodontic treatment alone.[27]

Facial height

The inferior one-third of the face, from Sn to Me, is divided into two unequal portions (Fig 11-10). The SN to upper stomion (USt) distance equals one-third of the distance from SN to Me. The lower stomion (LSt) to Me distance equals two-thirds of the Sn-Me distance. This

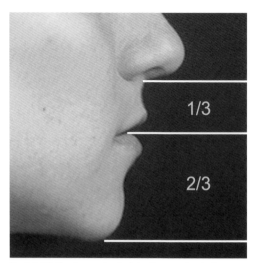 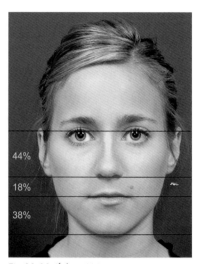

Fig 11-10 The lower third of the face is divided into two unequal portions: one-third of the distance from Sn to Me, and two-thirds of the distance from Sn to Me. If the inferior portion is more than two-thirds the total distance, it means the vertical is increased; if the superior portion is less than a third, it indicates a decreased vertical growth of that part.

Fig 11-11 If the N-Me measurement is 100% of the facial height, the N-Sn distance represents 44%, and the Sn-USt distance is 18%. The LSt-Me distance accounts for the remaining 38%.

inferior region also includes the interlabial gap, which is the vertical distance between the lips (USt-LSt) in a relaxed labial position. The ideal distance is 3 mm.[28]

Maxillary vertical
If the N-Me measurement is 100% of the facial height, the N-Sn distance represents 44%, and the Sn-USt distance is 18%. The LSt-Me distance accounts for the remaining 38%. A distance greater than 18% in the center third of the face represents an increased vertical (Fig 11-11).

The N–Sn region cannot be altered by orthodontics or routine jaw surgery, yet it has a huge impact on the lower face.[29]

Maxillary incisor exposure
Maxillary incisor exposure refers to the relationship between the maxillary incisors and the upper lip. Balanced facial esthetics requires correlation of several factors, including upper lip length and thickness, tooth size, degree of torque, incisor intrusion or extrusion, and vertical position of the maxilla. With the face at rest, 1 to 2 mm of the maxillary incisors should be visible through the lips. In a full smile, exposure of the full crown of the central incisors and up to 1 mm of gingiva is considered pleasant.[30] The crown length of the anterior teeth is therefore a very important esthetic factor, though the length and shape of premolars and molars also influence esthetics (Fig 11-12).

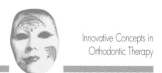

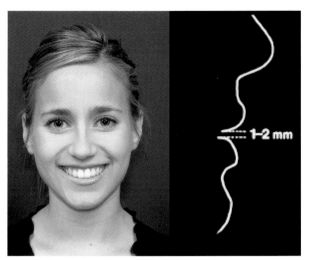

Fig 11-12 With the face at rest, 1 to 2 mm of the maxillary incisors should be visible through the lips. In a full smile, exposure of the full crown of the central incisors and up to 1 mm of gingiva is considered pleasant.

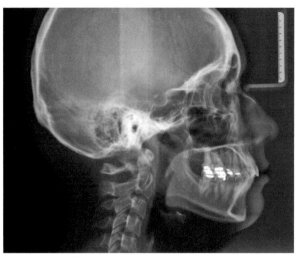

Fig 11-13 Maxillary cant in a 29-year-old patient is associated with facial asymmetry and TMJ issues.

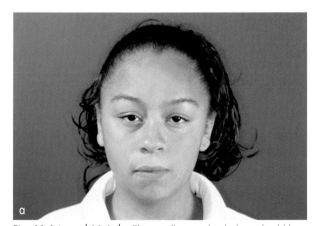

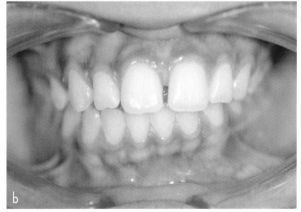

Figs 11-14a and 11-14b The maxillary occlusal plane should be parallel to the interpupillary line. An uneven maxillary occlusal plane may also point to a TMJ problem.

Maxillary occlusal plane

The aim of orthodontic treatment is to achieve good occlusion with anteroposterior (AP) facial balance. Any lateral mandibular displacement must be corrected by balancing the AP forces in addition to the skeletal right–left difference, or maxillary cant (Fig 11-13).

The maxillary occlusal plane should be parallel to the interpupillary line. An uneven maxillary occlusal plane may also point to a TMJ problem. Some authors report that the occlusal plane is elevated in the direction of mandibular displacement[19,31] (Fig 11-14).

Fig 11-15 *(left)* The presence of dark spaces in buccal corridors indicates a discrepancy between the arches.

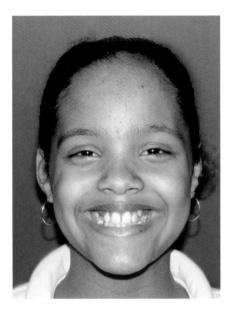
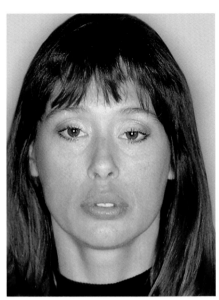

Fig 11-16 *(right)* Evaluation of the eyes must include ocular size in relation to other anatomic structures, eye shape, angles at the inner and outer canthi, globe prominence, position, and balance with respect to each other.

Midface transverse

Dark spaces in buccal corridors indicate a discrepancy between the arches (Fig 11-15). The mesiobuccal cusp of the maxillary first molar should be the most prominent tooth surface visible upon smiling. Maxillary and mandibular dental midlines should match the facial midline as closely as possible.

The eyes and orbital region

The eyes are such important facial features that in some patients they dominate other elements of the face. The size and balance of the eyes must be evaluated in relation to other anatomic structures and to each other (ie, whether one eye is higher than the other). The clinical assessment should also note *(1)* specific shape (eg, round, ovoid, narrow), *(2)* angles at the inner and outer canthi, *(3)* globe prominence, and *(4)* overall ocular position (Fig 11-16).

For the facial assessment, an anterior photograph is divided into vertical fifths, using the intercanthal distance as the central one-fifth (Fig 11-17). The location of the central vertical lines determines which of the following describes the patient:

- Wide-set eyes, which tend to give the face an open, youthful appearance
- Close-set eyes, which may appear dramatic or sultry
- Evenly spaced eyes, in which the intercanthal distance is 30 to 35 mm

The ideal location of the eyebrows differs between sexes. The male brow is located at the supraorbital rim and is fairly flat. The female brow lies slightly superior to the rim and has a more prominent arch located at the

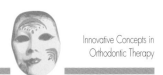

Innovative Concepts in
Orthodontic Therapy

level of the external lateral limbus (sclerocorneal). The brow should start medially at a vertical line that passes through the alar groove and medial canthus and continue laterally to end along an oblique line from the nasal ala through the lateral canthus at roughly the same height as the medial brow.

The eyelids may be too pronounced, normal, or too deep. Both upper and lower lids should be carefully examined, visually and manually, to determine shape and elasticity. If the eyelid is divided into vertical thirds, the upper lid margin should have its highest point at the junction of the center and medial thirds. The lowest point of the lower lid should be between the center and lateral thirds. The upper lid should cover 2 to 3 mm of superior iris; the lower lid margin usually approximates the inferior iris.

Nasal size and symmetry

Because the nose is typically the most prominent feature on the face and essential to facial symmetry, it is the most defining characteristic of the entire face. The nose is not only intimately connected to general appearance but also to heritage, ethnicity, facial character, and perceived strength. Orthodontic assessment and treatment must take the nose into account because nasal alterations can greatly improve appearance. In an esthetically pleasing face, the relationship between the width of the nose and the width of the mouth is equal to the golden ratio (1:1.618).

Breathing problems can be related to internal nasal shape. Noses that deviate internally often show concomitant external deviations or have a hump on the dorsum (the main bridge). To correct an external nasal deformity, it may be necessary to improve the nasal base, which functions much like the frame of a tent, with the fabric (skin) stretched over its structure. Expansion of the palate also has a large effect on nasal shape and can improve breathing.

The nose should be evaluated for dorsal deformities and appropriate width. Again, dividing the face into vertical fifths readily determines whether the lower nasal width is esthetically acceptable (see Fig 11-17). In white patients, the distance between alar creases should be equal to one eye-width (one-fifth); wider noses are acceptable in persons of Asian or African descent. The length of the nose is measured from N to tip (pronasale, or Pn), and the alar base width is approximately 70% of the nasal length.

Upper and lower lips

The location of the lips in relation to the nose and chin was discussed in the previous section on facial height. It must be remembered that surrounding facial structures, as well as the patient's dentition, will affect the appearance of the lips. Other considerations in the clinical evaluation of the lips include the width, the interlabial gap, and the amount of

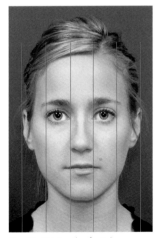

Fig 11-17 For the facial assessment, an anterior photograph is divided into vertical fifths, using the intercanthal distance as the central one-fifth.

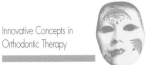

Innovative Concepts in Orthodontic Therapy

exposed incisor upon smiling. The oral commissures should touch vertical lines drawn from the medial limbus of each iris. The lower lip should be slightly fuller than the upper lip. When the lips are relaxed and the teeth are in occlusion, the maximum interlabial gap and amount of incisor visible should be 3 mm. Gingiva should not be seen in the smile, and no more than two-thirds of the maxillary incisors should be exposed.

The goal of an upper lip lift is to restore a proper amount of tooth exposure as well as to create a more youthful ratio of vermilion height to total lip height. In one study, labio-oral measurements were obtained in 55 attractive men and women. The average upper lip vermilion height (VS-USt) was determined to be 8.4 mm in men and 8.9 mm in women. The upper lip height (Sn-USt) was found to be 22 mm in men and 20 mm in women.[32] Another study that involved young white adults found the size of the upper lip vermilion to be 83% to 85% of that of the lower lip.[33]

The exact amount of lip resected will depend on the vertical height of the teeth and the current vertical height of the maxilla. Patients who have a longer upper lip in youth and those who lose more maxillary vertical height with aging will require a greater resection.

Hoefflin[34] states that the distance from the alar base horizontal to the upper lip vermilion should be the same as or shorter than the distance from the ocular supratarsal to the lower lid lash line. Because the periocular region may age at a different rate than the perioral region, however, the authors believe it is more accurate to use local landmarks. The following steps are required when a clinician photographs the patient in NHP:

1. Ask the patient to stand or sit comfortably with feet apart and weight evenly distributed.
2. Ask the patient to look straight into a mirror with eyes level.
3. Set the patient's lips in repose (ie, showing an interlabial gap with jaw and neck muscles relaxed).
4. Add a true vertical reference anterior to the patient's soft tissue profile.
5. Take a photograph of the bite in CO. If there is a big discrepancy, take two photographs: one that shows the bite in CO and one that shows the bite in CR.

Lateral view evaluation

The Sn vertical, constructed from the true horizontal while the patient is placed in NHP, is a good tool to assess the AP contour of the soft tissue profile.[34] A lateral picture or cephalogram should be recorded to apply this method to the evaluation, diagnosis, and treatment planning of orthodontic and orthognathic surgical cases.

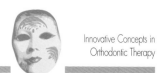

Innovative Concepts in
Orthodontic Therapy

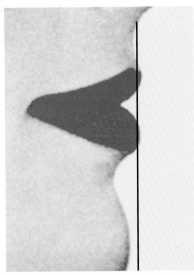

Fig 11-18 The Sn vertical, recorded in NHP, is a tool to determine the AP position of salient soft tissue points that reflect the underlying sagittal position of skeletal and dental structures.

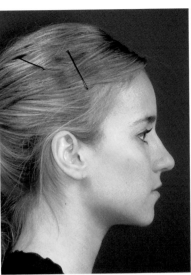

Fig 11-19 A balance must exist between nose, lips, and chin to achieve a pleasant profile.

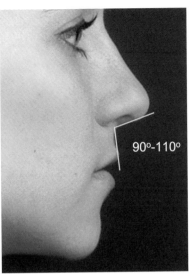

Fig 11-20 On profile view, the nasal projection, rotation, and length, in addition to the nasofrontal, nasofacial, and nasolabial angles, can be more closely evaluated.

To form a diagnosis, the Sn vertical is used to determine the AP position of salient soft tissue points that reflect the underlying sagittal position of skeletal and dental structures (Fig 11-18). This can reveal discrepancies such as maxillary protrusion or retrusion, mandibular protrusion or retrusion, or a combination of the two.[35,36]

The orthodontist may also incorporate the vertical plane into a visualized treatment objective based on an understanding of soft tissue response to tooth movement. Unlike other sagittal methods, the Sn vertical method of soft tissue assessment does not depend on the position of the chin.

Facial profile

Analysis of the facial profile focuses on the relationship between the nose, upper lip, lower lip, and chin.[37] These structures determine the overall harmony of the facial lateral view (Fig 11-19). The profile may be straight, concave, or convex. Convexity could result from labial protrusion or deficient chin projection.

Nose

A relatively large nose can give the impression of a retruded mouth and a convex profile. A snub nose will produce a more prominent nasolabial angle.[38]

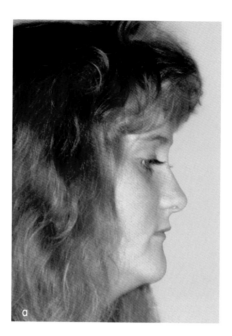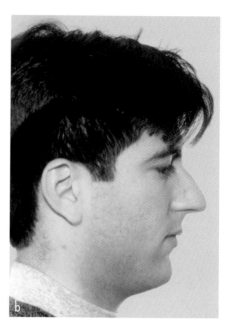

Figs 11-21a and 11-21b A normal nasolabial angle is between 90 degrees and 110 degrees.

On profile view, an evaluation is performed of the nasal projection, rotation, and length as well as the nasofrontal, nasofacial, and nasolabial angles (Fig 11-20). The nasofrontal angle is formed at the N by lines that extend from this point to the glabella (Gl) and to the nasal tip (Pn). Ideally, this angle will measure 120 degrees to 135 degrees. The position of the vertex of this angle (N) is also important because a higher or lower vertex indicates a longer or shorter nose, respectively. Its usual position is along the same vertical plane as the superior limbus of the eye.

Another method involves the nasofacial angle, which is formed by a line along the nasal dorsum that intersects a line from the Gl to the pogonion (Pg). The ideal nasofacial angle is 36 degrees. Nasal length, height, and projection may also be examined simultaneously by creating a right triangle between the alar groove, the PN, and the N. The projection, height, and length are represented in the triangle by sides with a ratio of 3:4:5, respectively.

Nasolabial angle

The average nasolabial angle, which is formed by lines along the columella and upper lip that intersect at the Sn, measures between 90 degrees and 110 degrees (Fig 11-21). Rotation of the nasal tip (lobule) can be assessed by evaluation of this angle. The ideal nasolabial angle for women is 100 degrees to 120 degrees; for men, it is 90 degrees to 105 degrees. Because dental or skeletal malformations of the maxilla influence this angle, it serves as a reference point to plan necessary corrections.[39]

An easy but often inaccurate method to determine nasal tip projection involves comparison of the nasolabial angle to the Sn-VS; the two should be roughly equal. The fault with this technique lies in the variabil-

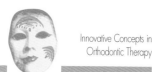

Innovative Concepts in
Orthodontic Therapy

ity of upper lip length. The alar and lobular lengths should be equal and 2 to 4 mm of columella should show. When viewed from below, the nose should have the shape of an equilateral triangle and the columella should be approximately twice as long as the lobule. The lobule should be 75% as wide as the alar base and the nostrils should be roughly pear-shaped.

Maxilla and mandible

The positions of the maxilla and mandible in sagittal view are evaluated with the patient in NHP. The relationship between the mandible and the maxilla is assessed with the mandible held back approximately 2 to 4 mm (Fig 11-22).

Lip outline

To evaluate the AP position of structures below the nose—eg, upper lip, lower lip, mentolabial sulcus, and Pg—all linear measurements are taken from a true vertical reference plane constructed perpendicular to the true horizontal through the Sn. This line has the smallest standard deviation among intracranial and extracranial assessment methods.[32]

Upper lip. The upper lip projects 3 to 5 mm anterior to the Sn vertical and is generally 0.5 mm more anterior in females than in males (Fig 11-23). This supports previous reports that female upper lips are naturally more protrusive than those of males.[37]

Lower lip. The lower lip is normally supported mainly by the maxillary incisors. In a balanced profile, it lies 2 to 3 mm posterior to the upper lip (see Fig 11-23).

Mentolabial sulcus

The mentolabial sulcus is located posterior to the Sn vertical in both males and females. The sulcus of females is about 2 mm anterior to that of males.[40]

Pogonion

In both sexes, the soft tissue pogonion (Pg) is posterior to the Sn vertical; the male Pg is about 0.5 mm more posterior than that of the female. The average for both sexes is between 1 and 5 mm behind the vertical (see Fig 11-23).

From the preceding comparisons, it may be concluded that, compared with males, females generally have slightly fuller lip regions, shallower labial sulci, and chins that are at least as relatively prominent. The latter observation is contrary to current clinical thinking. The male chin appears to be more prominent because the lips are not as full and the labial sulcus is more pronounced. Stated conversely, the female chin appears relatively less prominent because the female lips protrude more and the labial sulcus is shallower than those of males.[34]

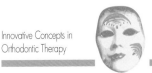

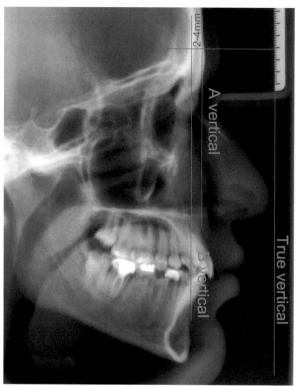

Fig 11-22 Linear maxillomandibular measurements as well as measurements of soft tissues from the lower part of the face are taken from a true vertical reference plane constructed perpendicular to the true horizontal through the Sn. This vertical reference line has the smallest standard deviation among intracranial and extracranial assessment methods.

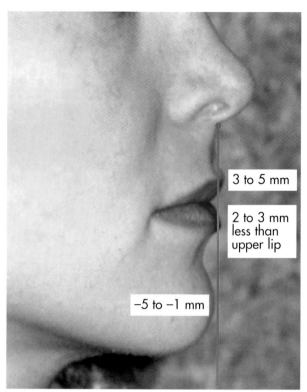

Fig 11-23 Women generally have slightly fuller lip regions and shallower labial sulci than men, and chins that are at least as relatively prominent as those of men. On average, the female upper lip extends 3 to 5 mm anteriorly past the vertical reference plane. The lower lip is 2 to 3 mm less anterior than the upper lip, and the chin is 1 to 5 mm posterior to the vertical.

Gonial angle

This sharp angle occurs where the masseter muscle attaches to the jaw. A square facial appearance can result from masseter muscle hypertrophy but can also be due to posterior projection and lateral flaring of the mandibular angle.

In 1972, Björk and Skieller reported that when superimposing on mandibular implants in low-angle Class II, division 2 cases, there tends to be considerable resorption of the inferior border of the mandible near the gonion (Go).[41] In theory, this would produce an *increase* in the gonial angle, yet clinically these are the cases where considerable *reduction* of the gonial angle is usually seen instead. This remains a conundrum and tells us that we have much to learn about the growth of the mandible.

Chin-neck angle

The typical range for the chin–neck angle is 80 degrees to 95 degrees. The exact angle is influenced by the quantity and shape of submental adipose tissue. When the chin is retracted, the submental tissues are more pronounced. When the chin comes forward, the opposite occurs. Profiles judged as more beautiful usually show an acute chin-neck angle.

Conclusion

The proper function of all living things is to preserve form and maintain quality of life. One of the challenges clinicians face is that although humans now live longer than ever before, they have not adjusted to the significance of function; rather, the current understanding of maxillofacial dysgnathias focuses on form, which changes with time and environmental factors. Future research must concentrate on the improvement of early treatment strategies that restore and prolong the dynamics of function for a healthier and longer life.

Specialists in orthodontics, oral surgery, and related dental fields should continue to evolve apace with contemporary technology and adapt to the fascinating changes and challenges of modern medicine. Dentistry has always strived to meet established yet theoretical goals, and the search for new treatments that result in more successful outcomes in all patients should persist so that concepts of ideal esthetics and function can be put into practice. Incorporation of techniques originally used in other medical fields, such as osteodistraction, has allowed breakthroughs in the treatment of maxillomandibular disharmony and other dysfunctions. An awareness of the elements that affect craniofacial esthetics, combined with an understanding of how form follows function in the lower face, will lead to more accurate diagnoses and treatment plans that provide patients with a healthy dentition for life. From day 1 of a clinician's education, such goals should exert a daily influence on how professional duties are performed.

If functional changes to the dentofacial complex that provide good occlusion and sound TMJs can be achieved orthodontically in a reasonable time and without compromise in facial esthetics, stability, or periodontal health, then surgery is not necessary. With dedication to research and attentive treatment planning, successful achievement of this goal is within the grasp of all clinicians.

Acknowledgment

The authors would like to acknowledge the contributions of Carlos F. Navarro IV, BS, to this chapter.

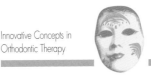

References

1. Burstone CJ. The integumental profile. Am J Orthod 1958;44:1–25.
2. Barker P, Goldstein BR. Theological foundations of Kepler's astronomy. Osiris 2001;16:88–113.
3. De Gandt F. Force and Geometry in Newton's Principia. Wilson C (trans). Princeton: Princeton University Press, 1995.
4. Field JV. Kepler's Geometrical Cosmology. Chicago: Chicago University Press, 1988.
5. Kepler J. The Six-Cornered Snowflake. Hardie C (trans). Oxford: Clarendon Press, 1966.
6. Grimm RE. The autobiography of Leonardo Pisano. Fibonacci Quarterly 1973;11(1):99–104.
7. Singh P. Acharya Hemachandra and the (so called) Fibonacci Numbers. Math Ed (Siwan) 1986;20(1):28–30.
8. Da Vinci L. Leonardo on the Human Body. O'Malley CD, Saunders JB de CM (trans). New York: Dover, 1983.
9. Da Vinci L. The Notebooks of Leonardo da Vinci. Richter JP (trans). New York: Dover, 1970.
10. Boyer CB, Merzbach UC. A History of Mathematics, ed 2. Hoboken: John Wiley & Sons, 1991.
11. Herzberg BL. Facial esthetics in relation to orthodontic treatment. Angle Orthod 1952;22(1):3–22.
12. Tweed CH. The Frankfort-mandibular incisor angle (FMIA) in orthodontic diagnosis, treatment planning and prognosis. Angle Orthod 1954;24(3):121–169.
13. Gregoret J, Tuber E, Escobar LHP, da Fonseca AM. Ortodoncia y Cirugía Ortognática: Diagnostico y Planificación, ed 2. Madrid: NM Ediciones, 2008.
14. Jacobson A. The proportionate template as a diagnostic aid. Am J Orthod 1979;75(2): 156–172.
15. Ricketts RM. Planning treatment on the basis of the facial pattern and an estimate of its growth. Angle Orthod 1957;27:14–37.
16. Neger M. A quantitative method for the evaluation of the soft-tissue facial profile. Am J Orthod 1959;45(10):738–751.
17. Merrifield LL. The profile line as an aid in critically evaluating facial esthetics. Am J Orthod 1966;52(11):804–822.
18. Wuerpel EH. On facial balance and harmony. Angle Orthod 1936;7(2):81–89.
19. Cole SC. Natural head position, posture, and prognathism: The Chapman Prize Essay. Br J Orthod 1988;15(4): 227–239.
20. González-Ulloa M, Stevens E. The role of chin correction on profileplasty. Plast Reconstr Surg 1968;41(5):477–486.
21. Jacobs JD. Vertical lip changes from maxillary incisor retraction. Am J Orthod 1978;74(4):396–404.
22. Burstone CJ, James RB, Legan H, Murphy GA, Norton LA. Cephalometrics for orthognathic surgery. J Oral Surg 1978;36(4):269–277.
23. Cabrera CAG, Cabrera M. Clinical Orthodontics. Curitiba, Brazil: Editora e Produções Interativas, 2004.
24. Peck H, Peck S. A concept of facial esthetics. Angle Orthod 1970;40(4):284–318.
25. Garner LD. Soft tissue changes concurrent with orthodontic tooth movement. Am J Orthod 1974;66(4):367–377.
26. Roth RH. The Roth Functional Occlusion Approach (course syllabus). Burlingame, CA: Roth-Williams Center for Functional Occlusion, 1999.
27. Echarri P. Diagnostico en Ortodoncia: Estudio Multidisciplinario. Barcelona: Quintessence, 1998.
28. Foster TD, Howat AP, Naish PJ. Variation in cephalometric reference lines. Br J Orthod 1981;8(4):183–187.
29. Riedel RA. An analysis of dentofacial relationships. Am J Orthod 1957;43: 103–119.
30. Angle EH. Treatment of Malocclusion of the Teeth: Angle's System. Philadelphia: S. S. White Dental Manufacturing Company, 1907.

Innovative Concepts in
Orthodontic Therapy

31. Fushima K, Inui M, Sato S. Dental asymmetry in temporomandibular disorders. J Oral Rehabil 1999;26(9):752–756.

32. Subtelny JD. The soft tissue profile, growth and treatment changes. Angle Orthod 1959;31(2):105–122.

33. Farkas LG, Katic MJ, Hreczko TA, Deutsch C, Munro IR. Anthropometric proportions in the upper lip-lower lip-chin area of the lower face in young white adults. Am J Orthod 1984;86(1):52–60.

34. Hoefflin SM. The labial ledge. Aesthet Surg J 2002;22(2):177–180.

35. Wylie WL. The mandibular incisor—Its role in facial esthetics. Angle Orthod 1955;25:32–41.

36. Hershey HG. Incisor tooth retraction and subsequent profile change in postadolescent female patients. Am J Orthod 1972;61(1):45–54.

37. Spradley FL, Jacobs JD, Crowe DP. Assessment of the anteroposterior soft-tissue contour of the lower facial third in the ideal young adult. Am J Orthod 1981;79(3):316–325.

38. Subtelny J. A longitudinal study of soft tissue facial structures and their profile characteristics, defined in relation to underlying skeletal structures. Am J Orthod 1959;45(7):481–507.

39. Stoner MM. A photometric analysis of the facial profile: A method of assessing facial change induced by orthodontic treatment. Am J Orthod 1955;41(6):453–469.

40. Burstone C. Lip posture and its significance in treatment planning. Am J Orthod 1967 Apr;53(4):262–284.

41. Björk A, Skieller V. Facial development and tooth eruption. An implant study at the age of puberty. Am J Orthod 1972;62(4):339–383.

Harmony of the Oral Components

12

Marco A. Navarro, DDS, MS

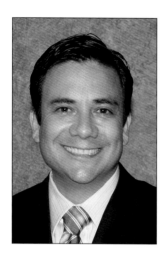

Marco A. Navarro, DDS, MS

Marco A. Navarro earned his DDS from the University of Nuevo Leon, Mexico in 1994 and his certificate in orthodontics and MS from the University of Detroit Mercy in 1999. He completed his advanced education in orthodontics (AEO) at the Roth-Williams Center in 2002. Dr Navarro is associate professor in the Graduate Orthodontic Program at the University of Nuevo Leon, Mexico. He maintains private orthodontics practices in Dallas, Texas, and in Mexico.

Email: marconavarro@mac.com

Harmony and timing—as all musicians well know—are essential to creating balanced and melodious acoustics. Each instrument in a musical ensemble, like each element of the stomatognathic system, plays a crucial role in the creation of the overall harmony in every performance. When one instrument is out of tune or one musician is out of rhythm, potential harmony becomes chaotic. The balance and synchronicity of the human body in homeostasis is a significantly complex and beautiful example of true harmonic functioning.

In the field of orthodontics, the harmonious balance of the stomatognathic system is the goal of every treatment. To achieve that goal, the clinician must completely understand the function of each part of the system so that it can be properly restored when its harmony has been compromised. A clinician must survey each part of the mouth as an individual element of the entire system and develop a treatment plan that specifically addresses the needs of each essential part to restore the system as a whole.

This chapter describes, with a clinical case as an example, how to achieve a healthy, functional stomatognathic system through orthodontics and interdisciplinary treatments. The relationship of support structures, function, and mastication are discussed in terms of how they contribute to a final schema. The orthodontic paradigm of balance and harmony and their connection with esthetics has changed; a new rhythm has been developed for the new millennium. It is important to maintain an open mind and consider new developments from the leaders of this specialty regarding treatment objectives, clinical research, and a unification of treatment criteria. Additional technology must be adopted and precise instrumentation used to create more accurate diagnoses of our patients. Simplified treatment mechanics using exotic alloys and auxiliaries such as miniscrew implants for cortical anchorage will result in infinite possibilities for improved treatment planning, reduced chair time, and increased comfort. These and other developments are currently being explored by numerous authors and reported in dental and orthodontic journals.

Concepts of Initial Diagnosis

The harmony and function of the stomatognathic system requires that no anatomic and supporting structures show signs of physical or structural damage if they are to work together with minimal stress during functional movements. Orthodontic specialists generally agree that the six keys of occlusion enumerated by Dr Andrews provide the goal for a static occlusion.[1] An ideal static occlusal relationship should result in an ideal functional occlusion, but this is not always the case. The functional aspects of the mouth tend to be overlooked.

The temporomandibular joints (TMJs), supporting bone, teeth, and muscles interact constantly and, given the ideal conditions, should last for a lifetime. When teeth do not have a protected occlusion during eccentric movements, signs and symptoms of dysfunction can start to appear. These symptoms depend on the type of disharmony and the patient's adaptive capacity and tolerance level.[2] It is important to remember that not all cases that look good function well.

Many authors have researched untreated ideal dental and facial esthetics and established cephalometric and dental guidelines to mimic what an ideal dental finished result should look like. The goal is to imitate the more beautiful and functional forms of nature, and almost everything has been studied across the various dental specialties. This ongoing research provides great amounts of data to incorporate into our clinical and theoretical knowledge.

While it is healthy for orthodontists to question some of the ongoing research projects, it is also necessary to incorporate new and existing technologies to create more esthetic and functional results. For example, the semiadjustable articulator has been used by other specialties for many years now, but orthodontists still reserve its use for only the "difficult" cases. This wonderful diagnostic tool allows clinicians to evaluate the static and functional (working and nonworking interferences) positions of the teeth during assessment of vertical dimension, anteroposterior positions, and transverse relations of the teeth and arches (Fig 12-1). But most importantly, the articulator provides a repeatable reference or starting point that can be used at any time during orthodontic treatment to reassess progress and treatment goals.[3] To achieve the best esthetic and functional result, its use should never be neglected. New technologies like cone beam computed tomography (Fig 12-2) allow advantages such as better interpretation of craniomandibular relationships, bone health, TMJs, and ideal location for cortical anchorage, with precision that orthodontists could have only dreamed of a few years ago. Archwires made from different alloys, in combination with self-ligating brackets, provide gentler and more directed forces to teeth with single or multiple roots. The use of these improvements in orthodontic materials provides gentler forces and less chair and treatment time. When all of this wonderful technology is combined with a sound diagnosis, treatment plans are usually transferred to clinical application with such precision that ideal outcomes can easily be predicted.

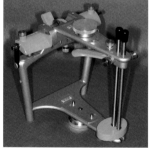

Fig 12-1 The relationship of teeth, TMJs, and neuromuscular systems is being increasingly recognized as an important factor in fixed prosthodontics. Currently, the need has increased among orthodontists for user-friendly articulators that simulate individual patient characteristics such as jaw movements.

Components of Jaw and Dental Function

In the visualization of an ideal finished case, one can imagine *(1)* beautiful dental anatomy; *(2)* ideal tooth crown lengths and widths with no signs of occlusal or incisal wear; *(3)* perfect gingival contour; *(4)* excel-

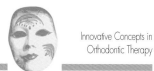

Innovative Concepts in
Orthodontic Therapy

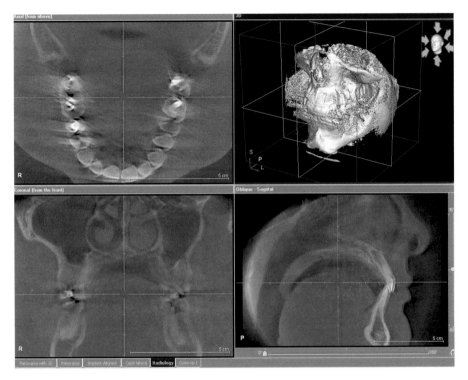

Fig 12-2 Cone beam computed tomography (CBCT) has many advantages over simple panoramic film and digital images, including accurate visualization of head and neck structures and reduction of x-ray doses. It has been rapidly adopted and is becoming the standard of care for several applications, and a preferred technique for others.

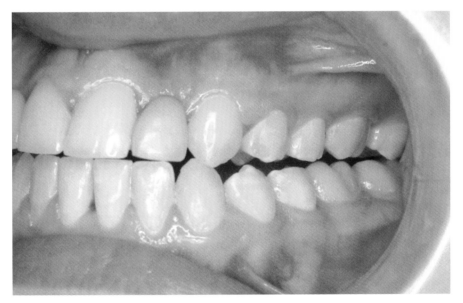

Fig 12-3 To achieve optimal functional occlusion, the teeth should be positioned so that they create what has been termed a mutually protected articulation. In this occlusal scheme, the posterior teeth protect anterior teeth from lateral stress at full closure, and the anterior teeth protect posterior teeth from lateral stress during mandibular movements, provided that the condyles are permitted a gliding movement along the eminentia. The anterior teeth and canines provide a gentle guide ramp that both allows the condyles to traverse the eminentia and discludes the posterior teeth on the working and balancing sides.

lent bone support; *(5)* a symmetric smile line; *(6)* splendid posterior intercuspation with anatomical sharp cusps that will provide great stability to their counterparts in occlusion; and *(7)* adequate anterior overlap and overjet that will provide at least 2 to 3 mm of posterior clearance during protrusive and lateral mandibular movement (ie, mutually protected articulation). This occlusal scheme, free of any maximal intercuspation–centric relation (MI-CR) discrepancies, avoids occlusal interferences during function (Fig 12-3). This allows the condyle to travel smoothly along the eminence and reduces adverse muscle activity. However, if a patient displays evidence of severe bruxism with periodontal problems and altered passive eruption, the ideal result for that particular patient is hardly the same as that previously described. This is the challenge that clinicians face when adults present for treatment. In previous years, most adults viewed orthodontic therapy as an extravagant cosmetic procedure. Recently, though, adults have begun to realize that a properly treated occlusion is just as beneficial for them as for teenagers.

When an adult patient does not have any of the adequate characteristics of a young dentition (ie, free of pathology, damage, or wear), it becomes increasingly important to understand that ideal tooth anatomy, ideal condylar position, and muscle balance play a crucial role in the attainment of an excellent result. Therefore, orthodontists must thoroughly comprehend how the harmony and balance of the stomatognathic system work before it can be treated.

In their static position, the condyles should be centered transversely against the articular eminence, with the disc interposed and as far upward as possible—this is now generally accepted as the stable condylar position. The maxillary teeth contact their opposing arch as the result of the functional movements of the mandible through muscular triggering, then the TMJs should be able to receive the load of the masticatory muscles without any excessive compression or being forced out of the glenoid fossa. The condyles should be able to move freely during function so that they glide with the discs against the articular eminence during mandibular movements from a static starting position. Ideal function can be disturbed if the dentition presents occlusal interferences or fulcrums that alter the lateral excursions of the mandible. It is well documented that these premature contacts can cause muscular imbalance. Proprioceptors located in the periodontal ligament can cause muscle splinting or cause the mandible to change or shift into an acquired muscular position to avoid these occlusal interferences.[4]

Longevity of the dentition has been connected to an ideal mutually protected occlusion, so restorative guidelines have been established with the following criteria to properly restore a dentition or perform orthodontic movements:

- 3 to 4 mm of overbite to provide for adequate anterior guidance
- 2 to 3 mm of overjet
- 1 mm of canine overjet with 4 to 5 mm of canine overbite
- Centric stops for all centric cusps
- Ideal anatomic form with sharp cusps and deep fossae

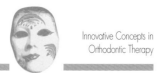

Innovative Concepts in
Orthodontic Therapy

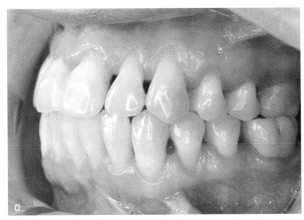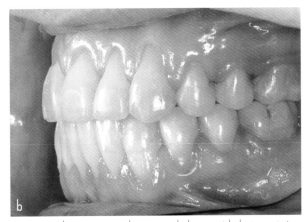

Figs 12-4a and 12-4b Interproximal reduction is indicated in nonextraction cases where some overbite is needed to provide better anterior guidance and where the crowns are overcontoured with an accurate amount of interdental bone and a good periodontal status. Lingual movement of the anterior mandibular teeth provides a deep enough overbite for adequate posterior clearance. This patient received periodontal therapy (before, a) and is ready for graft surgery (after, b).

This mutually protected articulation establishes that the anterior teeth protect the posterior teeth and the TMJ during eccentric movements, while the posterior teeth and the TMJ in turn protect the anterior teeth during mandibular closure. The canines prevent interferences during lateral movement of the mandible; their major role is to guide the mandible during the chewing stroke. During protrusive movement, the anterior teeth prevent posterior interferences in the mandible. Some authors suggest that the anterior teeth should have light or no anterior contact in MI position.[2]

Ideal posterior anatomy with good cusp heights provides adequate distribution of the occlusal forces through the periodontium and bone, resulting in better stability. Ideal anterior tooth anatomy facilitates the guidance of the mandible during protrusive and canine guidance. If the anterior teeth are worn, the amount of overjet is increased due to the passive eruption of the teeth, thus providing less space for the mandibular teeth. As an abraded tooth passively erupts to make contact with its counterparts, there is no longer a sharp cusp tip or sharp incisal edge. Depending on the degree of incisal wear, the buccolingual aspect of the tooth is now thicker, so the amount of posterior clearance from the contact point also is reduced. As a result, the mandibular incisors may be tipped lingually or the maxillary incisors displaced buccally. If the anterior teeth are intruded slightly, then the anterior guidance is compromised or nonexistent. If orthodontic treatment is to be performed without any restorative plan, only a good amount of interproximal reduction to move the mandibular anterior teeth lingually will provide a deep enough overbite for adequate posterior clearance. One should look to restore the dentition to its ideal anatomy to provide ideal harmony between functional and esthetic results (Fig 12-4).

As passive eruption occurs, a single tooth or group of teeth will migrate coronally, creating a contact from a cusp point to an area of contact. This will yield to a greater amount of force to be delivered to an opposing tooth, which leads to abfractions, tooth hypermobility, loss of attachment, or loss of supporting bone. The clinician then faces the dilemma of *(1)* a crown elongation with or without root canal treatment so that adequate space can be provided for the restoration that will recreate the anatomy or *(2)* intrusion of the tooth a certain distance to provide adequate space for an ideal preparation and subsequent ideal anatomic restoration.

From an esthetic point of view, irregular gingival margins, where a short tooth appears next to a longer one, are not pleasing to the eye, even with healthy periodontal tissues. Some cases (eg, passive eruption where gingival tissues migrate with the tooth) will necessitate gingivectomy with or without osseous removal, depending on crestal bone height. In other cases, a tooth that has been extruded due to incisal wear may display proper harmony with the supporting osseous structure, attached gingiva, and healthy periodontal ligaments but will still look short in relation to the adjacent teeth. This tooth may require orthodontic intrusion to accommodate and develop gingival symmetry to the gingival margins. Positive coronoplasty can restore the tooth or teeth to the anatomy required for ideal function and esthetics.

Adult patients pose a significant challenge to be treated only by the orthodontic specialist since most of these cases do not have ideal anatomy of the teeth or overall dental health, unlike the young adult or teen patients who present for treatment. Most of the time, adults present with missing teeth, gingival recession, bone loss due to periodontal problems, substantial wear, tooth mobility or migration, or discolored or stained teeth.

When adult patients are diagnosed and a treatment plan created, the clinician knows the results may be compromised either in function, esthetics, or stability. Therefore, the first steps in treating adults are to *(1)* evaluate the chief complaint, *(2)* ensure that the expectations of the patient can be met, *(3)* address the cause of the disease, and *(4)* seek the appropriate interdisciplinary consultation. One should strive for the best result possible and present an ideal treatment plan. It is ultimately the patient's decision whether or not to accept treatment.

Cases need to be evaluated with functional dental records so that the most stable position of the jaw can be located and tooth contact positions recorded (Fig 12-5). The only way to achieve this is to mount the case on an articulator, evaluate the amount of discrepancy from CR (stable condylar position) to MI, and then address the cusp-fossa relationship, vertical dimension of occlusion (VDO) or first contact during mandibular closure, and balancing or working side interferences during mandibular eccentric movement.

In cases where the amount of the discrepancy between CR and MI is large or myofascial pain is present, an occlusal splint will be necessary

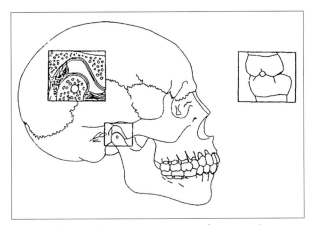

Fig 12-5 The mandible acquires a position of accommodation when a contact interference moves the condyles out of the fossae. Occlusion determines the condyle position. Occlusion and articulation are interdependent.

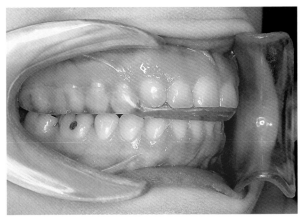

Fig 12-6 Splint therapy before orthodontic treatment is directed toward the realignment of the mandible to the skull, stabilization of the right and left TMJs, reduction of stress to the right and left TMJs, restoration to normal physiologic function, and reduction of muscle hyperactivity.

to relax the musculature and allow the condyles to achieve a stable condylar position (Fig 12-6). The orthodontic diagnosis should be made from this position once the mandible no longer appears to be repositioning after continuous use of splint therapy. This has to be corroborated or evaluated by the use of a condylar position indicator (CPI).

If the purpose of treatment is long-lasting function and esthetics, then a stable condylar position with coincident CR and MI should be the goal. Diagnosis and treatment planning should be performed from this position with proper mounted records that may allow for the following:

- Diagnostic cast setups
- Diagnostic wax-up of fractured or abraded teeth with genetic tooth form
- Negative coronoplasty
- Sectional casts
- Diagnostic model surgery
- Crown elongation, extrusion, or intrusion

The limitations of treatment are fewer when the orthodontist seeks an interdisciplinary approach with periodontists, prosthodontists, and maxillofacial surgeons who understand the gnathologic concepts of occlusion. Treatments should commence with a definite result in mind, rather than with the ideal result left to luck or chance. Every aspect of treatment has to be carefully diagnosed and reviewed by each member of the team. Once each clinician has a goal that has been agreed upon, treatment can begin. The possibilities have never been more numerous in dentistry, and specialists cannot limit themselves by neglecting to offer multidisciplinary treatment.

Tooth Anatomy and Its Relation to Ideal Function

Lee listed the primary functions of teeth as follows[2]:

1. Mastication
2. Swallowing
3. Speech
4. Expression
5. Psychologic well-being
6. Esthetics
7. Craniomandibular stabilization

Every one of these functions should be considered when planning treatment and examined in terms of how they are influenced by the anatomy of the teeth.

Occlusal wear in the adult patient has been misunderstood. Is it normal to have occlusal wear? What does "normal" mean? At what point does occlusal wear progress to a traumatic occlusion? What is the difference between tooth alignment treatment and a treatment looking for a functional occlusion? Intact tooth anatomy in the adult is necessary to achieve good esthetics as well as function. Teeth without excessive occlusal wear can reveal a wealth of information related to functional occlusion. The following description of the anatomy of some teeth does not purport to be complete but rather highlights some significant morphologic factors relating to oral function and esthetics that perhaps have been overlooked.

Mandibular incisors are a physiologic cornerstone for good occlusion. These teeth are essential to good anterior guidance; it is almost impossible to have a long-lasting, nontraumatic, functional occlusion without adequate clinical crown lengths of these teeth. Intact mandibular incisors, alone or in a mutually protected articulation, play a role in anterior guidance that could not be duplicated if they were abraded or if other teeth attempted to substitute (Fig 12-7).

Unworn incisal edges of mandibular teeth and the steep lingual aspects of maxillary anterior teeth produce greater clearance in protrusive excursions. This allows the posterior cusps freedom from interferences in physiologic movements and reduces the chances of wear of the posterior teeth.

The lingual fossa of the maxillary incisor also allows space for protrusive and lateral cycling movements of the mandibular incisors during mastication. In cases where the marginal ridges of these teeth are too pronounced, an enameloplasty has to be performed to obtain a proper overjet relationship, so the function will not be altered. The focus of this tooth's function in anterior guidance lies in the steepness of its lingual face and the torque of the crown. Because of its position as the most

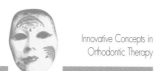

Innovative Concepts in
Orthodontic Therapy

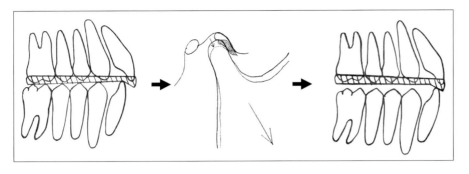

Fig 12-7 An occlusal splint helps to reproduce the performance of the anterior guide in a mutually protected articulation. The movement is coordinated between the tooth surfaces and the condyle-disc-eminence complex.

prominent anterior tooth, the maxillary incisor plays a fundamental role in esthetics. A tooth with correct crown length gives confidence to the patient when smiling.

It may be helpful to think of the canine and premolar teeth as the "canine area." The large buccal cusps of these teeth are important in medial guidance by the chewing side teeth: They guide the lateral mandibular movements in a more vertical manner in the coronal (anterior plane) and are the major factors in preventing harmful posterior contacts of the non–chewing side teeth (canine guidance).

Any alteration to tooth position and form that does not adequately follow the recommended interocclusal relationship may lead to traumatic occlusion, which would overload the system and eventually produce tooth wear, myofascial pain, or muscle spasm, among other consequences, all of which could jeopardize the patient's quality of life.

Traumatic Occlusion

Traumatic occlusion may be defined as any closure of the teeth that produces visible or nonvisible unphysiologic stress, damage, or overload of the teeth, joint, muscles, bones, periodontium, or nervous system. The signs and symptoms of traumatic occlusion include the following:

- Abrasion and fractures of teeth, dental restorations, or prostheses
- Craniofacial pain (myalgia)
- TMJ dysfunction
- Tooth migration or mobility
- Overload on the periodontium
- Exostoses

Of the border interferences, those on the nonworking side usually have the greatest impact on the neuromuscular system, resulting in excessive wear on anterior teeth from avoidance patterns. In addition to occlusal interferences, flat occlusal morphology in artificial crowns and natural teeth is also a cause of traumatic occlusion through overload.

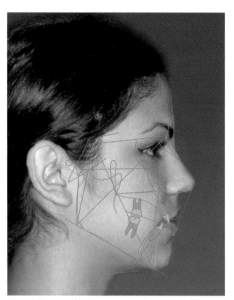

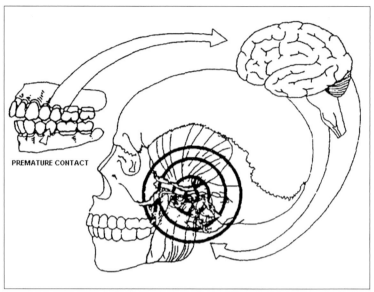

Fig 12-8 A profile picture was taken with the patient in MI; a cephalometric tracing was superimposed over the picture to reveal the centric occlusion to CR (CO-CR) discrepancy. The discrepancy was found in the mounted casts and was transferred to the cephalometrics through a procedure known as CO-CR conversion.

Fig 12-9 It has been demonstrated that any change in the occlusion produces a change in the proprioceptive input, which would be captured by periodontal proprioceptors. This is transmitted by the primary afferent neuron to the central nervous system (CNS), which in turn would change the neuromuscular response through motor neurons. This situation can be detected and recorded electromyographically.

Original natural tooth morphology per se is not the cause of traumatic occlusion. The majority of occlusal problems are created by the relationship of the mandibular teeth to the maxillary teeth as the jaws close. Poor relationships of the teeth may result from skeletal disharmonies, abnormal habits, missing teeth and subsequent tooth drift, worn teeth, iatrogenic causes, or other etiologies.

Most of the time, the mandible is in a position of accommodation (Fig 12-8). It is a hidden fact that the bearer of a malocclusion develops a pattern of neuromuscular protection to avoid interferences.[5] This pattern of protection is the result of feedback that begins in neuromuscular receptors located in the muscles of mastication, tendons, TMJs, and periodontium. The feedback communicates through the mesencephalic nuclei of the trigeminal nerve[6] (Fig 12-9). Of all these receptors, the most influential are the periodontal receivers. Shore states that 90% of the nerve endings responsible for proprioception are located inside the periodontal ligament, and these govern the jaw position.[7] According to Shore, the sensitivity of proprioceptors located in the periodontal ligament and muscles of mastication is so great that they are able to perceive differences of a fraction of a millimeter in thickness. Any abnormality or occlusal disturbance that alters the anatomical mandibular closure will initiate an immediate

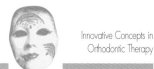

Innovative Concepts in
Orthodontic Therapy

response from the neuromuscular system. Consequently, occlusion determines condylar position. The interferences that cause this change are known as *occlusal prematurity*, and they can cause the mandible to reposition to avoid any premature contact. The resulting dental relationship seen clinically is dictated by the occlusion; therefore, it can be concluded that these occlusal prematurities can causes a neuromuscular response.

Among the consequences of a change in mandibular position are three main concepts to remember:

1. The mandible is no longer in its true position, and any diagnosis based on the new position will be wrong.
2. Extra jaw muscle activity is required to accommodate the mandible in its new position; when sustained, this extra activity can initiate muscle dysfunction.
3. The altered mandibular position will produce an abnormal relationship of the condyle-disc complex to the glenoid fossae, which has been considered a predisposing factor for TMJ dysfunction.

Sometimes, the mandible closes by passing through the occlusal prematurity, which will produce a sliding translational movement. Over time, the neuromusculature will "jump" the interference and move directly to the position of accommodation, producing a discrepancy between CR and centric occlusion (CO), the latter of which prevails. This is the relationship seen when patients are asked to bite in their usual position or when study casts are aligned by hand. Neither situation, however, gives any information on the position of the condyle-disc complex inside the glenoid fossae. It definitely does not indicate whether or not the mandible is in its true position.

This is just one benefit of mounting every single case on the articulator. Another benefit is that the articulator enables orthodontists to visually locate interference points or pathways of occlusal disharmony. If a clinician wants to evaluate an occlusion in CR, an articulator is a necessary means of diagnosis that permits evaluation of the condyle in the terminal closure position of the mandible during and after treatment. An occlusal disharmony cannot be studied or diagnosed in the mouth because the neuromusculature compensates for the mandible's disharmony in closing and in eccentric movements. To treat patients using CR as a basis, a diagnostic cast should first be made in CR so that the real mandibular position, previously camouflaged by neuromusculature, is revealed. Due to the articulator's lack of nerves, muscles, and ligaments, it is able to show malocclusions that otherwise could not be produced. This is perhaps the most important feature that an articulator can offer. It is possible that malocclusion is present in a majority of patients but is hidden by the neuromusculature.

Centric Relation

Vast written material about CR is available. Current knowledge indicates that CR occurs when the condyles are in their most superoanterior position in the articular fossae, resting against the posterior slopes of the articular eminence, with the articular disc properly interposed.[8–12] This position is determined by the muscles and has proved to be the most stable mandibular position.

Once the most orthopedically stable joint position has been located, the elevator muscles contract strongly (assuming no occlusal interferences) to maintain this stability. This position is therefore considered the most musculoskeletally stable position of the mandible. The articular surfaces and tissues of the joint are aligned so that forces applied by the musculature do not cause any damage.

The CR position has been found clinically to be the best location for MI.[3,13,14] Whenever MI does not occur at centric occlusion, there are always posterior occlusal interferences in lateral border mandibular movements with subsequent avoidance patterns.[15] Good posterior crown morphology and a proper anterior overbite reinforce the integrity of the discs of the TMJ each time the teeth are brought together in full occlusion in CR. This MI-CR relationship not only helps stabilize the condyle-disc complex in CR position in the fossa, it also helps maintain total craniomandibular stability.

Complete occlusion of the teeth is a specialized articulation of the craniomandibular system, and it can have a profound effect on the alignment and stability of the total craniomandibular articulation complex, including the maxillary and temporal bones and the TMJ. The teeth make full contact with the condyles in the CR position approximately 5,000 times per day. Swallowing helps to realign and stabilize the craniomandibular relationship into a state of biologic equilibrium, which is important for the comfort, function, and longevity of dental restorations.[16–18] A maxillary anterior guided occlusal splint that is properly constructed, adjusted, and maintained is probably the best tool to align and stabilize the mandible and its condylar relationship before the occlusion is treated and the true articulation of the teeth is identified.

In every case that the author plans, one goal is to create a treatment that results in an equal CO-CR relationship or that, at the very least, does not increase an existing CO-CR discrepancy. From a neuromuscular aspect, MI needs to occur with the condyles in their more orthopedic position (CR), or what could be called *centric relation occlusion* (CRO). When CRO is achieved, it is obvious that neuromuscular adaptation is not necessary if the position of the teeth allows an uninterrupted mandibular closure. In this way, unnecessary stress or overload is not introduced in the stomatognathic system, nor is its adaptability demanded.

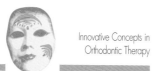

Innovative Concepts in
Orthodontic Therapy

Condylar and Anterior Tooth Guidance

A healthy occlusal anatomy functions in harmony with the TMJs and the anterior teeth, both of which determine the movement pattern of the mandible. During every movement, the unique anatomic relationship of these structures activates to dictate a precise, repeatable pathway. To maintain harmony of the occlusal condition, the posterior teeth must pass close to, but not contact, their opposing teeth during mandibular movements (Fig 12-10).

Condylar movements do not affect natural tooth morphology. Along with anterior overbite and the occlusal plane, condylar movements only influence the path of approach between the mandibular teeth and the maxillary teeth. Generally, the flatter the condylar paths, the greater the chance that posterior teeth will contact during eccentric movements.

The Bennett shift phenomenon can also affect the path of approach of the posterior teeth.[8,13,19] The greater the amount of Bennett movement (loose joints), the greater the chance of posterior eccentric contacts in protrusive and lateral jaw movements. With good canine overbite, the posterior teeth can usually be separated without reducing their genetic vertical profiles. Sometimes it is necessary to flatten the buccolingual profiles of second and third molars, however, to accommodate large amounts of Bennett movement.

Just as the TMJs determine or control the manner in which the posterior portion of the mandible moves, the anterior teeth determine how the anterior portion moves. As the mandible protrudes or moves laterally, the incisal edges of the mandibular teeth occlude with the lingual surfaces of the maxillary teeth. The steepness of these lingual surfaces determines the amount of vertical movement of the mandible. If the surfaces are very steep, the anterior aspect of the mandible will describe a steep incline path. If the anterior teeth have minimal vertical overlap, they will provide little vertical guidance during mandibular movements. The steeper the cusp, the larger the anterior overlap. To achieve good anterior guidance and avoid interference in protrusive movements, the ideal overlap should be 3 to 5 mm. If posterior cusps are flat, the amount could be less if adequate posterior clearance is provided by the joint eminence in any excursions.

During enunciation of certain sounds (eg, *s* sound), the condyles usually move forward down the eminences about 2 to 3 mm from the CR position depending on the amount of anterior horizontal overbite. The overbite becomes important because it allows the mandible to assume this forward posture comfortably, without the feeling of mandibular confinement. The horizontal overbite of the maxillary canines from the tips of the cusps to the labial surfaces of the mandibular canines is about 1 mm less than that of the incisors. The

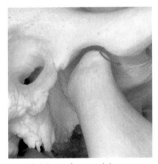

Fig 12-10 As the condyle moves out of the CR position, it descends along the articular eminence of the mandibular fossae. The rate angle at which it moves inferiorly as the mandible is protruded depends on the steepness of the articular eminence. If the surface is very steep, the condyle will describe a vertically inclined path. If it is flatter, the condyle will take a path that is less vertically inclined. The angle at which the condyle moves away from a horizontal reference plane is referred to as the *condylar guide inclination.*

canines do not need to match the overjet of the incisors because the mandible does not normally move laterally during periods of relaxation or speaking.

Occlusal plane

The plane of occlusion is important in functional movement only when combined with condylar paths and anterior overbite. These three factors (occlusal plane, anterior overbite, and condylar movements) interact to control the path and timing of the mandibular posterior teeth as they approach the maxillary posterior teeth. A steeper occlusal plane indicates that it will be more difficult to prevent eccentric posterior tooth interferences because the plane of occlusion more closely equals the path of the condyles and therefore increases their effect on occlusion.

The curve of Spee and the curve of Wilson are usually minimal in good natural occlusions. In an accentuated curve of Spee, each tooth has a different plane of occlusion. The occlusal plane of mesially inclined molars often approaches (or even exceeds) the descending paths of the condyles. This explains why it is often difficult to avoid protrusive and lateral interferences of second and third molars that have tipped anteriorly into a space created by an extracted adjacent tooth.

Vertical dimension

For many years, prosthodontics has taught that VDO is critical. It was explained that because of muscle length, interocclusal rest space, and rest position, one should never increase VDO. It was also believed that passive eruption of the teeth kept the VDO at its original level in worn dentitions, and if VDO was increased, it would inevitably return to its previous position.[20] Clinical experience has shown that VDO could be increased; nevertheless, it appears the range of results varies considerably from one patient to another. Considering that VDO is one of the least critical factors in rehabilitation of the occlusion, there is no advantage to increasing VDO any more than is necessary to restore good crown morphology on anterior and posterior teeth. If the anterior teeth are unworn and VDO is increased, orthodontics or orthognathic surgery is usually required to obtain good anterior relationships.

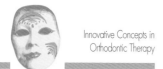

Innovative Concepts in
Orthodontic Therapy

Mastication and Occlusal Loading

Mastication consists of rhythmic and well-controlled separation of the maxillary and mandibular teeth. This activity is under the control of the central pattern generator, located in the brain stem. Each complete chewing stroke has a roughly tear-shaped movement pattern that can be divided into an opening phase and a closing phase. The closing movement has been further subdivided into the crushing phase and the grinding phase. During mastication, similar chewing strokes are repeated as food is broken down. Normal chewing strokes are well rounded. Generally, however, tall cusps and deep fossae promote a predominantly vertical chewing stroke. When the chewing strokes of persons with TMJ pain are observed, a common pattern emerges: The strokes are much shorter and slower and have an irregular pathway that appears to relate to the altered functional movement of the condyle that is the source of the pain.

The human body is subject to the physical laws of the universe. These laws have established that sharp tools (and therefore, sharp teeth) require less force and create less heat or friction and deformation compared with dull tools. It is well known that teeth do not actually contact during mastication and that patients can chew with either flat or sharp crowns, but ideally the posterior teeth have occlusal anatomy with substantial cusp height and fossa depth, and display vertical chewing strokes (approximately 70 degrees to the horizontal). Vertical chewing is less destructive than horizontal chewing because simultaneous contact points between inclined cusps surrounding cusp tips facilitate vertical force distribution through the teeth to the periodontium, thus preserving the cusp height. Since tooth anatomy is specific to individuals, it seems logical that it is the responsibility of the restorative clinician to give patients the best artificial tooth morphology possible, provided it does not inhibit condylar movements. The following case was treated based on this approach to meet the goals of anatomy and function described in this chapter.

Case Report

A 42-year-old man with a previous orthodontic treatment history was referred by the prosthodontist. The patient was willing to undergo restoration of his dentition because he did not like his smile. The prosthodontist was unable to make any more esthetic improvements because so much enamel had been worn away that it would be almost impossible to create adequate tooth length without the patient appearing to have vertical maxillary excess. As the abrasion had occurred, altered active eruption compensated for the amount of enamel lost (Figs 12-11a to 12-11e). Therefore, restoration would possibly require crown elongations and bone recontouring, in addition to endodontic procedures for all the teeth. Such an intrusive procedure holds a high risk of a poor crown-root ratio with excessively long maxillary incisors. Intraorally, one right and one left mandibular premolar and one maxillary left premolar had been extracted. Class I molar and Class II canine relationships were found on the right side, and Class II molar and canine relationships were found on the left side. An increased horizontal overjet of 6 mm was recorded. According to the cephalometric analysis, the patient had a retrognathic mandible, retroclined maxillary incisors, and proclined mandibular incisors (Figs 12-11f and 12-11g).

The mounted casts in CR show the increased overjet (Figs 12-11h to 12-11l). The previous orthodontic treatment apparently attempted to correct the skeletal discrepancy by orthodontic means only (mainly through Class II elastics and cervical headgear, as described by the patient). Consequently, the patient developed the habit of posturing his mandible forward to compensate for the mandibular deficiency and to avoid a CO interference caused mainly by the eruption of the maxillary left third molar. This displacement was depicted by the CPI as an important discrepancy between CO and CR. The multiple abrasions on his teeth in both arches, especially the incisors and canines, had led to an almost nonexistent functional occlusion. Working and balancing interferences were observed during all excursive movements because the teeth had lost most of their occlusal and incisal dental anatomy. His VDO was compromised. There were no significant crowding problems in either arch.

Orthognathic surgery was required to correct the patient's mandibular deficiency, so a consultation with the maxillofacial surgeon was scheduled. One of the concerns was the postoperative stability of the occlusion; most of the occlusal stability after a surgical splint is removed stems from correct tooth anatomy and adequate intercuspation. In this patient, there was no occlusal anatomy of the posterior teeth, and the mesiodistal width of the anterior teeth was diminished because of the severe abrasion that had created a large anterior Bolton discrepancy and little chance of a stable occlusal relationship. Coordination of both arches, however, did not represent a significant problem.

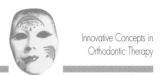

Innovative Concepts in
Orthodontic Therapy

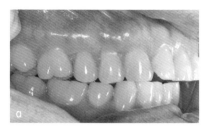
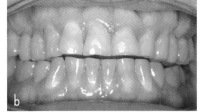
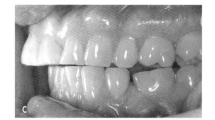

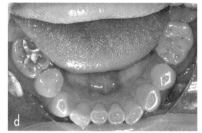
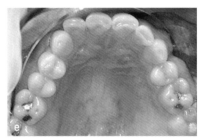

Figs 12-11a to 12-11e Intraoral photographs of a 42-year-old man referred to the author's practice. The pictures reveal significant abrasion of the enamel.

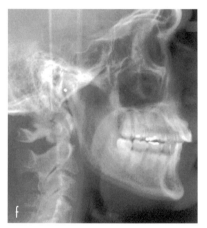
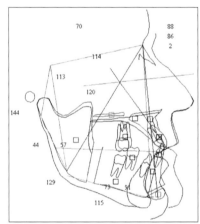

Figs 12-11f and 12-11g Cephalometric radiograph (f) and tracing (g).

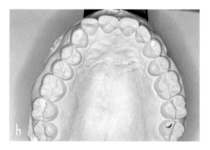
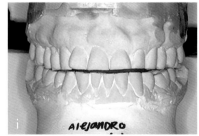
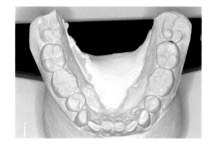

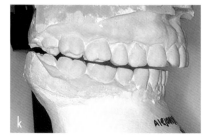
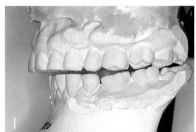

Figs 12-11h to 12-11l Mounted casts in CR with the first contact point in the lingual cusp of the maxillary left third molar.

Innovative Concepts in
Orthodontic Therapy

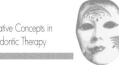

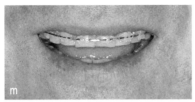 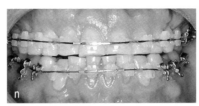 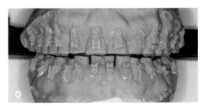

Figs 12-11m to 12-11o Sentalloy archwires (.020 × .020) on both arches. The extraction of the third molar eliminates the centric interference and allows an improved arc of closure from previously mounted casts.

Treatment goals

The interdisciplinary treatment plan involved the maxillofacial surgeon, prosthodontist, and orthodontist. The overall treatment goals were established with a focus on a simple approach and avoidance of crown elongations and bone recontouring, in addition to endodontic therapy for placement of posts and crowns on all teeth. These treatment goals included the following:

- Reestablish the correct dental anatomy with provisional resin composite restorations
- Reestablish the ideal vertical maxillary dental dimension with the correct relationship of incisal edge to lip line in repose, to avoid excessive show of the maxillary teeth
- Establish the correct anteroposterior and vertical maxillomandibular osseous relationship
- Correct the incisal and canine guidance with orthodontic, surgical, and prosthodontic treatment through placement of provisional crowns prior to final restorations

The specific orthodontic treatment plan included the following goals:

- Align and level both arches
- Establish a correct incisal torque
- Correct the upper and lower curve of Wilson
- Correct the gingival margin asymmetry
- Reduce the CO-CR discrepancy

Treatment progress

The four third molars were extracted to eliminate the centric interferences found in the evaluation of the casts. Mystique MB Roth (Dentsply) prescription brackets were bonded and .014-inch Sentalloy archwires (Dentsply) placed. The leveling process continued with .020 × .020 inch Bioforce archwires (Dentsply), .021 × .028 inch Sentalloy archwires, and .021 × .025 inch stainless steel archwires (Figs 12-11m to 12-11o).

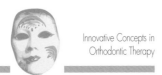

Innovative Concepts in
Orthodontic Therapy

After preoperative orthodontics was completed, a model was created with a wax-up of the full dentition to envision the correct dental anatomy for each tooth. This was placed on a semi-adjustable articulator set to the correct sagittal and vertical relationship. The full-mouth wax-up took into consideration the patient's arc of closure so that the VDO from the previous restorative procedure was recreated as closely as possible (Figs 12-11p to 12-11t). The result was a very large anterior open bite, so duplicate casts were made from the wax-up to perform all the clinical diagnostic objectives. In this way, the casts served as a working surgical setup to match a surgical treatment objective (STO). This setup would allow visualization of an ideal incisal and canine guidance in a mutually protected articulation, thereby giving the clinician a more realistic idea as to what would be required to create a correct overjet and overbite with the canines in a Class I functional relationship. It also would allow the surgeon to visualize the amount of maxillary intrusion required for some mandibular autorotation and therefore determine the approximate amount of mandibular advancement necessary. The prosthodontist advised the surgeon as to the length of the incisors needed to achieve the appropriate VDO with ideal esthetics in relation to the lip and smile line. The prosthodontist then calculated the correct length and width for all the anterior teeth, as well as the amount of material needed for the provisional reconstruction of the sharp occlusal dental anatomy of the posterior teeth. For proper postoperative stability with these provisional restorations, adequate interocclusal spacing should be planned so that the teeth can be prepped without the need for any endodontic procedures after removal of the provisional restorations.

When it was determined that the teeth were positioned correctly in the basal bone and the arches properly coordinated, then the patient was ready for the orthognathic procedure. The prosthodontist provisionally restored the dental anatomy proposed in the wax-up (Figs 12-11u and 12-11v). These provisional restorations included the correct dental anatomy in all posterior teeth to restore the patient's ideal dental dimensions. As had been visualized in the diagnostic mounting and wax-up, the restorations led to the development of a fulcrum that rotated the mandible posteriorly. This rotation created the expected anterior open bite (Figs 12-11w to 12-11bb). To help stabilize the patient's occlusion and neuromusculature before surgery, an occlusal splint was fabricated (Fig 12-11cc).

At this stage of treatment, the patient's dental anatomy was almost correct; the final functional resin composite restorations were to be added after a postoperative occlusal adjustment aided by a new wax-up. His VDO had been reestablished and his teeth leveled and aligned with the proper anterior and posterior torque. His osseous sagittal and vertical relationship would be corrected next.

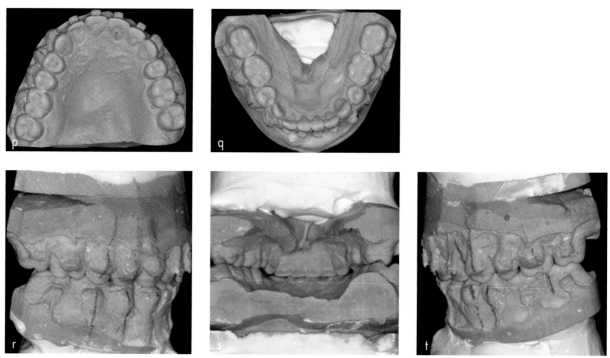

Figs 12-11p to 12-11t Wax-up to restore the anatomy on worn teeth. The wax-up was duplicated to perform all the clinical diagnostic objectives on the final surgical treatment objective (STO).

Figs 12-11u and 12-11v Postoperative reconstruction of both arches.

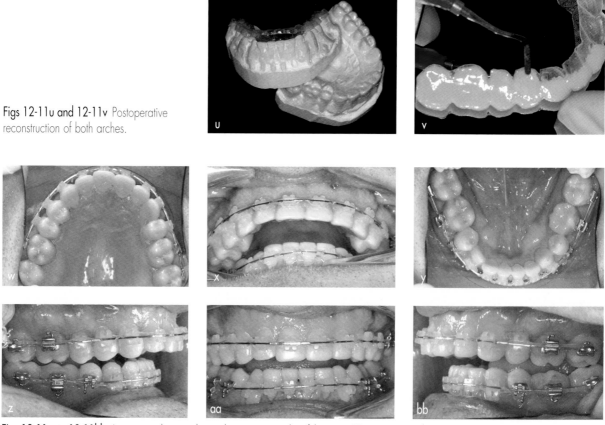

Figs 12-11w to 12-11bb As expected, once the teeth were restored, a fulcrum in CR was exposed.

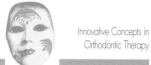

Innovative Concepts in
Orthodontic Therapy

The orthognathic procedure included a 5-mm impaction and 3-mm advancement of the maxilla in two pieces, combined with a bilateral sagittal split osteotomy (BSSO) advancement of the mandible (Figs 12-11dd to 12-11ll). Postoperatively, with the teeth restored to their ideal vertical dimension, the new orthodontic goal was to make final adjustments to the occlusal relationships, which were further adjusted through positive and negative coronoplasties. This stage allowed evaluation of the functional occlusion that resulted from changes to the anatomy of the teeth, as well as assessment of the patient's comfort once the ideal occlusal scheme was obtained. After it was determined that all the functional goals were achieved, the case was ready for the final step. Vertical elastics were attached to four miniscrew implants placed at the canine areas. The pressure applied would create an intrusive rather than extrusive force and would allow the teeth to settle. When all of the functional criteria were obtained and the patient was comfortable with his dental relationships, the orthodontic therapy was considered complete (Figs 12-11mm to 12-11pp).

One goal pursued throughout treatment was the reduction of the CR-MI discrepancy. It was necessary to recognize during the treatment planning that surgery would be required because this meant that several splints would have to be fabricated. A splint was used at each stage to help stabilize the patient's occlusion while the CO-CR discrepancy was gradually reduced. As the date of surgery approached, a repeatable CR position of the mandible was obtained prior to the surgery, and after the surgery the CO-CR discrepancy had been reduced so that it was almost nonexistent.

The most important indicator of success was that the patient was able to function without eroding or fracturing the composite restorations; this would only be possible if the patient's dental anatomy was free of working or balancing interferences so that the occlusal forces were in harmony. Proper functional occlusion prevents any muscular imbalance from causing disruption to the harmony of the oral components.

After the orthodontic treatment, the patient saw the prosthodontist for follow-up to prepare the crowns of all teeth based on the initial wax-up (Figs 12-11qq to 12-11tt). The definitive restorations consisted of zirconia crowns on both anterior and posterior teeth (Figs 12-11uu and 12-11vv).

The treatment resulted in a correct Class I occlusion with an ideal overjet and overbite (Figs 12-11ww to 12-11yy). The proper incisal and canine guidance was achieved, a mutually protected occlusion was restored, and the CO-CR discrepancy was fully reduced. The overall treatment goals in this case were met thanks to the cooperation of an interdisciplinary team with previously established objectives.

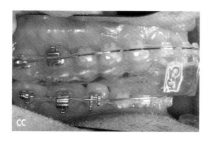

Fig 12-11cc Presurgical occlusal splint to stabilize the mandible.

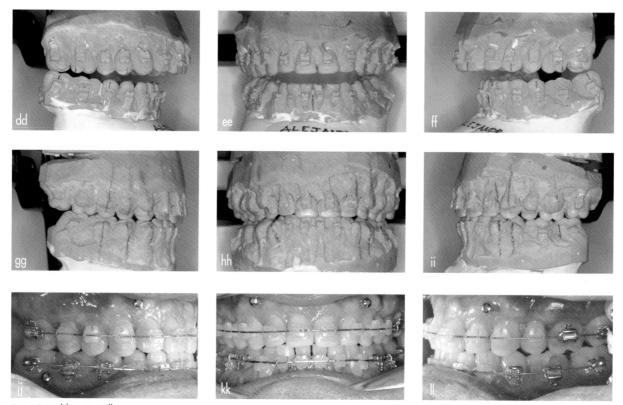

Figs 12-11dd to 12-11ll *Upper images:* Postoperative mounted casts. *Middle images:* New wax-up after surgery (positive coronoplasty). *Lower images:* New functional restorations are delivered and negative coronoplasty performed. Vertical elastics are attached to implants.

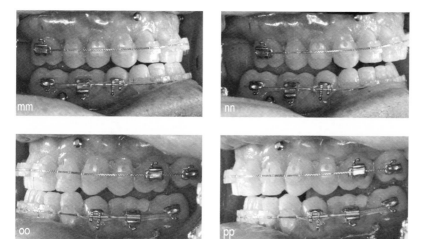

Figs 12-11mm to 12-11pp Mutually protected articulation. All of the postoperative occlusal adjustments and subsequent composite reconstruction are performed at the patient's orthodontic consultations.

Innovative Concepts in
Orthodontic Therapy

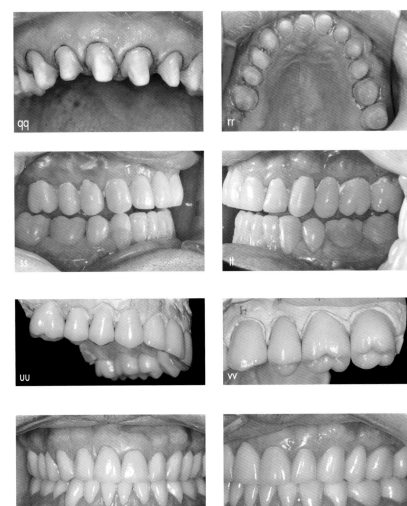

Figs 12-11qq to 12-11tt Crown preparations and provisional crowns.

Figs 12-11uu and 12-11vv Definitive zirconia restorations.

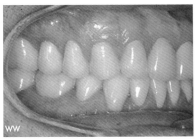

Figs 12-11ww to 12-11yy Final result.

Acknowledgments

The authors would like to acknowledge the contributions of Carlos F. Navarro IV, BS, and Jorge Villanueva, DDS, to this chapter. Thanks also to Raul Benavides, DDS, Lorena Molina, DDS, MS, and Albano Flores, DMD, MS, for the excellent restorative and surgical procedures performed. This quality of treatment would not have been possible without the interconsultation with these great dental practitioners.

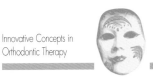

References

1. Andrews LF. The six keys to normal occlusion. Am J Orthod 1972;62(3):296–309.
2. Lee RL. Esthetics and its relationship to function. In: Rufenacht CR (ed). Fundamentals of Esthetics. Hanover Park: Quintessence, 1990:137–183.
3. Okeson JP (ed). Bell's Orofacial Pains, ed 5. Hanover Park: Quintessence, 1995.
4. Stallard H, Stuart CE. Concepts of occlusion. Dent Clin N Am 1963:591–606.
5. Ramfjord SP, Ash MM. Occlusion, ed 4. Philadelphia: Saunders, 1995.
6. Kawamura Y. Neurophysiologic background of occlusion. Periodontics 1967;5(4):175–183.
7. Shore NA. Disfunción Temporomandibular y Equilibrio Oclusal. Buenos Aires: Mundi, 1983.
8. Roth RH. Functional occlusion for the orthodontist. J Clin Orthod 1981;15(1):32–40, 44–51.
9. Roth RH. Functional occlusion for the orthodontist. Part II. J Clin Orthod 1981 Feb;15(2):100–123.
10. Roth RH. Functional occlusion for the orthodontist. Part III. J Clin Orthod 1981 Mar;15(3):174–179, 182–198.
11. Roth RH. Functional occlusion for the orthodontist. Part IV. J Clin Orthod 1981 Apr;15(4):246–265.
12. Roth RH. The Roth functional occlusion approach to orthodontics [course syllabus]. Burlingame, CA: Roth/Williams Center for Functional Occlusion, 1999.
13. Gibbs CH, Lundeen HC. The Function of Teeth: The Physiology of Mandibular Function Related to Occlusal Form and Esthetics. Gainesville, FL, L and G Publishers, 2005.
14. Angle EH. Treatment of Malocclusion of the Teeth. Philadelphia: S. S. White Dental Manufacturing Company, 1907.
15. Okeson JP (ed). Management of Temporomandibular Disorders and Occlusion, ed 3. St Louis: Mosby, 1993.
16. Utt TW, Meyers CE Jr, Wierzba TF, Hondrum SO. A three-dimensional comparison of condylar position changes between centric relation and centric occlusion using the mandibular position indicator. Am J Orthod Dentofacial Orthop 1995;107(3):298–308.
17. Wood DP, Korne PH. Estimated and true hinge axis: A comparison of condylar displacements. Angle Orthod 1992;62(3):167–175.
18. Lavine DS, Kulbersh R, Bonner PT, Pink FE. Reproducibility of the condylar position indicator. Semin Orthod 2003;9(2):96–101.
19. Lundeen HC: Centric relation records: The effect of muscle action. J Prosthet Dent 1974;31(3):244–253.
20. Thomas PK. Syllabus on full mouth waxing technique for rehabilitation: tooth-to-tooth cusp fossa concept of organic occlusion, ed 2. Instant printing services, 1967:1–10.

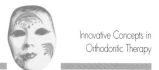

Innovative Concepts in
Orthodontic Therapy

Innovations in Three-Dimensional Imaging Techniques

13

Silvia Geron, DMD, MSc

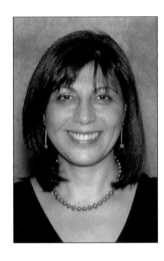

Silvia Geron, DMD, MSc

Silvia Geron is a specialist in orthodontics and dentofacial orthopedics. She received her DMD (dental surgeon) in 1980 and her MSc (cum laude majore) in 1991 from the Hebrew University Hadassah School of Dental Medicine, where she was a member of the orthodontic department from 1991 to 1996. She maintains a private practice limited to orthodontics, with an emphasis in lingual and adult orthodontics.

Dr Geron is currently the president of the Israel Orthodontic Society (IOS), the secretary and founding member of the World Society of Lingual Orthodontics (WSLO), examiner of the Israel Dental Association Scientific Council-Orthodontic Examination Committee, and reviewer for the *American Journal of Orthodontics and Dentofacial Orthopedics* and for the *Angle Orthodontics*. Dr Geron is director of lingual orthodontics for the international postgraduate orthodontic program at Tel-Aviv University and Tel-Hashomer Hospital, IDF, Israel.

Dr Geron was founder and editor of the *Journal of the Israel Orthodontic Society* and the founder and editor of the electronic *Adult and Lingual Orthodontics* journal (www.lingualnews.com). She is an active member of the European Society of Lingual Orthodontics (ESLO), WSLO, the American Association of Orthodontists (AAO), the World Federation of Orthodontists (WFO), the American Lingual Orthodontists Association (ALOA), and the IOS.

Dr Geron lectures extensively all over the world on the topics of adult multidisciplinary orthodontic treatment and lingual orthodontics.

Email: sigeron@gmail.com

Traditionally, orthodontists have collected panoramic and cephalometric radiographs, facial and intraoral photographs, and study casts for key diagnostic records. Recent advances in three-dimensional (3D) imaging technologies combine the best features of all these methods. Cone beam computed tomography (CBCT) allows assessment of dental and skeletal structures in three dimensions; laser- and optical-based surface imaging allow assessment of soft tissue relationships; and virtual study models enable automated visualization procedures and rigorous measurements. These diagnostic tools have introduced a new era in contemporary orthodontics and paved the way for 3D simulation and treatment planning, design, and production of corrective appliances. Clinical applications include *(1)* 3D fabrication of custom-made archwires, *(2)* virtual positioning of conventional appliances and production of transfer trays for indirect bonding, *(3)* design and production of custom attachments by reverse engineering, and *(4)* production of transparent aligners. The shift to 3D diagnosis appears to be irreversible since the 3D images have significant advantages over the previous two-dimensional (2D) technology. The opportunities to archive 3D craniofacial and dentofacial records for medicolegal purposes or for research also exceed anything currently possible with 2D records or traditional study casts.

This chapter provides an overview of contemporary 3D diagnostic tools available for orthodontists and explains the advantages, limitations, clinical applications, advanced uses for orthodontic appliance fabrication, interpretation, and legal aspects of these imaging modalities.

Radiographic Methods

Traditional periapical, panoramic, and cephalometric radiographs provide much important information for the clinician; however, the patient receives a large dose of radiation in the process of obtaining these records. To reduce this dose, larger radiographs (eg, panoramic and cephalometric radiographs) use an image intensifier instead of direct radiation onto the film. The image intensifier (a fluorescent lightboard) allows a fiftyfold decrease in the amount of radiation required. New technology for digital radiographs uses an image intensifier sensor that is even more sensitive and achieves a high-quality panoramic image with only 20% of the regular amount of radiation (Fig 13-1). The size of the resultant digital image can be adjusted to 1:1, although there is still some distortion of the image because of the different magnifications of objects at various distances from the sensor. This high-quality digital radiograph can be further improved by computer editing, such as contrast or brightness adjustments. Unfortunately, even this image is only a 2D outcome, while orthodontic diagnosis and treatment changes occur in the 3D world.

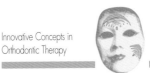

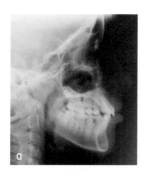
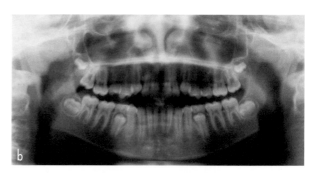
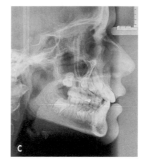
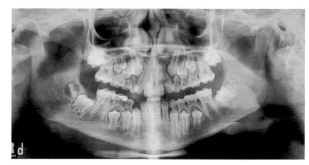

Figs 13-1a to 13-1d Conventional panoramic and cephalometric radiographs (a and b) versus digital radiographs (c and d), which are high-quality images that use only 20% the amount of radiation.

Various methods have been implemented to obtain 3D information from traditional 2D images. Baumrind et al[1] suggested combining two paired coplanar images; Grayson and coworkers[2] suggested combining several coronal and transverse perpendicular images. The exact 3D position of an object can be determined by geometric calculations. These techniques are difficult to interpret because some of the objects do not appear in both images and because of different magnification of the various structures in the images.

The CBCT technology available today is a radiographic image of the inner body organs that provides accurate 3D information of the dentofacial region to clinicians and researchers. CBCT reveals the shape of the roots and their locations, the relationship between various hard and soft tissue structures, root resorption, or different pathologies (Fig 13-2). It is possible to see the structures peeled off the bone (Fig 13-3), to show only the soft tissue or only the airways (Fig 13-4), or to produce a panoramic or cephalometric view at different levels. At the same time, this modality uses a significantly smaller amount of radiation and eliminates the need for repeated radiographs to localize anatomical structures because all of this information is obtained in one scan. CBCT provides many clinical application possibilities and views that were not previously feasible.

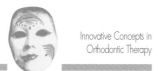

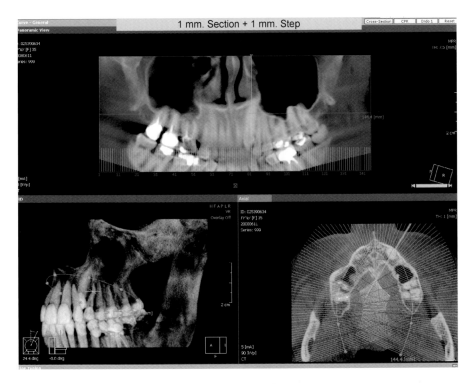

1 mm. Section + 1 mm. Step

Fig 13-2 CBCT is a 3D radiograph that provides accurate information about the shapes of the roots and their locations, the relationship between various structures, root resorption, or various pathologies.

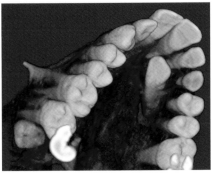

Fig 13-3 CBCT enables the clinician to see the impacted canine pulled off the bone. (Courtesy of Dolphin Imaging, Chatsworth, CA.)

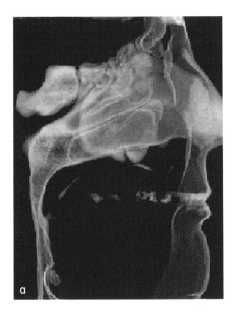
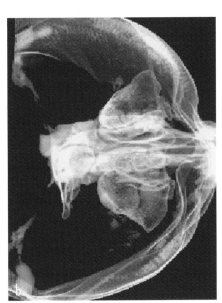

Figs 13-4a and 13-4b CBCT can show the airway only, without the surrounding soft or hard tissues.

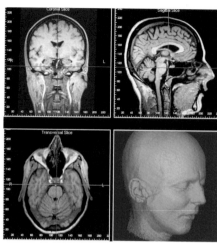

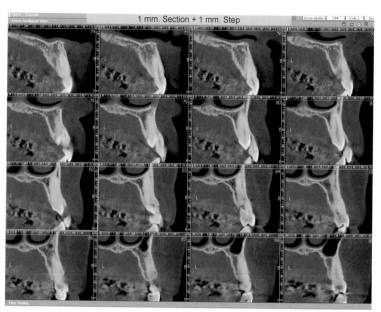

Fig 13-5 MRI provides greater contrast between the different soft tissues of the body, making it especially useful in brain, musculoskeletal, cardiovascular, and oncologic imaging. (Courtesy of Dolphin Imaging, Chatsworth, CA.)

Fig 13-6 CT produces a large series of 2D radiographs (slices) taken around a single axis of rotation. These slices can be manipulated and reformatted in various planes to demonstrate various structures based on their ability to block the x-ray beam.

Dental CBCT versus medical CT

The imaging methods used in medical fields today are magnetic resonance imaging (MRI) and computed tomography (CT). MRI provides greater contrast between the different soft tissues of the body, making it especially useful in brain, musculoskeletal, cardiovascular, and oncologic imaging (Fig 13-5).

CT was introduced to the medical field in 1971 and was implemented in clinical practice in the 1980s. It produces a large series of 2D radiographs that spiral around a single axis of rotation, which can be manipulated and reformatted in various planes to demonstrate, as a set of consecutive slices, various structures based on their ability to block the x-rays.[3] The application of CT within dentistry has been limited due to the high levels of radiation to which the patient is exposed and the high cost of scanning (Fig 13-6).

CBCT scanners have been available for craniofacial imaging since 1998[4]; lately there has been a surge of interest in this method, and as a result, several new CBCT scanners have been introduced to the market. CBCT scanners use a cone-shaped x-ray beam, rather than a conventional linear fan beam, to provide images of the bony structures of the skull. The cone beam performs only one revolution to capture the entire section. In this method, the amount of radiation is approximately 20% that of the regular spiral CT. The CBCT scanner is composed of an anode

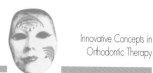

Innovative Concepts in
Orthodontic Therapy

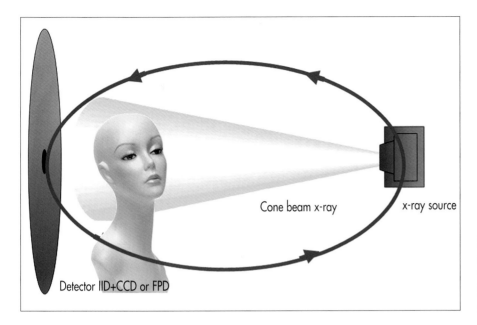

Cone beam x-ray   x-ray source

Detector IID+CCD or FPD

Fig 13-7 The CBCT scanner is composed of an anode (x-ray source) at one end and a detector mounted on the other end to capture the cone-shaped beam.

(x-ray source) positioned on one end and a detector mounted on the other end to capture the cone-shaped beam (Fig 13-7). The detector is one of two types:

- Image intensifier detector (IID): typically a phosphor-photocathode screen paired with a charge-coupled device (CCD).
- Flat-panel detector (FPD): typically a cesium-iodine array scintillator coupled with a photo-sensor array. This is the more recently developed technology that offers less distortion and a uniform brightness of the scanned image.[5]

CBCT scanners differ in the field of view; the larger scanner, whose field ranges from nasion to gnathion and from zygoma to zygoma, is more suitable than the smaller versions for orthodontic applications.

Unlike CT, which is well suited for medical applications, CBCT is specific to dentistry. It is faster and more convenient, with higher resolution and better image quality. The scanner's compact size, its ability to allow the patient to remain in a vertical position, and the relatively low radiation dose makes the CBCT ideally suited to image the craniofacial region, including dental structures. On the other hand, CBCT is not calibrated for density; therefore, the values assigned cannot be used directly to estimate bone density.

The volume data of the CBCT scan are collected while the anode-detector complex rotates 360 degrees around the patient's head. A radiograph (projection) is taken at each degree of the rotation. Images are created by short x-ray pulses during the scan, which significantly reduce the total exposure time.

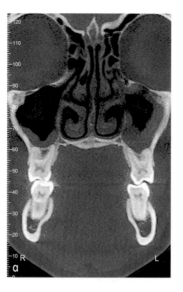

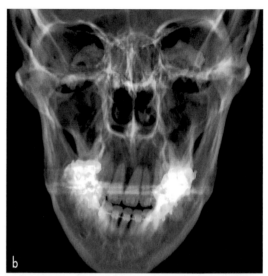

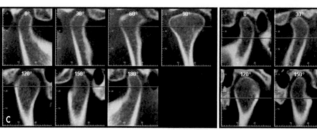

Figs 13-8a to 13-8d The original data received from the projections of a single scan are reconstructed by an algorithm to reproduce images in different views. Frontal cross section (a). Frontal cephalogram (b). Group of temporomandibular joint (TMJ) slices (c). Select TMJ slice position and parameters (d). (Courtesy of Dolphin Imaging, Chatsworth, CA.)

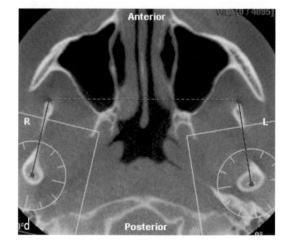

Each projection is corrected for geometric and dynamic distortions and stored in the computer. Subsequently, reconstruction software is applied to the volume of data to produce a stack of 2D grayscale level images of the anatomy, and all projections are reformatted with a filtered back-projection algorithm to generate the 3D data, which can be viewed from every aspect (Fig 13-8). The original data received from the projections of one scan are reconstructed by the algorithm to reproduce images in coronal, sagittal, and axial views, in addition to panoramic

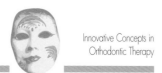

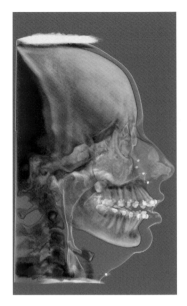
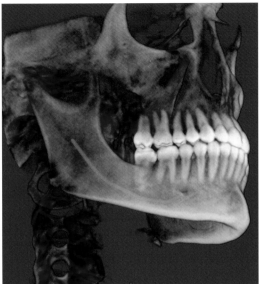

Fig 13-9 *(left)* CBCT image demonstrating translucent soft and hard tissues. (Courtesy of Dolphin Imaging, Chatsworth, CA.)

Fig 13-10 *(right)* CBCT view of the teeth stripped of soft tissues and bone, with marked nerve. (Courtesy of Dolphin Imaging, Chatsworth, CA.)

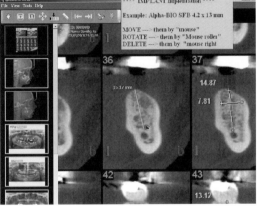

Fig 13-11 Accurate measurements for implant insertion are made on 2D slices of a CBCT image.

views and lateral or frontal cephalometric views. These data also make it possible to *(1)* see translucent soft and hard tissue images (Fig 13-9), *(2)* view the teeth from all angles without soft tissues and bone, *(3)* mark any special structure in the image (Fig 13-10), and *(4)* see the airways stripped of all soft and hard tissues (see Fig 13-4). The algorithm also allows the slices to be combined to create 3D images from any angle. The 3D image facilitates the visual assessment of anatomical parts but cannot be used for quantitative measuring. The ratio of the picture to the object in each 2D slice is 1:1, however, and therefore accurate measurements can be made in this view (Fig 13-11).

CBCT images versus conventional radiographs

Conventional panoramic and cephalometric radiographs are affected by distortion and magnification errors caused by the distance of the examined object to the film and x-ray source, and by different magnification

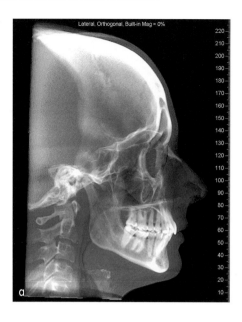

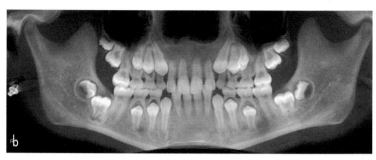

Figs 13-12a and 13-12b Cephalometric and panoramic views derived from CBCT have no distortion, no overlapping, and no superimposition of the contralateral side or the spinal column. (Courtesy of Dolphin Imaging, Chatsworth, CA.)

of bilateral structures. The CBCT, on the other hand, is produced by tracing an outline in the 3D image, so the panoramic or cephalometric images (Fig 13-12) can be processed using visualization techniques such as the maximum intensity projection (MIP) algorithm and raycast, which enable separate representation of the right and left side of the skull, or virtual excision of all nonpertinent structures (eg, the parietal bone on one side for a view into the skull).

CBCT image quality depends on the detector and number of projections, the noise, and the image contrast. An increased radiation dose reduces the noise and improves voxel quality, but the risks of a higher dose should be carefully considered in terms of what it can contribute to the specific case treatment decisions and treatment plan.

Accuracy of CBCT

The accuracy of CBCT measurements and spatial distortion was studied by comparing different settings of the CBCT scanner with direct digital caliper measurements from a cast.[6] CBCT measurements were made on a DICOM viewer (Digital Imaging and Communications in Medicine, which is the standard for distribution of any medical images). The results showed no statistically significant differences among the 3D images. When compared with the CBCT measurements, the direct digital caliper measurements showed a statistically significant difference, but the absolute difference was 0.1 mm and is not likely significant for most clinical applications. The author concluded that the CBCT machine used in the study has clinically accurate measurements and acceptable resolution. Other studies had similar findings.[7,8] The data rendered with CBCT are just as accurate as the gold standard of direct physical measures.

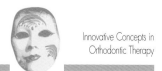

Innovative Concepts in
Orthodontic Therapy

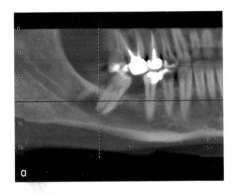
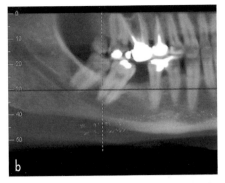

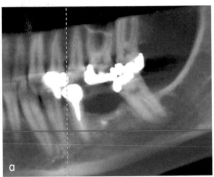
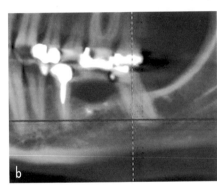

Fig 13-13a Reconstruction artifact obscures objects distal to the first molar.

Fig 13-13b The corrected view shows the second molar. (Courtesy of Yigal Ganot, Panolote-Galor, Israel.)

Fig 13-14a If the patient is put into a less-than-ideal position during image acquisition, data can be misinterpreted. The teeth distal to the missing teeth appear tipped, which may lead to an inaccurate path of implant insertion.

Fig 13-14b The correct inclination of the teeth. (Courtesy of Yigal Ganot, Panolote-Galor, Israel.)

Considerations in CBCT use
Artifacts

Some imaging artifacts are inherent in CBCT units because of the nature of the image acquisition and reconstruction process. Some are more pronounced in CBCT scans than in their CT counterparts because of the different processes through which the images are acquired.[9] These artifacts can lead to inaccurate or false diagnoses. For example, soft tissue in a CBCT image tends to appear black, and bones tend to appear white. Thin bones, however, might have a lower density (brightness) than a thick soft tissue and may appear black or not show up at all. The brightness depends on tissue density, the interference of certain artifacts like partial object effect or beam hardening, and the reconstruction algorithm.

Figure 13-13a shows an example of a reconstruction artifact in which the CBCT panoramic view does not show any tooth distal to the first molar because of the wrong outline from which the panoramic image was taken. The corrected image shows the second molar that was absent in the previous panoramic view (Fig 13-13b).

Motion artifacts are common in CBCT and are attributable to improper patient stabilization. A malpositioning error during image acquisition can lead to misinterpretation of the data; for example, the angle of the teeth in Fig 13-14a distal to the missing teeth may lead to inaccurate direction of implant placement, but the correct inclination of the teeth is shown in Fig 13-14b.

Metal artifacts occur when the attenuation values of objects behind the metallic object are incorrectly high. Bright and dark streaks appear in the images and significantly degrade the image quality. Metallic streak artifacts occur in all directions from the high-attenuation object because of the cone-shaped beam (Fig 13-15). The effect of metal artifacts in the soft tissue region is magnified in CBCT because the soft tissue contrast is usually lower in these images.[10]

Radiation dose

Radiation dose is an important concern in radiographic examination. It has been reported that the patient effective dose from CBCT scans ranges from 45 to 650 μSv (1 microsievert [μSv] = 100 microroentgens [μR]). This large range was attributed to variations among equipment, exposure protocols, and applied methodology.[11,12] It also has been reported to affect the resulting image quality for various exposure protocols.[13,14]

In some reports, the recorded radiation dose for a CBCT scan was 50 μSv. This is low in contrast to a full-mouth series (150 μSv), a panoramic radiograph (about 50 μSv), and a conventional dental CT[15] (about 2,000 μSv). In other studies,[16] the radiation dose for a CBCT scan with a NewTom 9000 scanner (AFP Imaging) was reported as 50.3 μSv, which is higher than amounts recorded for the full-mouth series (33 to 84 μSv) or the panoramic radiograph (2.9 to 9.6 μSv). Ludlow et al[11] reported that CBCT radiation is high relative to conventional radiographic methods but very low relative to medical CT. Using the BERT index (background equivalent radiation time), a NewTom 3G (AFP Imaging) scan is equivalent to 4 to 6 days of average per capita background (environmental) radiation.

Although the radiation dose of CBCT is generally lower than that of CT, the repeated use of CBCT may increase the collective radiation dose given for medical purposes that is disproportionate to the frequency of its justified use. Since the amount of radiation in CBCT is higher in comparison with panoramic and cephalometric radiographs, referral to CBCT should be carefully considered in relevant cases. On the other hand, the clinician should consider the capacity of one scan to generate an infinite number of reformatted images from all angles and therefore greatly reduce the need for additional radiographs, combined with its capacity to achieve a vast amount of information in higher definition. The CBCT should therefore be used in cases where 3D information is necessary to assist in treatment decisions and improve treatment results. If one strictly adheres to the ALARA (as low as reasonably achievable) principle, then one should try to optimize image quality at reasonably low radiation levels.[17]

Orthodontic uses of 3D radiographic imaging

Various 3D cephalometric measurements, absolute and angular, can be made on the 3D CBCT image (Fig 13-16). Superimposition of the 3D

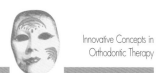

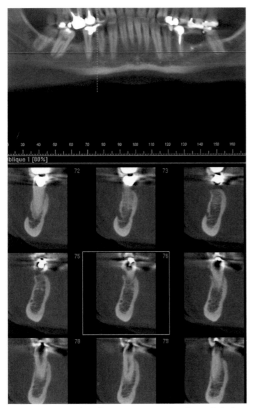

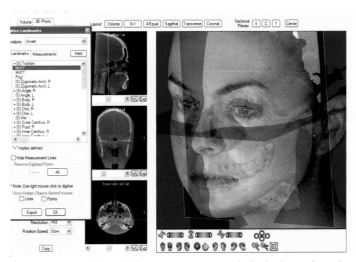

Fig 13-16 Various 3D cephalometric measurements, both absolute and angular, can be made on the 3D CBCT image. Cephalometric points can be digitized on the volume or on any of the slices. (Courtesy of Dolphin Imaging, Chatsworth, CA.)

Fig 13-15 Metal artifacts appear as bright and dark streaks in the images in all directions because of the cone-shaped beam.

model can also be done for *(1)* follow-up of treatment progress, *(2)* comparison to the normal, *(3)* evaluation of airway competency, *(4)* evaluation of soft tissues, and *(5)* treatment prognosis. CBCT allows differentiation of the dental changes from the skeletal changes.[18,19]

CBCT technology makes it possible to clearly determine the boundaries between soft tissue and air and to demonstrate the paranasal sinuses, nasal cavities, and the nasopharyngeal area.

Temporomandibular disorders (TMDs) are difficult to diagnose with panoramic radiographs, and if additional radiographs are needed, the patient receives an increased radiation dose. CBCT has the advantage of 3D visualization of temporomandibular joint (TMJ) anatomy and pathologies. A blinded observational cross-sectional in vitro study examined the diagnostic accuracy of TMJ images made with CBCT, panoramic radiography, and linear tomography. The CBCT images provided superior reliability and greater accuracy than TOMO and TMJ panoramic projections in the detection of condylar cortical erosion.[20]

Another study investigated the complex relationships between TMJ function and craniofacial morphology using a four-dimensional

Innovative Concepts in
Orthodontic Therapy

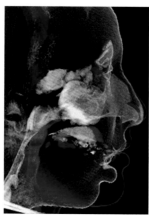

Fig 13-17 CBCT scans can be used for superimpositions to evaluate growth changes and orthodontic treatment progress and results, and for treatment planning, simulation, and prediction of treatment outcomes. (Courtesy of Dolphin Imaging, Chatsworth, CA.)

analysis. This study combined a 3D CBCT of the cranium and mandible, a 3D laser scan of the dental surface, and a recording of mandibular movement data. The method described performs dynamic simulations of condyle-to-fossa distances and occlusal contacts during mandibular function that may be useful in diagnosis of TMDs in patients with mandibular deformities and malocclusions.[21]

Temporary anchorage device (TAD) placement presents another application for CBCT. CBCT enables analysis of bone thickness at the insertion site to improve placement of miniscrew implants (MSIs) and minimize the risks of root injury.[22]

Kim et al described a method to precisely transfer the radiographic information to the surgical site.[23] CBCT images were used to replicate dental casts on which surgical guides were fabricated for the proper insertion of MSIs. The accuracy of MSI placement aided by a 3D surgical guide was evaluated and compared to the accuracy of placement in conventional procedures.[24] The results showed that the 3D surgical guide provided for precise MSI placement.

CBCT scans can be used to measure and quantify bone remodeling, skeletal expansion, and alveolar tipping during orthodontic expansion of the jaws. They are also useful for studying the effects of expansion on the bony sutures, teeth, and periodontal tissues.[25–27]

It is possible to make bones transparent in the scan images, which allows visualization of *(1)* developing permanent teeth, *(2)* the position of teeth and roots, *(3)* impacted and supernumerary teeth, *(4)* bone width and morphology for orthodontic MSI placement, *(5)* bone regions for orthognathic surgery, and *(6)* diagnosis of pathologies such as root resorption, hyperplasias, and anomalies of the condyle.

3D imaging is important for primary diagnosis; for superimposition to evaluate growth changes, orthodontic treatment progress, and results; and for treatment planning, simulation, and prediction of treatment outcomes (Fig 13-17).

Imaging can also simplify communication of the treatment plan and results with colleagues and explanation of the treatment options and expected outcome to the orthodontic patient. Simulations created with 3D imaging techniques that show treatment examples are also a very powerful marketing tool.

Case applications: Location of impacted canines and supernumerary teeth

Two brief case studies demonstrate how CBCT can serve as an important diagnostic tool in the diagnosis and treatment planning of impacted and supernumerary teeth.

The patient in Case 1 had bilateral maxillary impacted canines and a right maxillary second molar impaction, both of which were evident on

Innovative Concepts in Orthodontic Therapy

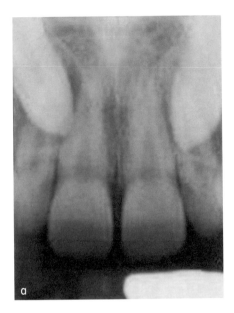
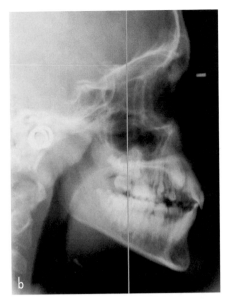
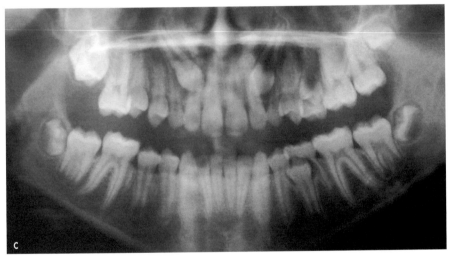

Figs 13-18a to 13-18c Case 1: Conventional panoramic and periapical radiographs reveal bilateral maxillary impacted canines and a maxillary right second molar impaction.

routine panoramic and periapical radiographs (Fig 13-18). It was possible to locate the impacted canines seen in these radiographs using either the vertical or horizontal parallax method; the vertical parallax method was chosen.[28] In this method, the panoramic beam originates from a lower angle relative to the periapical radiograph. The labially impacted canine is expected to appear superior in the panoramic radiograph, while the palatally impacted canine should appear in an inferior position. The clinician was unable to obtain a definite location of the impacted canines with this method, however, and the cephalometric radiograph was used in an attempt to obtain additional information about the mesiodistal position of the impacted canines. The CBCT slices and the 3D image gave much more definitive information regarding the position of the canines and the right second molar (Fig 13-19).

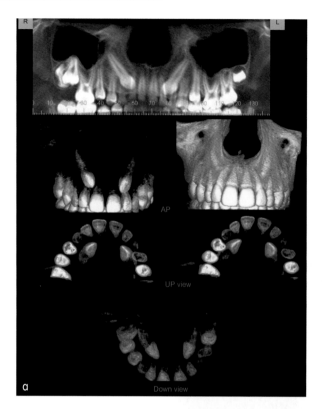

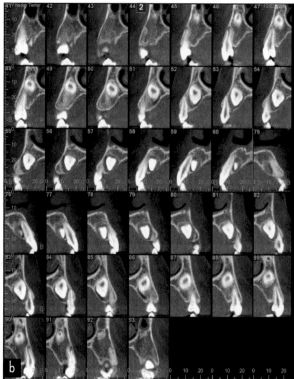

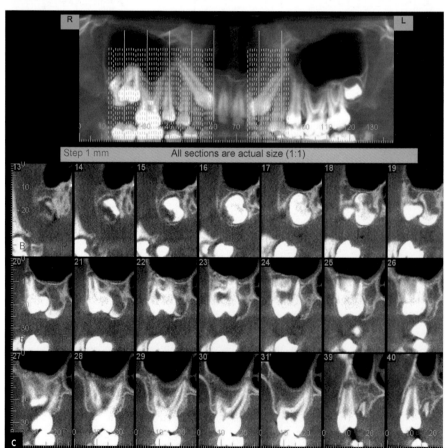

Figs 13-19a to 13-19c Case 1: CBCT slices and 3D images provide more definite information regarding the position of the canines and the second molar.

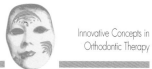

Innovative Concepts in
Orthodontic Therapy

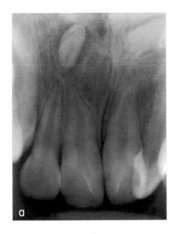
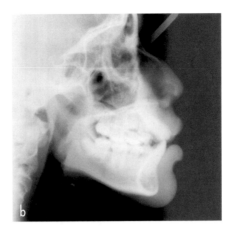
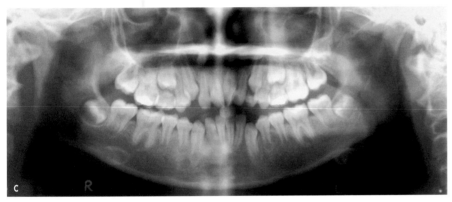

Figs 13-20a to 13-20c Case 2: Maxillary supernumerary teeth are seen in a radiograph. The parallax method could not be used to locate the supernumerary teeth since they were in a very high location and did not overlap other teeth.

The patient in Case 2 presented with supernumerary maxillary teeth (Fig 13-20). The parallax method could not be used to locate the supernumerary teeth because their positions were very high and they did not overlap other teeth. The CT slices and the 3D image accurately revealed the position of the supernumerary teeth, which was essential knowledge for successful surgery (Fig 13-21).

Smooth transition from two dimensions to three dimensions

The shift from 2D to 3D images seems to be irreversible; however, the shift to exclusive use of 3D images will not happen immediately. A full understanding of the potential clinical uses and the ability to completely interpret the data have yet to be achieved.

As the profession moves from traditional 2D cephalometric analysis to new 3D techniques, it is often necessary to compare 2D with 3D data. CBCT provides simulation tools that can help bridge the gap between image types. CBCT acquisitions can simulate panoramic, lateral, and posteroanterior cephalometric radiographs so that they can be compared with preexisting cephalometric databases. CBCT-derived 2D lateral cephalograms were proved to be more accurate than conventional lateral cephalograms for most linear measurements.[7]

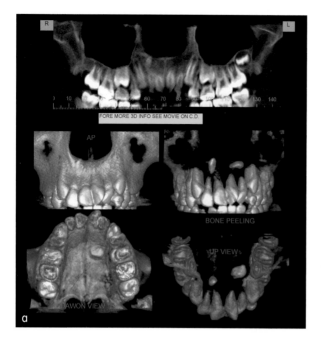

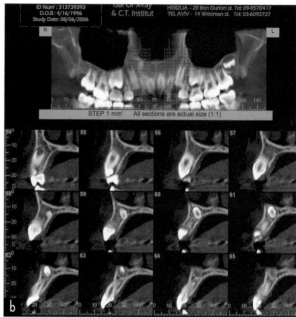

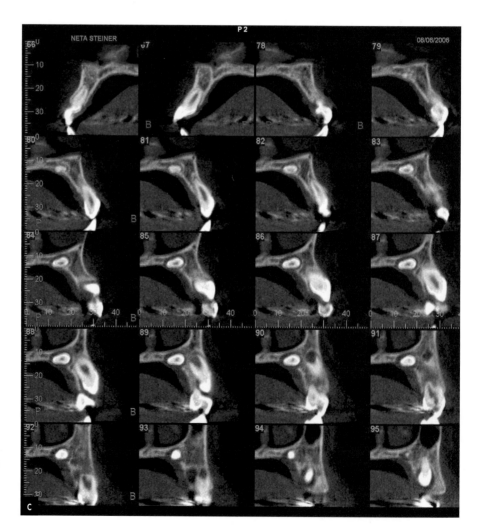

Figs 13-21a to 13-21c Case 2: The CT slices and the 3D images provide accurate information about the position of the supernumerary teeth.

Kumar et al[29] demonstrated on dry skulls that CBCT-generated lateral cephalometric images could be used successfully to make cephalometric measurements, similar to the conventional cephalometric radiograph, and that the raycast technique is superior to MIP for visualization of structures needed for cephalometric measurements. This suggests that the transition from an existing database based on 2D cephalograms to 3D analysis can be done gradually with CBCT-generated cephalometric images and therefore can be more easily accepted by clinicians.

Interpretation of CBCT and legal aspects

Ideally, a radiologist should perform the assessment of CBCT findings. This is not always practical or feasible, however, and the orthodontist should be able to assess the findings, interpret most of the skull anatomy, and identify pathology. If questionable information is uncovered, the next step should be to consult a radiologist. Presently, this technology is relatively new and is therefore ahead of the learning curve and the potential liability exposure curve.

In a study of CBCT scans of 500 consecutive patients, incidental findings were found in 123 patients. The responsibility when these findings lead to pathologic consequences is significant.[30] The problem of liability regarding CBCT was discussed by Jerrold,[31] who consulted different practitioners with dual degrees—general practitioner dentist–attorney, orthodontist-attorney, and periodontist-attorney—and asked for their opinions on questions such as the following:

1. What is the orthodontist's liability for misreading or not fully reading CBCT scans?
2. Is the orthodontist required to read all scans, although only a few of the hundred or so that can be viewed are relevant to treatment?

Based on their answers, Jerrold concluded that the orthodontist is liable to interpret the images used for diagnostic and therapeutic purposes. All cuts viewed must be evaluated in the same manner and at the same level of detail as conventional panoramic or cephalometric radiographs. There were mixed opinions on whether that responsibility applies to the entire volume data or only to the slices used for the intended purpose. Ultimately, the responsibility of the orthodontist is absolute: If pathology is evident on the scan, the clinician has the duty to recognize it and either treat it or refer it for further diagnosis.

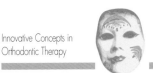

3D Surface Imaging

Conventional orthodontic analysis places more emphasis on the relationship of the hard tissues (bone and teeth) than on the relationship of soft tissues. Conventional diagnostic tools show the hard tissues much better than the soft tissues, and the orthodontist primarily aims to affect the hard tissues—ie, move the teeth and change the bone shape. In addition, 3D CBCT has limited resolution of facial soft tissues. However, orthodontists are now more aware that the treatment outcome and the evaluation of success are directly affected by the esthetics of the soft tissues, in static and dynamic stages.

3D surface images may be used for diagnosis, analysis, treatment monitoring, and outcome evaluation. This information, once obtained, is available for the orthodontist without the need to recall the patient for further evaluation, since the patient's face is captured at every angle in these images, and the information can be shared with colleagues. Two main technologies, laser-based scanning and optical-based scanning, are currently available for 3D imaging of facial soft tissues.

Laser-based technology for 3D surface imaging

Laser-based imaging technology, compared to CBCT, provides a less invasive method of capturing the face. It uses straightforward geometric triangulation to determine the surface coordinates of the target object. In this method, a laser beam (spot or stripe) scans the surface area of the target object. The object scatters the light, which is then collected at a known triangulation distance from the laser. Through trigonometry, the x, y, and z coordinates of a surface point are calculated.

Several reports evaluated facial soft tissue changes before and after orthodontic treatment using a 3D laser scanner. Baik et al[32,33] suggested a 3D coordinate system and measurement items for the analysis of Korean facial soft tissues to acquire averaged values and suggest data that could serve as guidelines for the 3D evaluation of the facial image. From these data, a template could be formed for orthodontic diagnosis and treatment planning.

The laser-based technologies have several shortcomings for facial scanning. The slowness of the method makes it difficult to use on patients, especially children, who are instructed to sit without movement or breathing during the scanning process, as any small movement may create distortion of the image. Other disadvantages include safety issues related to exposure of the eyes to the laser beam, especially in growing children, and the inability to capture the soft tissue surface texture and color[34] (even with the new white-light laser approach).

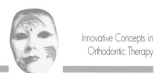

Innovative Concepts in
Orthodontic Therapy

Optical-based technologies for 3D surface imaging

Optical-based imaging technologies include the structured light method and stereophotogrammetry. The structured light method (for which only one camera is needed) is adequate for smaller capture areas and less accurate for a 3D model of a human subject's face from ear to ear. This technique is used for intraoral scanning of the teeth with the OraScanner (OraMetrix). The stereophotogrammetry technique is a sophisticated software approach based on the fundamental principle that two pictures taken of the same object, at a distance similar to the distance between a person's eyes, creates a stereo pair of images that can be used to record depth. The patient sits in front of the 3D camera on which the operator records a single 3D data set. From this, any 2D photographic view can be generated—left and right lateral, frontal, or left and right oblique.[35]

After the scan is taken, the subject's face is converted mathematically and expressed as a series of coordinates with an x, y, and z definition. The data can be coordinated with CBCT data to provide a thorough view of the patient's external and internal structures (Fig 13-22).

Optical-based 3D surface imaging provides added value for diagnosis in terms of texture and color. The process of imaging a patient in this 3D format can be simpler and quicker than traditional photography, and images can be taken as frequently as needed because these systems are noninvasive. This technique can also be used for simulation of the possible outcomes of the chosen treatment plan.

3D facial models are very valuable media for locating subjectively the source of deformity and its magnitude. For objective assessment of facial morphology and facial changes following orthodontic treatment, different analyses have been proposed. The results of facial analysis can be presented in different ways (eg, landmark displacement, color millimetric maps, or volumetric changes). The current variety of presentations reflects the need to standardize the methods of assessment.

Digital Models

The plaster cast of the dental arches is a very useful tool for orthodontic diagnosis and treatment planning; however, plaster casts are fragile and consume valuable physical storage space. Virtual models of the dental arches have been available for several years now and provide an alternative (Fig 13-23). These models have advantages over physical casts in terms of storage (8 to 10 megabytes per model) and retrieval (network availability); the orthodontist can access these records at any time to analyze or reanalyze the patient and continually monitor the condition during treatment. Multiple studies have compared the traditional study casts with the digital and virtual models, with good results.[36–38]

Silvia Geron

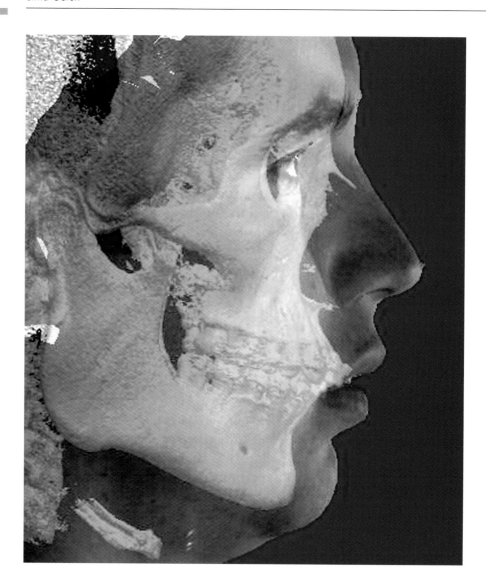

Fig 13-22 Surface optic scanning, merged with CBCT data, provides a thorough view of the patient's soft and hard tissues. (Courtesy of Dolphin Imaging, Chatsworth, CA.)

The electronic records enable analytic features, point-to-point measures, Bolton analyses, and measurement of overjet, overbite, and arch length discrepancies. Intra- and inter-arch relationships, as well as transverse relationships and the occlusion, can be examined more easily and with much more precision (Fig 13-24). It is also a simple process to send the model or part of it by email, to print it to simplify communication, to link it to the patient's file, and to create a backup. The virtual models can be used for simulation of tooth movements. They are also helpful for fabrication of archwires using specific robotics after the bracket positions are set up on the virtual dental arches,[39] or fabrication of active orthodontic appliances such as clear aligners.

The 3D intraoral models can be produced either by laser or CT scans of the silicone impression and registration bite taken by the orthodontist,[40] or by intraoral optic scanning[41] (structured light technique/OraScanner). The physical cast need only be produced if required and

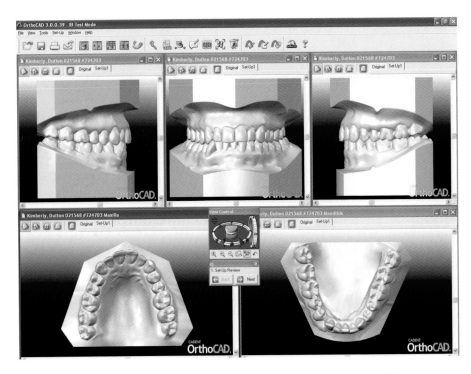

Fig 13-23 Virtual models of the dental arches. (Courtesy of Cadent, Fairview, NJ.)

can be created by various reverse engineering (RE) and rapid prototyping (RP) systems.

Software

Several software applications (eg, Orapix [Orapix], DigiModel [OrthoProofUSA], and OrthoCAD [Cadent]) have been developed to enable the orthodontist to view, manipulate, measure, and analyze 3D digital study models. The models can be reviewed separately or together from any direction and in any desired magnification onscreen. Ortho-CAD software comes with several diagnostic tools such as measurement analysis, Bolton analysis, arch width and length, midline analysis, inter-occlusal contacts, overjet, and overbite. Any view can be printed or sent to a colleague as an email attachment (see Figs 13-23 and 13-24).

Virtual setup is also possible with OrthoCAD (Fig 13-25). The software enables virtual bracket positioning using a feature called IQ that is based on the virtual setup. After the clinician approves the simulated treatment model and selects the brackets and tubes, the virtual brackets are positioned on the simulation and transferred to a physical cast by RE. A transfer tray for indirect bonding is then fabricated by OrthoCAD and sent to the orthodontist.

A new function recently added to the software, iTero, takes intra-oral scans to record digital impressions for dental restorations and then transmits the information to the laboratory, where the restoration is manufactured.[42] Recently, new software was developed that enables the use of iTero intraoral scans for orthodontic models.

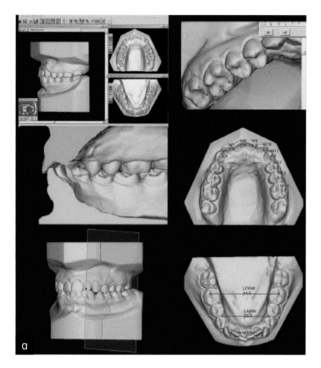

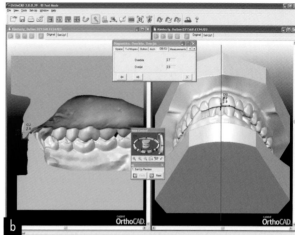

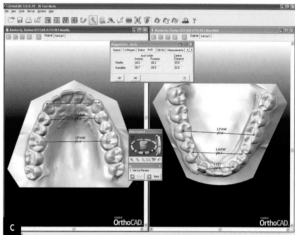

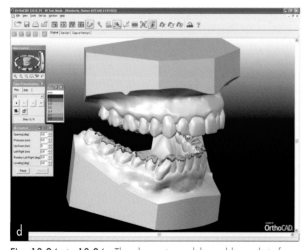

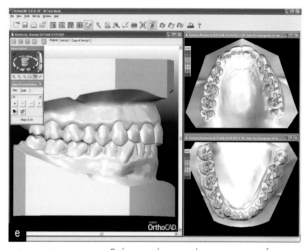

Figs 13-24a to 13-24e The electronic models enable analytic features, point-to-point measures, Bolton analysis, and measurement of overjet, overbite, and arch length discrepancies. (Courtesy of Cadent, Fairview, NJ.)

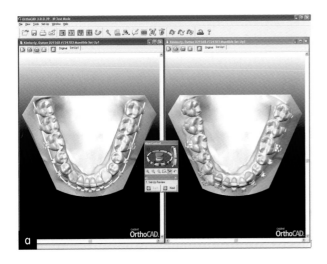

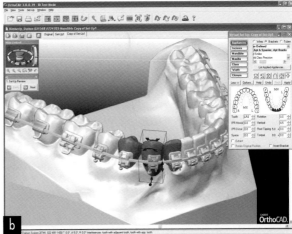

Figs 13-25a and 13-25b Virtual setup is processed. (Courtesy of Cadent, Fairview, NJ.)

Fabrication of active orthodontic appliances

Various RE techniques allow the digital models to be used in the creation of active orthodontic appliances. After the virtual design and simulation of orthodontic operations has been reviewed, RP manufactures physical casts that can be used for further treatment planning and functional tests.[43] These systems can replace stages in orthodontic processes currently performed by hand, such as the design and manufacture of corrective appliances.[44]

One such corrective appliance is the Invisalign (Align Technology) appliance for orthodontic tooth movement. It is a thin overlay sequential appliance[45] based on the treatment plan, the records, and the models that are sent to Align Technology. A CT scan is made from the dental impressions to produce a 3D digital model. CAD (computer-aided design) software is then used to simulate the movement of teeth during treatment. The treatment plan is reviewed, modified, and approved before the aligners are created. Invisalign then uses advanced stereolithography to build precise models of the teeth at each stage of treatment. Individualized clear aligners are made from these models and sent to the office.

Patient-specific appliances (PSAs) are another example of an active orthodontic appliance. With fabrication of the PSAs, it is imperative to match treatment to the patient's needs as closely as possible, which decreases the reliance on hand-eye coordination. Insignia (Ormco) is a PSA for the labial technique.[46] The silicone impressions are digitized to form a precise mathematical model of the patient's anatomy; then the individual teeth are segmented from the whole arch and the final occlusion constructed. Over this setup the appliances are designed: brackets, wire forms, and precision placement devices. iBraces/ Incognito (Lingualcare) is a system that generates individual brackets for the lingual technique at a computer workstation. The brackets are

Innovative Concepts in Orthodontic Therapy

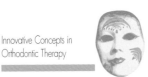

constructed from a wax-like material on a prototyping machine and cast in gold. The finished brackets are then fixed onto the malocclusion model, and a bonding tray is fabricated. The highly complex geometries resulting from this individualization are programmed into the archwire through bending technology.

The combination of different imaging and RE technologies can provide fascinating virtual possibilities and clinical applications for orthodontics. For example, Faber et al[47] described the clinical application of CBCT combined with RP for diagnosis, treatment planning, and appliance production in a case of maxillary canine impaction. A 3D model that displays not only the crowns but also the individual roots and craniofacial structures was presented by Macchi et al.[48] The model currently in use, whether plaster or virtual, is limited to the display of the crowns only, without root morphology and the surrounding bone, and it cannot show the true size, location, or relationship of the roots to the teeth and other anatomical structures. A combination of CT scans of the craniofacial structures and laser scanning of the dental arches provides high-resolution 3D images with relatively low radiation exposure. This combined model could greatly help the clinician in diagnosis and treatment planning to *(1)* determine various treatment options (setups), *(2)* monitor changes over time, *(3)* predict and display final treatment results, and *(4)* measure treatment outcomes accurately.

Conclusion

3D imaging techniques in orthodontics are rapidly spreading and changing the face of the future of the specialty. These techniques enable the clinician to present a physical object as a virtual, computerized picture that may be used for records, diagnosis, or treatment planning. RE by RP or stereolithography reverses the traditional process by converting the virtual 3D image to a concrete object.

The interpretation of the CT image is very important and depends on a solid comprehension of the inherent limitations of the machine and the software—and the different possible artifacts—which may lead to misdiagnosis. Understanding the deficiencies of CT images prevents misinterpretations and false diagnoses.

In the near future, 3D imaging and RE techniques in different combinations will undoubtedly become everyday tools in orthodontic diagnostics, treatment planning, and production of appliances. This technology makes it possible to collect and store a vast amount of data, generate a variety of hard and soft tissue analyses that combine to create a virtual patient, and fabricate patient-specific appliances for convenience and accuracy.

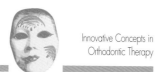

Innovative Concepts in
Orthodontic Therapy

Acknowledgment

I wish to thank Mr Amnon Leitner of the Panorama Institute, Naharia, Israel, for his generous assistance with the images that appear in this chapter.

References

1. Baumrind S, Moffitt FH, Curry S. The geometry of three-dimensional measurement from paired coplanar x-ray images. Am J Orthod 1983;84:313–322.
2. Grayson B, Cutting C, Bookstein FL, Kim H, McCarthy JG. The three-dimensional cephalogram: Theory, technique, and clinical application. Am J Orthod Dentofacial Orthop 1988;94:327–337.
3. Hounsfield GN. Computerized transverse axial scanning (tomography). 1. Description of system. Br J Radiol 1973;46:1016–1022.
4. Mozzo P, Procacci C, Tacconi A, Martini PT, Andreis IA. A new volumetric CT machine for dental imaging based on the cone-beam technique: Preliminary results. Eur Radiol 1998;8:1558–1564.
5. Cattaneo PM, Melsen B. The use of cone-beam computed tomography in an orthodontic department in between research and daily clinic. World J Orthod 2008;9:269–282.
6. Ballrick JW, Palomo JM, Ruch E, Amberman BD, Hans MG. Image distortion and spatial resolution of a commercially available cone-beam computed tomography machine. Am J Orthod Dentofacial Orthop 2008;134:573–582.
7. Moshiri M, Scarfe WC, Hilgers ML, Scheetz JP, Silveira AM, Farman AG. Accuracy of linear measurements from imaging plate and lateral cephalometric images derived from cone-beam computed tomography. Am J Orthod Dentofacial Orthop 2007;132:550–560.
8. Stratemann SA, Huang JC, Maki K, Miller AJ, Hatcher DC. Comparison of cone beam computed tomography imaging with physical measurements. Dentomaxillofac Radiol 2008;37(2):80–93.
9. Lee RD. Common image artifacts in cone beam CT. AADMRT Newsletter. Summer 2008.
10. Zhang Y, Zhang L, Zhu R, Lee AK, Chambers M, Dong L. Reducing metal artifacts in cone-beam CT images by preprocessing projection data. Int J Radiat Oncol Bio Phys 2007;67(3):924–932.
11. Ludlow JB, Davies-Ludlow LE, Brooks SL, Howerton WB. Dosimetry of 3 CBCT devices for oral and maxillofacial radiology: CB Mercuray, NewTom 3G and i-CAT. Dentomaxillofac Radiol 2006;35(4):219–226.
12. Tsiklakis K, Donta C, Gavala S, Karayianni K, Kamenopoulou V, Hourdakis CJ. Dose reduction in maxillofacial imaging using low dose Cone Beam CT. Eur J Radiol 2005;56(3):413–417.
13. Loubele M, Jacobs R, Maes F, et al. Radiation dose vs. image quality for low-dose CT protocols of the head for maxillofacial surgery and oral implant planning. Radiat Prot Dosimetry 2005;117(1–3):211–216.
14. Guerrero ME, Jacobs R, Loubele M, Schutyser F, Suetens P, van Steenberghe D. State-of-the-art on cone beam CT imaging for preoperative planning of implant placement. Clin Oral Investig 2006;10:1–7.
15. Halazonetis DJ. From 2-dimensional cephalograms to 3-dimensional computed tomography scans. Am J Orthod Dentofacial Orthop 2005;127(5):627–637.
16. Becker A. Radiographic methods related to the diagnosis of impacted canines. In: Becker A (ed). The Orthodontic Treatment of Impacted Teeth, ed 2. London: Informa Healthcare, 2007:11–28.

17. Loubele M, Bogaerts R, van Dijck E, et al. Comparison between effective radiation dose of CBCT and MSCT scanners for dentomaxillofacial applications [published online ahead of print July 16,2008]. Eur J Radiol.

18. Cevidanes LH, Styner MA, Proffit WR. Image analysis and superimposition of 3-dimensional cone-beam computed tomography models. Am J Orthod Dentofacial Orthop 2006;129(5):611–618.

19. Hwang HS, Hwang CH, Lee KH, Kang BC. Maxillofacial 3-dimensional image analysis for the diagnosis of facial asymmetry. Am J Orthod Dentofacial Orthop 2006;130(6);779–785.

20. Honey OB, Scarfe WC, Hilgers MJ, et al. Accuracy of cone-beam computed tomography imaging of the temporomandibular joint: Comparisons with panoramic radiology and linear tomography. Am J Orthod Dentofacial Orthop 2007;132(4);429–438.

21. Terajima M, Endo M, Aoki Y, et al. Four-dimensional analysis of stomatognathic function. Am J Orthod Dentofacial Orthop 2008;134(2):276–287.

22. Deguchi T, Nasu M, Murakami K, Yabuuchi T, Kamioka H, Takano-Yamamoto T. Quantitative evaluation of cortical bone thickness with computed tomographic scanning for orthodontic implants. Am J Orthod Dentofacial Orthop 2006;129(6):721.e7–721.e12.

23. Kim SH, Choi YS, Hwang EH, Chung KR, Kook YA, Nelson G. Surgical positioning of orthodontic mini-implants with guides fabricated on models replicated with cone-beam computed tomography. Am J Orthod Dentofacial Orthop 2007;131(4, suppl):82S–89S.

24. Suzuki EY, Suzuki B. Accuracy of miniscrew implant placement with a 3-dimensional surgical guide. J Oral Maxillofac Surg 2008;66(6):1245–1252.

25. Habersack K, Karoglan A, Sommer B, Benner KU. High-resolution multislice computerized tomography with multiplanar and 3-dimensional reformation imaging in rapid palatal expansion. Am J Orthod Dentofacial Orthop 2007;131(6):776–781.

26. Garrett BJ, Caruso JM, Rungcharassaeng K, Farrage JR, Kim JS, Taylor GD. Skeletal effects to the maxilla after rapid maxillary expansion assessed with cone-beam computed tomography. Am J Orthod Dentofacial Orthop 2008 Jul;134(1);8.e1–8.e11.

27. Phatouros A, Goonewardene MS. Morphologic changes of the palate after rapid maxillary expansion: A 3-dimensional computed tomography evaluation. Am J Orthod Dentofacial Orthop 2008;134(1):117–124.

28. Armstrong C, Johnston C, Burden D, Stevenson M. Localizing ectopic maxillary canines—Horizontal or vertical parallax? Eur J Orthod 2003 Dec;25(6):585–589.

29. Kumar V, Ludlow JB, Mol A, Cevidanes L. Comparison of conventional and cone beam CT synthesized cephalograms. Dentomaxillofac Radiol 2007;36(5):263–269.

30. Cha JY, Mah J, Sinclair P. Incidental findings in the maxillofacial area with 3-dimensional cone-beam imaging. Am J Orthod Dentofacial Orthop 2007;132(1):7–14.

31. Jerrold L. Litigation, legislation, and ethics. Liability regarding computerized axial tomography scans. Am J Orthod Dentofacial Orthop 2007;132(1):122–124.

32. Baik HS, Jeon JM, Lee HJ. Facial soft-tissue analysis of Korean adults with normal occlusion using a 3-dimensional laser scanner. Am J Orthod Dentofacial Orthop 2007;131(6):759–766.

33. Baik HS, Lee HJ, Lee KJ. A proposal for soft tissue landmarks for craniofacial analysis using 3-dimensional laser scan imaging World J Orthod 2006;7:7–14.

34. Hajeer MY, Millett DT, Ayoub AF, Siebert JP. Applications of three-dimensional imaging in orthodontics: Part I. J Orthod 2004;31(1):62–70.

35. Lane C, Harrell W Jr. Completing the 3-dimensional picture. Am J Orthod Dentofacial Orthop 2008;133(4):612–620.

36. Garino F, Garino GB. Comparison of dental arch measurements between stone and digital casts. World J Orthod 2002;3(3):250–254.

37. Zilberman O, Huggare JA, Parikakis KA. Evaluation of the validity of tooth size and arch width measurements using conventional and three-dimensional virtual orthodontic models. Angle Orthod 2003;73(3):301–306.

Innovative Concepts in
Orthodontic Therapy

38. Santoro M, Galkin S, Teredesai M, Nicolay OF, Cangialosi TJ. Comparison of measurements made on digital and plaster models. Am J Orthod Dentofacial Orthop 2003;124(1):101–105.

39. OraMetrix website. Available at www.orametrix.com. Accessed 1 June 2009.

40. Hajeer MY, Millett DT, Ayoub AF, Siebert JP. Applications of three-dimensional imaging in orthodontics: Part II. J Orthod 2004 Mar;31(1):154–162.

41. Mah J, Bumann A. Technology to create the three-dimensional patient record. Sem Orthod 2001;7(4):251–257.

42. CRA Foundation Newsletter, November 2007.

43. Ciuffolo F, Epifania E, Duranti G, De Luca V, Raviglia D, Rezza S, Festa F. Rapid prototyping: A new method of preparing trays for indirect bonding. Am J Orthod Dentofacial Orthop 2006;129(1):75–77.

44. Gracco A, Mazzoli A, Raffaeli R, Germani M. Evaluation of three-dimensional technologies in dentistry. Prog Orthod 2008;9(1):26–37.

45. The Invisalign website. http://www.invisalign.com. Accessed June 2009.

46. Ormco Insignia website. http://www.insigniabraces.com. Accessed June 2009.

47. Faber J, Berto PM, Quaresma M. Rapid prototyping as a tool for diagnosis and treatment planning for maxillary canine impaction. Am J Orthod Dentofacial Orthop 2006;129(4):583–589.

48. Macchi A, Carrafiello G, Cacciafesta V, Norcini A. Three-dimensional digital modeling and setup. Am J Orthod Dentofacial Orthop 2006;129(5):605–610.

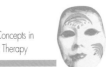

14

Class II Maxillomandibular Protrusion Correction: Creating Soft Tissue Profile Harmony

P. Emile Rossouw, BSc, BChD, BChD, MChD, PhD, FRCD(C)

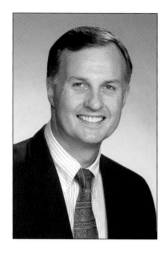

P. Emile Rossouw,
BSc, BChD, BChD, MChD, PhD, FRCD(C)

P. Emile Rossouw earned his BSc (chemistry and physiology), BChD (dentistry), BChD (honors in children's dentistry), MChD (orthodontics, cum laude), and PhD (dental sciences) from the University of Stellenbosch, South Africa. He became professor and head of the Department of Orthodontics, Faculty of Dentistry, University of Stellenbosch, until he was recruited as head of the Discipline of Orthodontics, Faculty of Dentistry, University of Toronto, Toronto, Canada (1993–2000). Dr Rossouw was subsequently appointed director of the Burlington Growth and Research Centre at the University of Toronto (until 2002). From 2002–2004, he was professor and clinic director in the Department of Orthodontics, Baylor College of Dentistry, a division of The Texas A & M University System in Dallas, Texas. Presently, Dr Rossouw is professor and chairman of the Department of Orthodontics at Baylor College of Dentistry. He became a Fellow of the Royal College of Dentists of Canada during a convocation ceremony in 1999 and has since been serving this college as an examiner for orthodontics.

His published works range through the areas of clinical orthodontics, biomaterials, jaw growth, and long-term stability. Dr Rossouw has contributed more than 100 publications to the dental literature, which include scientific articles, chapters in books, and abstracts.

Dr Rossouw has lectured nationally and internationally. He is a member of many associations and societies, among them the American Association of Orthodontics and the well-respected Tweed Foundation, where he served as clinical instructor. He serves on the review panels for various orthodontic and general dentistry journals.

Email: ERossouw@bcd.tamhsc.edu

Approximately 15% to 30% of American children have Class II malocclusions,[1,2] comprising roughly 20% to 30% of all orthodontic patients.[3] These individuals typically have retrusive or retrognathic chin positions, and the skeletal Class II pattern is generally not self-correcting.[4,5] Analysis of the average patient with a Class II malocclusion generally reveals the following:

- Class II molar relationship
- Skeletal Class II
- High Frankfort–mandibular plane angle
- Retrusive mandible
- Open bite tendency
- Maxillomandibular protrusion

Orthodontists face the challenge of correcting these skeletal Class II malocclusions in everyday practice (Figs 14-1 and 14-2). This chapter explains how, along with traditional headgear and extraction therapies, miniscrew implants (MSIs) can be used to correct Class II maxillomandibular protrusions. MSIs assist in anchorage control during correction, and they play a crucial role in vertical control during orthodontic treatment. When combined with conventional fixed appliance treatment, MSIs promote the outcome of a dentofacial structure that demonstrates ideal smile characteristics and soft tissue profile attractiveness.

Treatment Options for Class II Malocclusions

Orthodontic techniques commonly used to correct Class II malocclusions include *(1)* extraction therapy with headgear anchorage, *(2)* nonextraction headgear treatment with maintenance of the maxillary position and/or distalizing maxillary molars, and *(3)* functional appliances that assist in correction of the Class II relationship by addressing the protrusion or forward position of the mandible. Headgear used with either extraction or nonextraction regimens creates orthopedic changes in the maxilla[6–8] in addition to orthodontic tooth movement and has been the appliance of choice for this type of therapy in the past (Fig 14-3).

In compliant patients, headgear treatment predictably attains an ideal dental Class I molar and canine relationship, proper overbite and overjet, and significant anteroposterior improvement. However, it does not generally result in significant improvements in the anteroposterior relationship of the chin.[9] In fact, a number of studies have reported unfavorable backward rotation of the mandible following headgear therapy.[8,10–12]

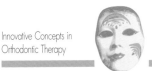

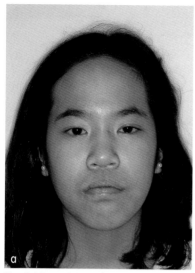
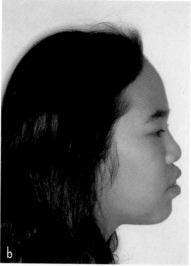
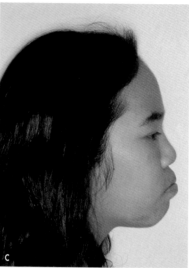

Figs 14-1a to 14-1c This patient presented with a typical Class II maxillomandibular malocclusion. Pretreatment facial photographs demonstrate a full lower soft tissue profile (protrusive lip position), lip strain, and retrognathic or retruded chin position.

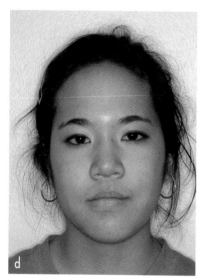
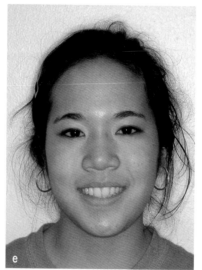
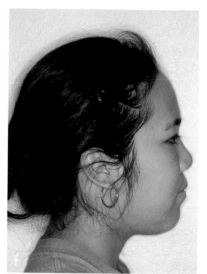

Figs 14-1d to 14-1f Corrective therapy utilized miniscrew implants (MSIs) for maximum anchorage, which resulted in enhanced soft tissue balance and an esthetic smile with an ideal smile line and no dark buccal corridors.

A recent study evaluated the effect of extraction headgear, nonextraction headgear, and Herbst treatments. The results showed that contemporary treatments do not adequately address mandibular deficiencies, and the authors of that study concluded that future treatments must incorporate true mandibular rotation into the Class II skeletal correction to obtain long-term successful patient outcomes.[13]

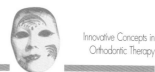

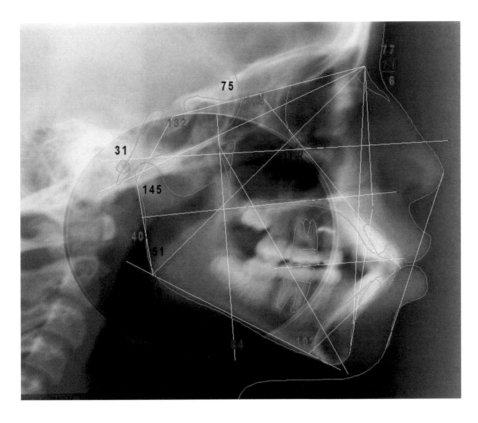

Fig 14-2 Cephalometric analysis of a patient with a skeletal Class II maxillomandibular protrusion reveals a protrusive lower soft tissue profile.

Considerations in Treatment Planning

As mentioned above, the orthodontic treatment of Class II maxillomandibular protrusion generally consists of premolar extraction combined with anchorage, either extraoral or intraoral, that provides leverage for tooth movement. If crowding is present, the extraction protocol may include only maxillary first premolar extraction. In a majority of treatments, however, a combination of either maxillary and mandibular first premolars or maxillary first and mandibular second premolars are extracted as part of therapy. The extraction sequence provides space to resolve the crowding but it also allows for the protrusion to be more effectively reduced, which results in a harmonious balance of the hard and soft tissues. In addition to extractions, it is imperative that the clinician consider several other factors when treatment planning a Class II malocclusion case. A treatment that maintains or improves hard and soft tissue esthetics and also addresses function provides the best opportunity for patient satisfaction.

Soft tissue profile

Orthodontic patients frequently seek treatment in an effort to correct facial disharmony.[14] The smile ranks second only to the eyes as the most important feature in facial attractiveness. Dentofacial attractiveness has

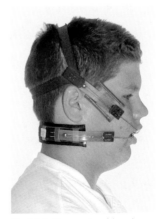

Fig 14-3 Conventional headgear therapy is an orthodontic solution that provides necessary anchorage and vertical control. Compliance is the main limitation of this appliance.

Innovative Concepts in Orthodontic Therapy

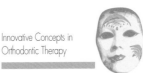

been shown to be a major determinant of overall physical beauty, and providing a symmetric smile greatly enhances the perception of symmetry and harmony in the rest of the face (see chapter 11).[15] Self-esteem tends to be heavily influenced by the awareness of one's level of physical attractiveness, which also plays a large role in how one is treated by others in society.[16] Therefore, it is not surprising that the correction of a physical imbalance such as a malocclusion that also addresses the soft tissue profile can result in increased confidence and improved interpersonal relationships.

The chin is an important component of the profile, yet it is rarely addressed by contemporary treatment modalities. It has been shown that individuals with straighter profiles and a more prominent chin are judged as more attractive than individuals with a retruded chin position.[17,18]

If the rotation of the mandible is a primary reason for the deficient profile, then it becomes clear that true rotation must be addressed in an attempt to produce greater anterior chin projection. Techniques that focus on correction of a Class II relationship through a greater amount of true mandibular rotation (eg, anchorage with MSIs) should produce more noticeable improvements in chin projection, thus providing patients with a more ideal facial change and posttreatment profile (Fig 14-4). Perception of profile, and especially smile attractiveness, may differ depending on the age or sex of the viewer; while some studies have found a difference in men's and women's assessments of smiles, others have not. Evidence is limited and controversial, but overall, orthodontists and laypeople seem to prefer smiles with smaller buccal corridors that show teeth beyond the canines during smiling[19] (see Figs 14-1 and 14-5).

Vertical control

Vertical control is another important consideration during treatment planning and execution of orthodontic correction of Class II malocclusions. Studies have shown that chewing exercises, performed for approximately 4 weeks to as long as 2 years, can increase masticatory function and can produce 2 to 2.5 degrees of closure in the mandibular plane angle.[20–22] The mandibular plane angle can also be reduced by posterior bite blocks, which have been shown to intrude posterior teeth and decrease the mandibular plane angle,[23,24] and vertical chin cups with or without headgear wear, which can redirect condylar growth and increase posterior facial height.[25,26] Removable molar intrusion appliances have been proposed as a method to intrude maxillary molars and allow favorable forward rotation.[27] While these methods produce favorable results, most are dependent on excellent patient cooperation.

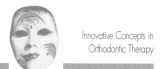

Innovative Concepts in Orthodontic Therapy

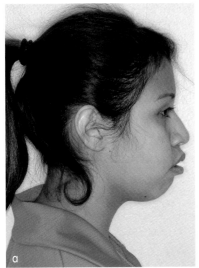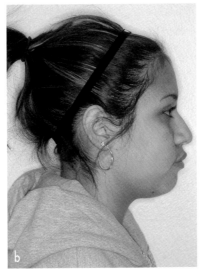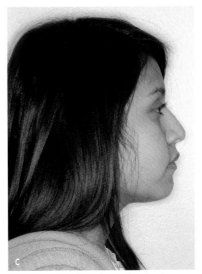

Figs 14-4a to 14-4c A pretreatment Class II disharmony (a), the subsequent progress (b), and posttreatment result (c) shows the development of dentofacial harmony. This patient is an example of successful treatment planning with maximum anchorage utilizing MSIs to allow forward mandibular rotation.

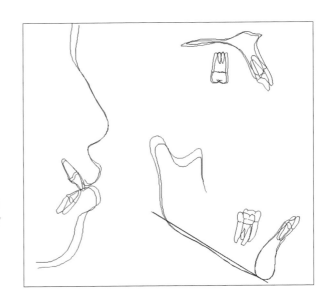

Fig 14-4d Cephalometric superimposition of the two treatment stages (pretreatment, black; posttreatment, green) clearly shows the ideal outcome; vertical control (note stable position of the maxillary first molar) and mandibular forward rotation have been achieved and create a more orthognathic, or straight, profile. Retraction of the anterior teeth into the space provided by the extraction of premolar teeth enhanced the treatment outcome.

Anchorage

Successful orthodontic and dentofacial orthopedic treatment is identified by a healthy, functional, and stable result. An ideal orthodontic treatment plan should always include consideration of appropriate anchorage, as it is fundamental to success. Anchorage requirements may range from simple to complex and may involve a wide range of forces to accomplish treatment objectives. The teeth or sources external to the teeth provide a base on which anchorage can be secured to provide resistance for tooth movement. Moreover, lack of anchorage often leads to compromised treatment options. Tweed[28,29] developed a technique based on the principles of the edgewise arch to improve treatment

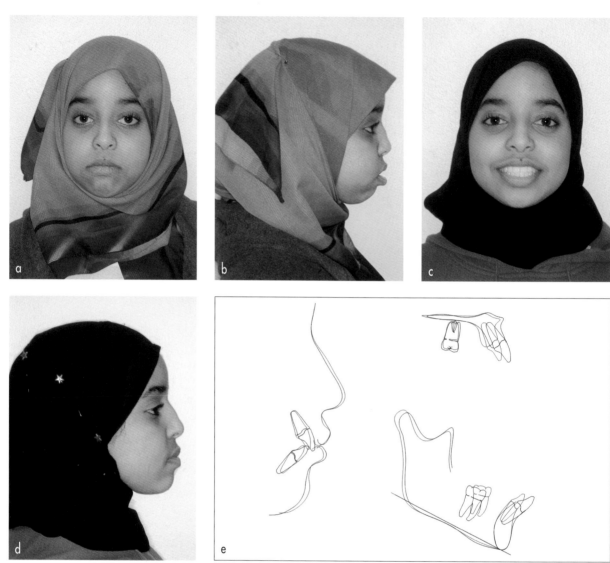

Figs 14-5a to 14-5e Pretreatment (a and b) and posttreatment (c and d) frontal and profile images. Superimposition cephalometric analysis (e) showing adequate soft tissue outcome following a treatment protocol of premolar extraction with the help of MSI anchorage (pretreatment, black; posttreatment, green). Note molar stability and forward mandibular rotation, a result of adequate vertical control. Moreover, appropriate treatment planning utilizing a protocol of MSI anchorage ensures an esthetic soft tissue profile and smile, irrespective of the extraction regimen.

outcome of Class II malocclusions. His philosophy for success included a sound diagnosis, study of the problem, appropriate treatment goals, and preparation of proper anchorage. As far back as 1939, Wright[30p152] declared that "successful orthodontic management is dependent upon a definite plan formulated from careful case analysis. Some treatment failures are due to incorrect analysis. Others may be traced to the inability to carry out a treatment plan, but often they are the result of lost or insufficient anchorage. Thus anchorage is one of the major problems in orthodontia and is worthy of careful study."

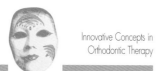

Planning for appliances that provide the necessary amount of anchorage demands an evaluation of the active and reactive tooth movements. The reactive tooth movements are usually responsible for any failure to achieve the planned goals, as Newton's third law applies to all orthodontic forces. In an effort to combat these reactive tooth movements, Tweed[31] described three types of anchorage:

- Type A: Treatment objectives require that no or very little anchorage be lost (ie, no forward movement of anchor units). This is typically referred to as *maximum anchorage*.
- Type B: Anchorage is not critical. Space closure is performed by reciprocal movement of both active and anchorage segments. The anchorage movement of one or more dental units is balanced against the movement of another on which the reactive forces are placed. This is typically referred to as *moderate anchorage*.
- Type C: Anchorage loss is desirable during closure of space; thus, optimal biomechanics requires considerable anterior movement of the anchorage segment. In other words, anchorage loss, normally an undesirable movement of the reactive anchorage segment, now occurs as a planned side effect of the movement of the active segment. This is typically referred to as *minimum anchorage*.

Miniscrew Implants

In 1945, Gainsforth and Higley's study on screw implants in the rami of dogs introduced the concept of intraosseous anchorage to orthodontics.[32] Subsequent research failed to find successful clinical applications of this anchorage, however, until 1983, when Creekmore and Eklund[33] showed the potential of intraoral implant anchorage use in their report of the intrusion of anterior teeth. Since then, a number of researchers have explored the possible clinical applications of intraoral implant anchorage and built a solid foundation for its predictable use in a variety of treatment approaches.

Contemporary orthodontic treatment continually seeks methods that eliminate the variable nature of patient compliance yet provide simultaneous anchorage and vertical control during the orthodontic treatment process to ensure consistently successful outcomes (see Figs 14-4 and 14-5). MSIs, or temporary anchorage devices (TADs), currently provide orthodontists with a predictable, compliance-free method to inhibit or reduce dentoalveolar development of malocclusions. Animal studies and clinical case reports have shown that mini-implants, MSIs, and titanium miniplates can intrude molars a minimum of 0.5 mm each month to a total of 5 mm over the course of treatment; this movement usually reduces the mandibular plane angle.[27,34–36] Through closure of the mandibular plane angle, MSIs allow the mandible to rotate forward and create favorable improvements in the soft tissue profile. MSIs offer several advantages over other removable appliances: *(1)* the implants require no patient compliance; *(2)* they provide absolute anchorage with no reciprocal forces; and *(3)* less force is needed for absolute anchorage.

As discussed above, anchorage is an essential element to help control various levels of forces during treatment. *Webster's International Dictionary* defines *anchorage* as "a secure hold sufficient to resist a heavy pull." This implies a source of attachment that is absolutely stable and rigid. Therefore, it can be deduced that, intraorally, there is no true dental anchor available to sufficiently resist active forces. Hence, MSIs have grown in popularity throughout the years as orthodontists have become more familiar with the many biomechanical advantages of using these devices for anchorage in an ever-increasing proportion of cases.

Treatment planning

A sound protocol of treatment planning ensures a successful dentofacial outcome. The Holdaway soft tissue visual treatment objective (VTO) plays an important role in treatment planning because it provides a picture of how the dental objectives can be achieved in harmony with the soft tissue goals after the intraoral crowding and space requirements are addressed.[37] The author currently includes a VTO as a component of each orthodontic treatment plan.

In addition, the following elements should be determined at the treatment planning stage:

- Level of anchorage required by the proposed orthodontic treatment.
- Ideal position and amount of space for MSIs, identified through radiographs and clinical examination (Figs 14-6 and 14-7). It is occasionally necessary to create space in this area through separation of the roots prior to MSI placement. Pre- and postinsertion radiographs are essential to verify proper placement.
- Size of the mini-implants required for correct anchorage utilization.
- Whether the patient gives informed consent for the placement and use of MSI anchorage.

Guidelines for placement

MSIs adequately fit between the roots of teeth (see Figs 14-6 and 14-7). However, it is essential to take note of zones that combine adequate bone quantity with bone quality, where MSIs can be inserted with minimal complications for successful anchorage. A radiologic study of the interradicular bone zones by Poggio et al[38] listed "safe zones" to guide interradicular MSI placement. In the study, volumetric tomographic

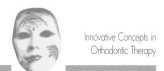

Innovative Concepts in
Orthodontic Therapy

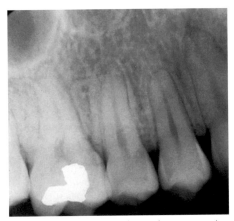

Fig 14-6a A periapical radiographic image indicating adequate space for MSI placement.

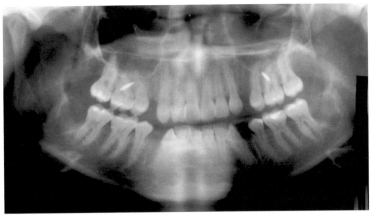

Fig 14-6b Postinsertion panoramic radiograph.

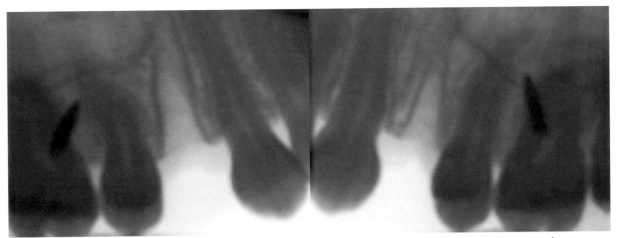

Fig 14-6c Periapical radiographic images. These, along with the panoramic radiograph (see Fig 14-6b), show the position of MSIs as recommended in the literature.[38,39]

images were taken with the NewTom System (AFP Imaging) and examined to determine maxillary and mandibular locations for safe implant placement. The interradicular maxillary buccal space between the first molar and second premolar (5 to 8 mm from the alveolar crest) can be considered a safe zone. Thus this site was chosen to enhance anchorage through MSIs in Figs 14-8 to 14-10. Schnelle et al[39] indicated that the attached gingiva may not be an ideal site for MSI placement because of a lack of interradicular bone, as evidenced by the assessment of panoramic radiographs. Thus it may be necessary to occasionally insert the MSI higher up in the vestibule and to ensure that a comfortable MSI head is available to prevent soft tissue irritation in this area. Periapical radiographs further enhance this examination.

Innovative Concepts in
Orthodontic Therapy

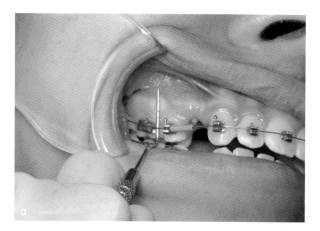
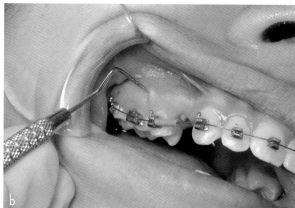
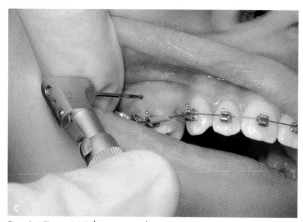
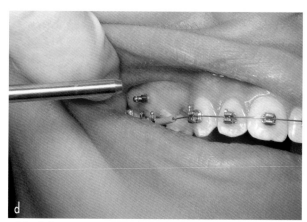

Figs 14-7a to 14-7d Initiation of maximum anchorage with the insertion of the 1.8 mm × 8 mm MSIs between the maxillary first molar and second premolar. The insertion site requires adequate bone quantity for primary stability of the implants. Determine the mesial and distal roots of the neighboring teeth by clinical inspection after a radiographic assessment (a). A periodontal probe works well for this step. The area identified for the MSI insertion in the attached gingiva at the mucogingival border is an ideal location (b). Only topical anesthetic and, in rare instances, minimal local infiltration is required. Pilot hole preparation is done with a 1.1-mm fissure bur or a small round bur (c) (smaller than the implant diameter), if required. This is followed by insertion of the MSI. Force is applied with a slow but deliberate forward-direction screw action (d). It is imperative to insert the MSI without lateral movements (wiggling), as these may affect the primary stability of the MSI.

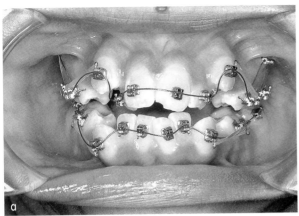
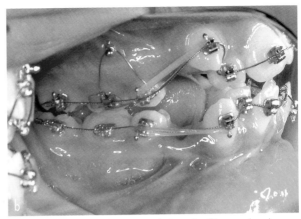

Figs 14-8a and 14-8b Frontal (a) and lateral (b) occlusal views of the initiation of treatment with 0.018-inch Speed self-ligating brackets (Strite Industries) and 1.8 mm × 8 mm MSIs (IMTEC) in position. The anchor units are suspended by a 0.01-inch stainless steel ligature wire, which provides anteroposterior and vertical control during active treatment. Note the glass-ionomer cement bite raisers on the molars that aid in elimination of dental interferences as the anterior crossbite is corrected. The glass-ionomer cement is a relatively soft material that gradually wears away without damage to the opposing teeth and ultimately leaves very little to be removed by the orthodontist. Moreover, it serves as a fluoride reservoir that protects against decalcification.

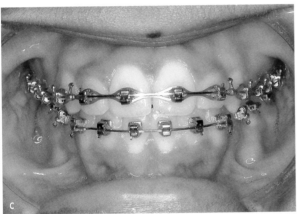
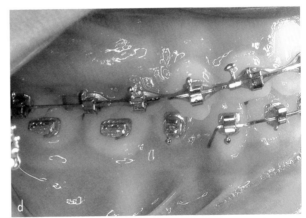

Figs 14-8c and 14-8d Frontal (a) and lateral (b) occlusal views at the end of active treatment prior to appliance removal showing the attainment of a Class I occlusal relationship. Note that the MSIs have been removed previously, and healing was uneventful.

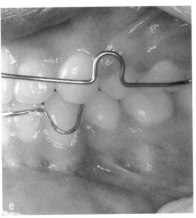
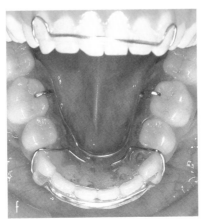
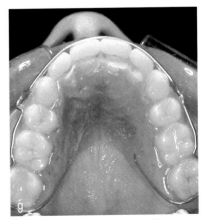

Figs 14-8e to 14-8g Lateral occlusal (e), maxillary (f), and mandibular (g) views of the initiation of the retention phase. Note the Class I occlusal relationship with removable upper and lower retainers in place.

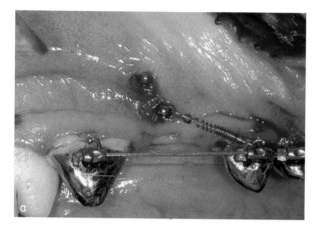
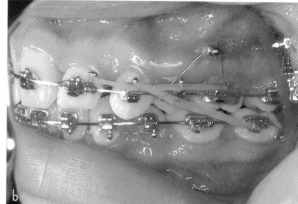
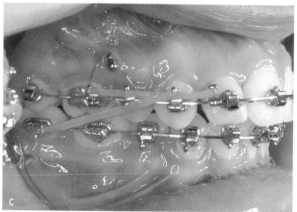
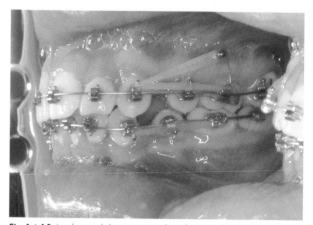

Figs 14-9a to 14-9c Implant drifting occurs in some cases due to a variety of factors. Note the drifting of the loaded implant versus the control in this experimental project (a). Similar observations were made in the clinical treatment (b). However, MSIs can remain clinically usable for anchorage, irrespective of this drifting. Compare the stable implant (b) with the contralateral implant, which has drifted inferiorly (c).

Fig 14-10 Implant stability is essential to direct and indirect anchorage, both of which are illustrated in this photograph. Direct anchorage is obtained through traction from the tooth to the MSI. Indirect anchorage is evident in the Class I traction between the tooth being retracted into the extraction space and the suspended anchor unit (note the ligature wire between molar and premolar to the MSI).

Personal observations from clinical experience and the literature have allowed the creation of several important guidelines regarding the placement of MSIs[40–44]:

- It is the author's preference to prepare a small pilot hole that guides implant penetration during placement, regardless of whether a drill-free implant is used (IMTEC manufactures both). The drill-free mini-implant has a sharp tip that could potentially damage the root.[43]
- An overdrilled pilot hole leads to inadequate primary stability. It is imperative to use absolute handpiece stability during the pilot hole preparation and implant placement. However, drill-free MSIs are available if preferred.
- Use sufficient irrigation to avoid heat buildup during pilot hole drilling.[40]

Innovative Concepts in
Orthodontic Therapy

- Adequate bone should be available at the site (see Fig 14-6). Cortical bone thickness is important because MSIs depend mostly on cortical anchorage.
- Medullary bone appears to be less important; however, a histomorphometric analysis of the mini-implant bone contact area during experimental mini-implant projects showed this area should be considered for anchorage.[45] In addition, no significant differences were shown in a project that tested the behavior of the MSIs when they were *(a)* loaded immediately; *(b)* subjected to 25 versus 50 g of force; *(c)* located between mesial or distal bone-to-implant contact, regardless of the amount or timing of the load; or *(d)* located between the maxillary or mandibular bone-to-implant contact.[46]
- Minimize surgical trauma; insert the MSI slowly and precisely to allow release of pressure within the bone.

An optimal MSI orthodontic anchorage system (see Fig 14-10) meets the following requirements:

- Stable during use
- Small dimensions
- Minimal surgical morbidity
- Easy placement and removal
- Simple and reliable attachment
- Capable of immediate loading
- Economical
- Broad area of application (not site specific)
- Able to withstand loads greater than clinically required

Implant stability

Studies conducted in the Department of Orthodontics at Baylor College of Dentistry have shown very high levels of mini-implant stability in the experimental animal model and in prospective human studies. These implants provide exceptionally stable long-term anchorage. Moreover, the mini-implants can be utilized for direct or indirect anchorage (see Fig 14-10).

Histologic examination[45] has shown adequate bone-to-implant contact, which conforms to the concept of osseointegration as defined by Brånemark,[40,46] with placement of conventional dental implants (Fig 14-11). If an MSI comes into minimal contact with the roots of adjacent teeth, uneventful healing could occur; however, deeper penetration toward the pulp chamber could lead to necrosis. Ultimately, a lack of healing in this situation could lead to loss of the tooth or, at minimum, endodontic treatment. Disadvantageous sequelae could include resorption and ankylosis.[47,48]

P. Emile Rossouw

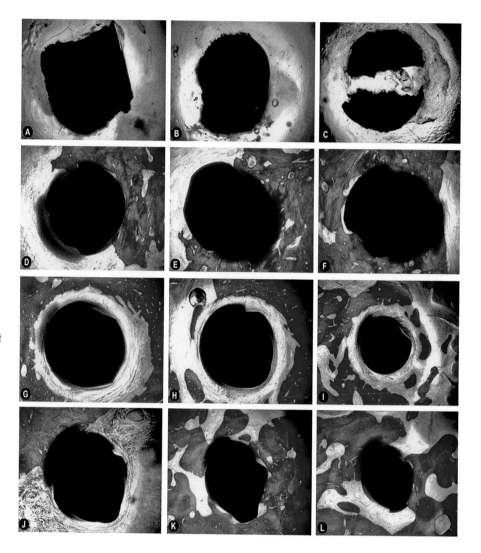

Fig 14-11 Bone-to-implant contact (osseointegration) is important to ensure that the MSI will provide the required stability for anchorage. Images A, B, and C (maxilla) and G, H, and I (mandible) show mobility due to lack of bone-to-implant contact, whereas images D, E, and F (maxilla) and J, K, and L (mandible) show stability where adequate bone-to-implant contact has been measured.[45]

The intentional removal of MSIs can be accomplished without complication after treatment is complete. Most MSIs may be removed without anesthetic; where necessary, the clinician should apply topical anesthetic similar to that used at the initial MSI placement.

Delayed mobility

Delayed mobility or movement of an MSI can occur days or months after placement[49] (see Fig 14-9) and could be caused by such factors as overloading, trauma, parafunctional habits, mastication, or toothbrush trauma. It is doubtful that underloading would cause failure. It is important to inform patients of this possibility; patient education will ensure proper care.

The following is a procedure for management of delayed mobility of mini-implants:

1. Assess the mobility of the MSI.
2. Remove the etiology behind the mobility.
3. Reinforce the rigidity by a re-screw action if possible.
4. Immobilize the MSI to prevent further vertical or horizontal movement.
5. Replace the MSI only if:
   a. The noted sequence of action fails.
   b. The patient experiences sensitivity or pain when force is applied.
   c. Gingivitis or peri-implantitis persists.

Patient Satisfaction

Patient and orthodontist surveys report positive responses to the use of the MSI for anchorage.[50] Patients may express concern prior to treatment and may anticipate pain. However, no complaints such as pain or irritation of soft tissue were recorded with respect to MSI placement during the prospective clinical studies at Baylor College of Dentistry. Most patients adapt to the implants within days and note at the end of the treatment that they would recommend this treatment to others. One of the most important factors in patient satisfaction with this treatment is that it is not obtrusive, unlike external headgear appliances mostly used for similar anchorage effects. In addition, the esthetic soft tissue outcomes meet the prescriptive parameters published in the literature and provide patients with esthetic solutions to the problems that initially directed them to the orthodontist for treatment.

Conclusion

MSIs are undoubtedly a very successful and tremendous adjunct to the orthodontic armamentarium for noncompliant patients. The shift toward treating patients with these appliances versus extraoral headgear could be considered a modern-day milestone of our discipline. Soft and hard tissue goals such as proportional chin projection or rotation of the mandibular plane angle can be adequately attained when this clinical protocol is followed. The ability of mini-implants, through stable anchorage, to apply the correct amount of force necessary for true correction of skeletal Class II maxillomandibular protrusion without invasive procedures is a significant functional advantage of these devices.

As this technique continues to evolve and develop within orthodontic practice, numerous unanswered questions remain; hence, the author and colleagues plan to further enhance this exciting and important area of orthodontics in present and future studies. Some of our

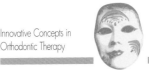

present clinical and laboratory studies related to anchorage are focused on *(1)* damage and healing of tissue during and following MSI use; *(2)* three-dimensional volumetric cone beam computed tomography evaluation of bone quality to assess differences in adult and adolescent cortical thickness as indicator for MSI stability; *(3)* segmental intrusion using MSIs in the maxilla and mandible to enhance forward mandibular rotation to complement the esthetic profile changes described in this chapter; and *(4)* answering questions with respect to the effect of tooth intrusion on root resorption. The data obtained will contribute significantly to our efforts in evidence-based clinical treatment.

References

1. Proffit WR, Fields HW Jr, Moray LJ. Prevalence of malocclusion and orthodontic treatment need in the United States: Estimates from the NHANES III survey. Int J Adult Orthodon Orthognath Surg 1998;13:97–106.
2. Proffit WR. The orthodontic problem. In: Proffit WR, Fields HW Jr (eds). Contemporary Orthodontics, ed 3. St Louis: Mosby, 2000:9–13.
3. Burkhardt DR, McNamara JA, Baccetti T. Maxillary molar distalization or mandibular enhancement: A cephalometric comparison of comprehensive orthodontic treatment including the pendulum and the Herbst appliances. Am J Orthod Dentofacial Orthop 2003;123:108–116.
4. Baccetti T, Franchi L, McNamara JA Jr, Tollaro I. Early dentofacial features of Class II malocclusion: A longitudinal study from the deciduous through the mixed dentition. Am J Orthod Dentofacial Orthop 1997;111:502–509.
5. Chung CH, Wong WW. Craniofacial growth in untreated skeletal Class II subjects: A longitudinal study. Am J Orthod Dentofacial Orthop 2002;122:619–626.
6. Elms T, Buschang PH, Alexander RG. Long-term stability of Class II, Division 1 nonextraction cervical face-bow therapy: II. Cephalometric analysis. Am J Orthod Dentofacial Orthop 1996;109:386–392.
7. Firouz M, Zernik J, Nanda R. Dental and orthopedic effects of high-pull headgear in treatment of Class II, division 1 malocclusion. Am J Orthod Dentofacial Orthop 1992;102:197–205.
8. Baumrind S, Korn EL, Isaacson RJ, West EE, Molthen R. Quantitative analysis of the orthodontic and orthopedic effects of maxillary traction. Am J Orthod 1983;84:384–398.
9. Taner-Sarisoy L, Darendeliler N. The influence of extraction orthodontic treatment on craniofacial structures: Evaluation according to two different factors. Am J Orthod Dentofacial Orthop 1999;115:508–514.
10. Schiavon Gandini MR, Gandini LG Jr, Da Rosa Martins JC, Del Santo M Jr. Effects of cervical headgear and edgewise appliances on growing patients. Am J Orthod Dentofacial Orthop 2001;119:531–538.
11. Fischer TJ. The cervical facebow and mandibular rotation. Angle Orthod 1980;50:54–62.
12. Wieslander L, Buck DL. Physiologic recovery after cervical traction therapy. Am J Orthod 1974;66:294–301.
13. LaHaye MB, Buschang PH, Alexander RG, Boley JC. Orthodontic treatment changes of chin position in Class II division 1 patients. Am J Orthod Dentofacial Orthop 2006;130:732–741.
14. Herzberg BL. Facial esthetics in relation to orthodontic treatment. Angle Orthod 1952;22:3–22.
15. Jenny J, Cons NC, Kohout FJ, Jacobsen JR. Relationship between dental aesthetics and attributions of self-confidence. J Dent Res 1990;69:204.

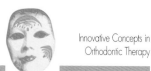

Innovative Concepts in
Orthodontic Therapy

16. Dion K, Berscheid E, Walster E. What is beautiful is good. J Pers Soc Psychol 1972;24:285–290.

17. Czarnecki ST, Nanda RS, Currier GF. Perceptions of a balanced facial profile. Am J Orthod Dentofacial Orthop 1993;104:180–187.

18. Spyropoulos MN, Halazonetis DJ. Significance of the soft tissue profile on facial esthetics. Am J Orthod Dentofacial Orthop 2001;119:464–471.

19. Martin AJ, Buschang PH, Boley JC, Taylor RW, McKinney TW. The impact of buccal corridors on smile attractiveness. Eur J Orthod 2007;29:530–537.

20. Kiliardis S, Tzakis MG, Carlsson GE. Effects of fatigue and chewing training on maximal bite force and endurance. Am J Orthod Dentofacial Orthop 1995;107:372–378.

21. Ingervall B, Bitsanis E. A pilot study of the effect of masticatory muscle training on facial growth in long-face children. Eur J Orthod 1987;9:15–23.

22. Kawazoe Y, Kobayashi M, Tasaka T, Tamamoto M. Effects of therapeutic exercise on masticatory function in patients with progressive muscular dystrophy. J Neurol Neurosurg Psychiatry 1982;45:343–347.

23. Woods MG, Nanda RS. Intrusion of posterior teeth with magnets. An experiment in growing baboons. Angle Orthod 1988;58:136–150.

24. Melsen B, McNamara JA, Hoenie DC. The effect of bite-blocks with and without repelling magnets studied histomorphometrically in the rhesus monkey *(Macaca mulatta)*. Am J Orthod Dentofacial Orthop 1995;108:500–509.

25. Buschang PH, Sankey W, English JD. Early treatment of hyperdivergent open-bite malocclusions. Semin Orthod 2002;8:130–140.

26. Majourau A, Nanda R. Biomechanical basis of vertical dimension control during rapid palatal expansion therapy. Am J Orthod Dentofacial Orthop 1996;106:322–328.

27. Gurton AU, Akin E, Karacay S. Initial intrusion of the molars in the treatment of anterior open bite malocclusions in growing patients. Angle Orthod 2004;74:454–464.

28. Tweed CH. The application of the principles of the edgewise arch in the treatment of Class II, Division 1, part I. Angle Orthod 1936;6(3):198–208.

29. Tweed CH. The application of the principles of the edgewise arch in the treatment of Class II, Division 1, part II. Angle Orthod 1936;6(4):255–257.

30. Wright CF. A consideration of the anchorage problem. Angle Orthod 1939;9(4):152–159.

31. Tweed CH. Clinical Orthodontics, vol 1 and 2. St Louis: Mosby, 1966.

32. Gainsforth BL, Higley LB. A study of orthodontic anchorage possibilities in basal bone. Am J Orthod Oral Surg 1945;431:406–417.

33. Creekmore TD, Eklund MK. The possibility of skeletal anchorage. J Clin Orthod 1983;17(4):266–269.

34. Chang YJ, Lee HS, Chun YS. Microscrew anchorage for molar intrusion. J Clin Orthod 2004;38:325–330.

35. Kuroda S, Katayama A, Takano-Yamamoto T. Severe anterior open-bite case treated using titanium screw anchorage. Angle Orthod 2004;74:558–567.

36. Yao CJ, Wu CB, Wu HY, Kok SH, Chang HF, Chen YJ. Intrusion of the overerupted upper left first and second molars by mini-implants with partial-fixed orthodontic appliances: A case report. Angle Orthod 2004;74:550–557.

37. Holdaway RA. A soft-tissue cephalometric analysis and its use in orthodontic treatment planning. Part II. Am J Orthod 1984;85(4):279–293.

38. Poggio PM, Incorvati C, Velo S, Carano A. "Safe zones": A guide for miniscrew positioning in the maxillary and mandibular arch. Angle Orthod 2006;76:191–197.

39. Schnelle MA, Beck FM, Jaynes RM, Huja SS. A radiographic evaluation of the availability of bone for placement of miniscrews. Angle Orthod 2004;74:832–837.

40. Albrektsson T, Eriksson A. Thermally induced bone necrosis in rabbits: Relation to implant failure in humans. Clin Orthop Relat Res 1985;195:311–312.

41. Cope JB. Temporary anchorage devices in orthodontics: A paradigm shift. Sem Orthod 2005;11:3–9.

42. Dalstra M, Cattaneo PM, Melsen B. Load transfer of miniscrews for orthodontic anchorage. Orthod 2004;1:53–62.

Innovative Concepts in
Orthodontic Therapy

43. Heidemann W, Terheyden H, Gerlach KL. Analysis of the osseous/metal interface of drill free screws and self-tapping screws. J Craniomaxillofac Surg 2001;29:69–74.
44. Huja SS, Litsky AS, Beck FM, Johnson KA, Larsen PE. Pull-out strength of mono-cortical screws placed in the maxillae and mandibles of dogs. Am J Orthod Dentofacial Orthop 2005;127:307–313.
45. Woods PW, Buschang PH, Owens SE, Rossouw PE, Opperman LA. The effect of force, timing, and location on bone-to-implant contact of miniscrew implants. Eur J Orthod 2009;31(3):232–240.
46. Owens SE, Buschang PH, Cope JB, Franco PF, Rossouw PE. Experimental evaluation of tooth movement in the beagle dog with the mini-screw implant for orthodontic anchorage. Am J Orthod Dentofacial Orthop 2007;132:639–646.
47. Brisceno CE, Rossouw PE, Carrillo R, Spears R, Buschang PH. Healing of the roots and surrounding structures after intentional damage with miniscrew implants. Am J Orthod Dentofacial Orthop 2009;125:292–301.
48. Hembree M, Buschang PH, Carrillo R, Spears R, Rossouw PE. The effects of intentional damage of the root and surrounding structures with miniscrew implants. Am J Orthod Dentofacial Orthop 2009;135:280.1e–9e.
49. Liou EJ, Pai BC, Lin JC. Do miniscrews remain stationary under orthodontic forces? Am J Orthod Dentofacial Orthop 2004;126:42–47.
50. Buschang PH, Carrillo R, Ozenbaugh B, Rossouw PE. 2008 survey of AAO members on miniscrew usage. J Clin Orthod 2008;42(9):513–518.

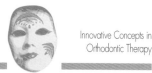

Esthetic Proportions of the Smile

15

Georges L.S. Skinazi, DDS,
PhD, Prof HDR hon, CIEH

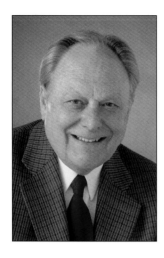

Georges L. S. Skinazi, DDS, PhD, Prof HDR hon, CIEH

Georges L. S. Skinazi is honorary professor of dentofacial orthopedics at the University of Paris-Descartes, France. He earned his DDS and PhD from the University of Paris V, his Dr of Sciences from the University of Paris VII, CIEH Paris V, HDR. Prof Skinazi is an honorary member of the French Society of Dento-facial Orthopedics and the European Orthodontic Society, a founding member of the Angle Society of Europe, and a member of the American Association of Orthodontists, among others. He is international co-editor of *Seminars in Orthodontics* and *Journal of Clinical Orthodontics*, a consultant for *Angle Orthodontist*, and a former visiting professor at the University of California at San Francisco as well as the University of Richmond, Virginia. He maintains a private practice in Paris.

Email: skinaziorth@wanadoo.fr

Objectively speaking, a smile is merely a position of the mouth and lips created by a more or less intense muscular contraction that results in a certain level of exposure of the dentition. In light of this, the author has created an analysis of the smile that provides a new perspective to esthetic appraisal called the *Skinazi Smile Analysis*. An assessment of a patient in a rest position as well as in a broad smile reveals important information regarding the dynamics of the hard and soft tissues and how the resulting facial expression is esthetically perceived.

The field of orthodontics has already established objective systems, such as cephalometric analysis and exploration of casts, to measure a patient's features and ratios and determine the ideal treatment plan. An additional analysis of the smile that quantitatively considers the proportions of facial and soft tissue structures and their role in the smile may add an important factor to the treatment planning process. Through data collected from a variety of patient populations and extensive clinical experience, the Skinazi Smile Analysis is a system by which one can gain a better sense of a patient's current esthetic state and where improvements may be made during treatment. This chapter identifies representative aspects of the smile that can be objectively measured and discussed with patients, and explains the role of these measurements in orthodontic diagnosis and treatment planning.

Elements of Objective Analysis

The first step in the creation of a new method of assessment is to confirm which components of the dentofacial anatomy should be taken into consideration and how to measure them. The proportionate depth of the mouth and the lips, at rest and in profile, was included as one set of measurements; the focal point of the evaluation is a standard set of lines that form a trapezoid-shaped region between the nose and chin. The frontal view of the mouth in a wide smile was noted as another element that could provide valuable information. The following anatomical features were identified as the four main parts of the smile:

1. Upper lip
2. Lower lip
3. Visible teeth
4. Exposed gingiva

Each of these features can be measured as a percentage of surface area of the smile, and the total smile can be measured as a proportion of the overall face.

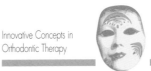

To develop the Skinazi Smile Analysis, the author examined two groups of patients who were generally defined by a group of orthodontists and lay people as attractive. The patients all had a Class I occlusion; the combined mean values of measurements and proportions obtained for both sexes, detailed below, are intended as a standard for the evaluation of other patients.

Images of the faces of young men and young women found in magazines and various ads were used as a reference to compare to the sample patient photographs. The people in the magazine pictures were often celebrities with especially attractive smiles whose faces and attitudes have a tendency to influence patients' and practitioners' tastes and definitions of beauty and serve as the ideal to which patients may sometimes unrealistically aspire. Although these images cannot be considered to be standardized with the same rigorous selection criteria as that used for the patient populations, the data collected from this group were considered important. Indeed, the sample patients who were judged to be more attractive had smile measurements that were closer in value to these public figures. Therefore, positive facial expressions in a lively, unposed face in people who are considered to be attractive by the general public are all the more representative of "ideal" expressions that are commonly desirable to patient populations.

Evaluation of the full range of motion of mouth and lips at both profile and full frontal view gives the clinician a sense of the many possibilities in this relatively small area and how changes to these structures may affect a specific patient. Two extreme positions can be taken by the lips compared with the central rest position where they lie easily upon and in contact with the vestibular part of the back teeth. In order to try to evaluate these extreme expressions, the faces of control subjects were photographed while making these expressions (Figs 15-1 to 15-4).

1. Retracted: There is a strong contraction of the corners of the mouth. This is what happens when there is a grin. In this position, the lips are highly retracted, and there is a maximum amount of dental surface exposed.
2. Pushed forward: Both lips are forcefully pushed forward due to maximal contraction of the orbicularis muscle. The lips are completely puckered and look like they are disappearing into a cone.

Knowledge of how a patient's natural range of expressions appears when demonstrating a full range of motion based on individual musculoskeletal makeup leads to treatment plans for solutions that are ideal for that particular person.

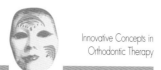

Innovative Concepts in
Orthodontic Therapy

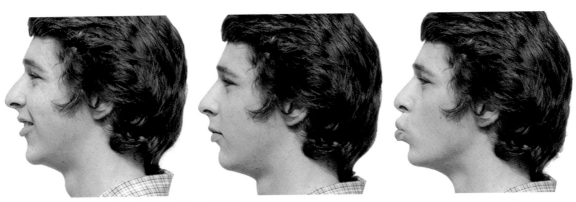

Fig 15-1 Young man, in profile, with three different labial positions.

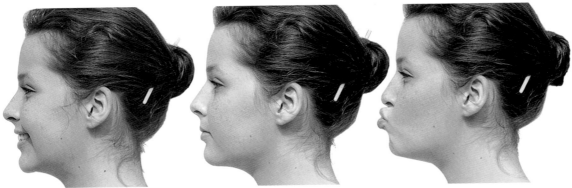

Fig 15-2 Young woman, in profile, with three different labial positions.

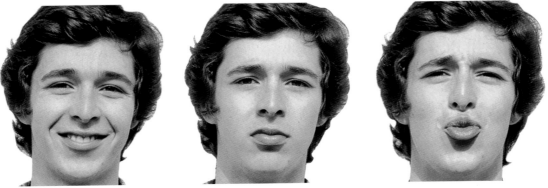

Fig 15-3 Young man, frontal view, with the three different labial positions.

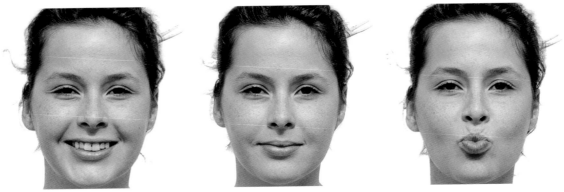

Fig 15-4 Young woman, frontal view, with the three different labial positions.

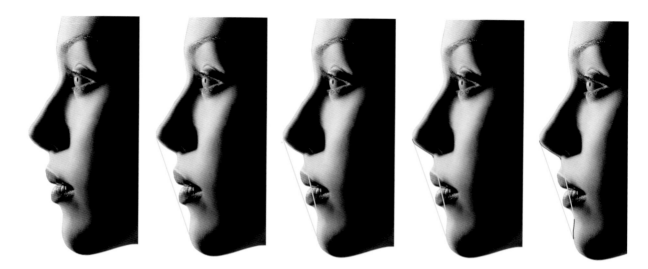

Fig 15-5 Drawing the trapezoid.

Measurement of the Relief of the Lips in Profile
Trapezoidal area

To perform an analysis of a patient's proportions based on the profile of the face, photographs and radiographs should first be taken with labial musculature at rest. The soft tissue contours of the head, face, and lips should be perfectly visible on the profile radiograph and match the size of the face on the photograph (1:1 ratio).

Using the outline of the profile, a trapezoidal polygon could be drawn for each patient based on the following (Fig 15-5):

1. A tangent line drawn from the tip of the nose (pronasale) to the tip of the chin (pogonion) (Ricketts E-line, or esthetic plane)
2. A tangent line drawn from the bottom of the labionasal groove (subnasale) to the bottom of the labiomental groove (supramentale) (Canut plane)
3. An outline of the lower part of the nose
4. An outline of the upper part of the chin

The shape formed by these lines represents an interesting area of the face because it shows the "playground" of the mouth and lips between the nose and the chin, the two most significant areas of relief in a cutaneous profile of the face. This area is where most of the changes occur during smile and other expressions.

Qualitative criteria

To assess whether the facial profile is in harmony, review the photograph and radiograph to see whether the patient's lips are closed and touching with no creases or contractions when they are at rest. A more attractive

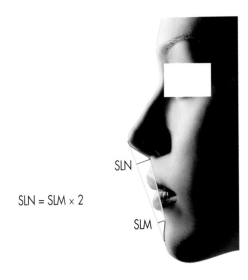

SLN = SLM × 2

Fig 15-6 The labiomental groove is half the labionasal groove.

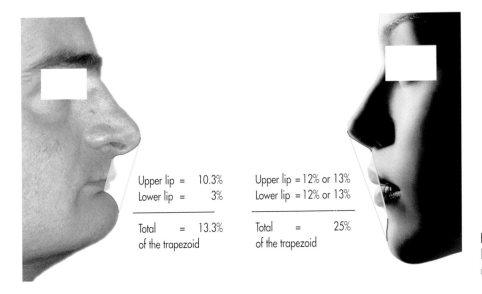

Upper lip =   10.3%
Lower lip =   3%
_____
Total   =   13.3%
of the trapezoid

Upper lip = 12% or 13%
Lower lip = 12% or 13%
_____
Total   =   25%
of the trapezoid

Fig 15-7 The percentages of the labial surfaces are different for different patients.

mouth should have an upper lip that is tangent to the E-line, or slightly pulled back from it. The anteriormost edge of the lower lip is slightly behind the upper lip.

Quantitative criteria

The trapezoidal shape drawn on the photograph can be used to quantitatively determine whether a patient's lips fall within an acceptable range for a balanced profile. The distance between the bottom of the labiomental groove of the esthetic plane is equal to approximately half of the distance separating this same plane from the bottom of the labionasal groove (Fig 15-6). The two resting lips in the image should fill approximately 25% of the trapezoid area. In a well-balanced profile, each lip should represent 12% to 13% of the space (Fig 15-7).

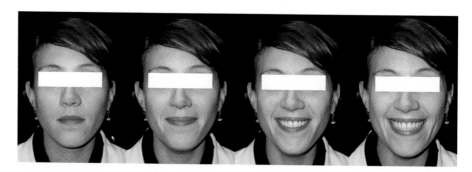

Fig 15-8 The four different expressions.

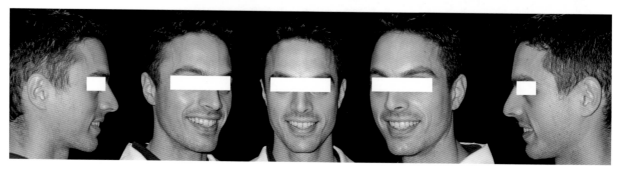

Fig 15-9 The five points of view.

Evaluation of the Frontal Wide Smile

Process

To evaluate the esthetic proportions of the wide smile, the face of the patient should be photographed with *(1)* the facial muscles completely at rest, *(2)* a small smile, *(3)* an average smile, and *(4)* a wide smile (Fig 15-8). Each of these expressions is to be photographed from five different points of view (Fig 15-9):

1. Right profile
2. Three-quarter right profile
3. Full face
4. Three-quarter left profile
5. Left profile

The clinician should always take care to place the subject and the photographer in the same position on spots marked on the floor.

An outline of the entire face is then drawn to emphasize the four parts of the smile (upper lip, lower lip, exposed teeth, and exposed gingiva). When present, the buccal corridors and tongue are drawn also. It is then possible to measure all visible surfaces. Because it would be too time-consuming and too subject to human math error for the clinician to use a ruler to estimate the area of each of the four main elements, it is recommended to scan or import the images into graphic software (ACDSee Canvas 9, ACD Systems) that can more precisely measure the surfaces in square millimeters and provide percentages.

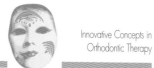

Innovative Concepts in
Orthodontic Therapy

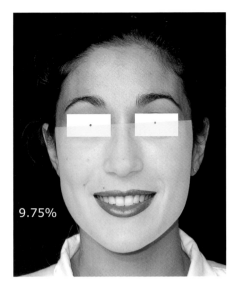 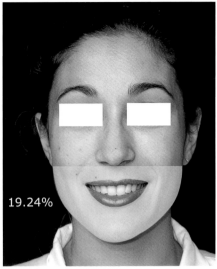

9.75%

19.24%

Fig 15-10 *(left)* The surface of the smiling mouth in relation to the large surface of the face (bipupillary line).

Fig 15-11 *(right)* The surface of the smiling mouth in relation to the lower part of the face (subnasale point).

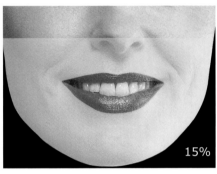

15%

Fig 15-12 The surface of the smiling mouth of celebrities subnasale point in relation to the lower part of the face.

Measurements of the mouth

To evaluate the ratio of the mouth to the face, two proportions can be recorded.

- The proportional surface of the mouth in a wide smile frontal view in relation to the surface of the face: A line can be drawn horizontally on the photograph along the bipupillary plane, and the mouth area cut out of this shaded area, which should run to the chin. The average value for both sexes (rounded to the nearest whole number) is 10% (Fig 15-10).
- The proportional surface of the mouth in a wide smile frontal view in relation to the surface of the face from the subnasale point to the chin: A line can be drawn horizontally through the tip of the nose rather than the bipupillary plane. The average value of the smile within this area for both sexes (rounded to the nearest whole number) is approximately 19% (Fig 15-11). The value for women is slightly higher compared to that for men, and the percentages measured in the reference photographs of celebrities show a slightly lower value (15% on average) (Fig 15-12).

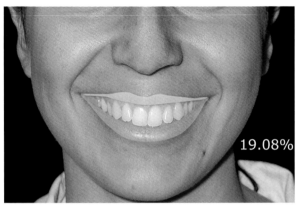

Fig 15-13a The surface of the upper lip in relation to the total smiling mouth.

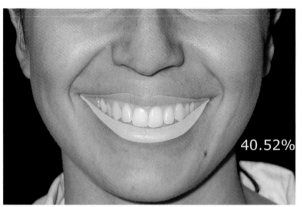

Fig 15-13b The surface of the lower lip in relation to the total surface of the smiling mouth.

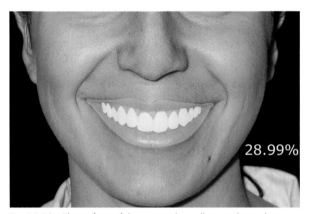

Fig 15-13c The surface of the exposed maxillary teeth in relation to the total smiling mouth.

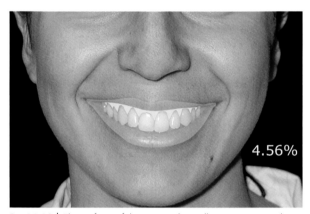

Fig 15-13d The surface of the exposed maxillary gingiva in relation to the total smiling mouth.

The four main parts of the smile

The surface of the four parts of a smiling mouth are compared to the total surface of the smile by drawing an outline of the upper lip, exposed teeth, lower lip, and exposed gingiva on the image of the face. The average proportions, rounded to the nearest whole number, have been shown to vary between an attractive patient and a celebrity, as follows:

Healthy attractive patient

1. Upper lip. Average both sexes combined: 19% (Fig 15-13a)
2. Lower lip. Average both sexes combined: 41% (Fig 15-13b)
3. Maxillary tooth exposure. Average both sexes combined: 29% (Fig 15-13c)
4. Gingival exposure. Average both sexes combined: 5% (Fig 15-13d)

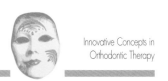

Innovative Concepts in
Orthodontic Therapy

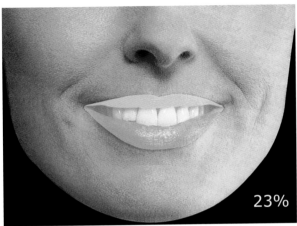

Fig 15-14a The surface of the ideal upper lip in relation to the total smiling mouth.

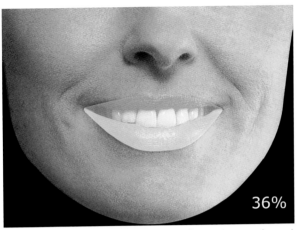

Fig 15-14b The surface of the ideal lower lip in relation to the total smiling mouth.

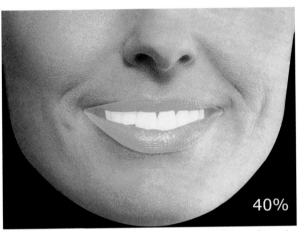

Fig 15-14c The surface of the ideal exposed maxillary teeth in relation to the total smiling mouth.

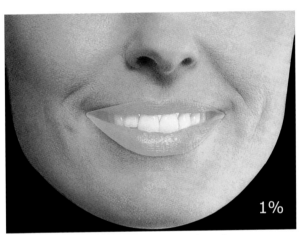

Fig 15-14d The surface of the ideal exposed maxillary gingiva in relation to the total smiling mouth.

Celebrity/attractive public figure

- Upper lip. Average both sexes combined: 23% (Fig 15-14a)
- Lower lip. Average both sexes combined: 36% (Fig 15-14b)
- Maxillary tooth exposure. Average both sexes combined: 40% (Fig 15-14c)
- Gingival exposure. Average both sexes combined: 1% (Fig 15-14d)

Women have a slightly higher percentage than men of upper lip, about equal proportions of lower lip and gingival exposure, and slightly less show of the maxillary teeth.

Negative Factors

The preceding analysis shows that a frontal view of a wide smile is very attractive based on the exposure of three essential components: the upper lip, the lower lip, and a large portion of the maxillary teeth in particular. The gingival tissues only appear very discreetly to show that the gums are well attached to the teeth.

Several other components can be identified as factors in the attractiveness of a wide smile. It would be an exaggeration to say that one of these components could completely and totally destroy the harmony of a smile. It is more realistic to say that each of them plays a role in slightly visually detracting from a wide smile that would otherwise generally be considered attractive. Thus, these 10 negative factors also must be evaluated and analyzed qualitatively to determine the strength of their effects on the harmony of the wide smile. Through identification of these factors and their extent, the clinician may be able to plan an orthodontic treatment that addresses these directly.

In this step, the entire face is taken into account with a large natural smile, and each element of the following list is scored according to the number of points possible. Several observers, individually or in a group, can discuss these scores to reach a consensus. The grades are then added together to obtain an "emotional score" on a scale of 0 (very good) to 100 (very poor) (Fig 15-15). Although this is obviously subjective, it provides an idea of the level of severity of the case under consideration.

1. The maxillary teeth are unattractive, malaligned, or have an unattractive shape, texture, or color.
2. There is excessive exposure of the maxillary gingiva. The lips go too high upon smile and create a gingival wall that gives the smile a "horsey" look.
3. The mandibular teeth are too exposed and take up too much space compared to the maxillary teeth; this often occurs naturally in older patients as the integument undergoes ptosis, compounded by the effect of gravity over time.
4. The mandibular teeth are not only visible but also show irregularity and/or missing teeth, or they are covered with plaque and/or calculus.
5. Black buccal corridors expose two large dark triangles, sometimes made worse by a history of poor dental treatment, teeth that appear mutilated, or extraction sites.
6. A protruding tongue has a tendency to push forward into the spaces between the teeth.
7. An asymmetric mouth creates unbalanced facial volumes.
8. Exposed mandibular gingiva gives the impression that the mouth has completely collapsed.
9. Wrinkles and skin folds interfere with the smile.

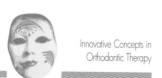

Innovative Concepts in
Orthodontic Therapy

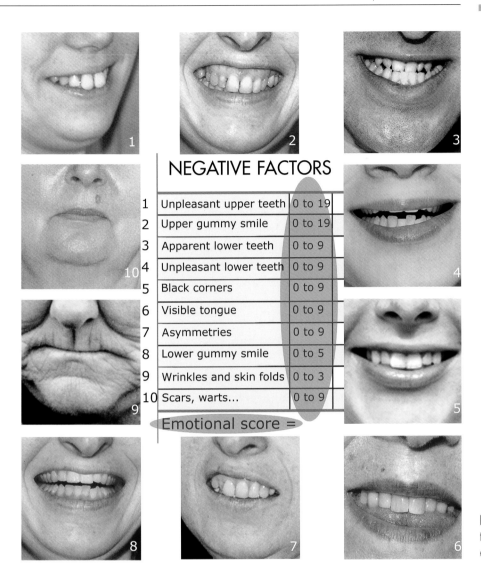

Fig 15-15 The 10 negative factors and their values in the total emotional score.

10. Skin marks such as papilloma, scars, or cheloids inhibit movement of the mouth or otherwise distract the viewer from the smile.

Data on these negative effects were gathered from all groups, and average responses to the effect of the negative factor on the whole appearance of the smile were calculated. While celebrity smiles were considered to have no negative factors interfering with the smile (emotional score of 0%), a more realistic rate of occurrence of negative factors would be 5% to 7%, even in patients considered attractive. The most frequent factors that may be encountered are black corridors, a forward-positioned tongue, crowded incisors, and exposure of the mandibular gingiva.

The question of the role of dynamic lip movements (orbicularis oris) in evidence of negative factors must also be considered. Indeed,

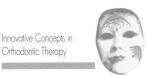

while speaking, eating, drinking, chewing, swallowing, or during all types of social exchange, the mouth, the lips, and all of the orofacial musculature go through a multitude of movements.

Conclusion

The aim of this Skinazi Smile Analysis is to provide a useful tool to evaluate the esthetics of the face and the smile. A certain amount of data and a certain number of measurements and percentages concerning intermediary facial expressions related to gender or to particular subgroups were not analyzed in the study leading to the current recommendations and will be evaluated in further studies. All data that were studied are statistically significant (SD ≤ 0.1).

It can be assumed that the volume of the mouth has an extensive effect on the overall appearance and esthetics of the smile. The management of the contents of the mouth (the teeth) should also take into account the mouth and lips that surround and support the intraoral structures. Based on assessment of the smiles of celebrities who embody society's esthetic ideals, the optimal proportions of smile components should be considered when a patient's frontal smile is evaluated: The upper lip should preferably make up about 24% of the smile, more than what an average patient may present, and the lower lip should likely take up less space of the overall smile compared with what is seen in normal patients. The gingiva should be seen upon smiling, but at a minimal percentage.

When patients come for orthodontic treatment, they have usually imagined how treatment might improve their appearance. They rarely desire to look like everyone else but rather are searching for a better version of themselves. It is therefore useful to be able to show each patient a set of objectified average, harmonious mouth and smile proportions for comparison to the current situation and a better understanding of what issues could be addressed by orthodontic treatment. It is also important to consider the baseline esthetics of a patient prior to treatment planning to identify additional areas of improvement. For example, the more that teeth are exposed in a smile, the more positive feedback the smile receives. Thus, a patient who naturally shows more teeth will be more interested in having something attractive to show off and may invest in esthetic restorations.

If the practitioner and the patient take an approach that combines desires and expertise, they will be able to imagine creative alternatives that go beyond the "basic" structures of the mouth, teeth, and smile to reach solutions that would otherwise have remained unthought of. Thanks to the use of these scales and objective measurements, a real compromise between function and esthetics can be obtained in treatment.

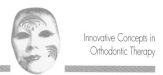

Innovative Concepts in
Orthodontic Therapy

Bibliography

Aboucaya WA. Le sourire dento-labial et la beauté faciale [thesis]. Paris: Université Paris VI,1973.

Ackerman MB. Buccal smile corridors. Am J Orthod Dentofacial Orthop 2005;127:528–529.

Ackerman JL, Ackerman MB, Brensinger CM, Landis JR. A morphometric analysis of the posed smile. Clin Orthod Res 1998;1(1):2–11.

Begin M, Skinazi GLS. Quelques repères pour sourire jeune. Inf Dent 2006;88:547–550.

Cozzani G. Giardino Della Orthodonzia Ed Martina Bologna. CSO Editore-La Spezia Anno 2000:7–10.

Dong JK, Jin TH, Cho HW, Oh SC. The esthetics of the smile: A review of some recent studies. Int J Prosthodont 1999;12(1):9–19.

Goldstein CE, Goldstein RE, Garber DA. Imaging in Esthetic Dentistry. Hanover Park, IL: Quintessence, 1998.

Heiss M. "Göttliche proportionen" des attraktiven Gesichtes (thesis). Giessen, Germany: Justus Leibig Universität, 2002;1–5.

Hui Bon Hoa L. Des sourires et de leurs proportions. Mémoires CECSMO Université Paris V 2006;10–97.

Induni S. Profil cutané et vieillissement (thesis). Paris: Université Paris V, 1997:121.

Nafziger YJ. A study of patient facial expressivity in relation to orthodontic/surgical treatment. Am J Orthod Dentofacial Orthop 1994 Sep;106(3):227–237.

Julieron M. La concavité sous-nasale(thesis). Paris: Université Paris V, 1978:92.

Kessel SP. Smile analysis. Am J Orthod Dentofacial Orthop 2003;124(6):11A.

Kokich V. Esthetics and anterior tooth position: An orthodontic perspective. Part II: Vertical position. J Esthet Dent 1993;5(4):174–178.

Kokich V. Esthetics and anterior tooth position: An orthodontic perspective. Part II: Vertical position. Part III: Mediolateral relationships. J Esthet Dent 1993;5(5):200–207.

Le Beherec J. Rapports labio-dentaires: Choix d'une ligne de reference verticale: NB/ND (thesis). Paris: Université Paris V, 1981:52.

Matthews TG. The anatomy of a smile. J Prosthet Dent 1978;39(2):128–134.

Migault O. Contribution à l'appréciation du nez dans le profil cutané. Mémoires CEC-SMO. Paris: Université Paris V, 1994:5–61.

Miller CJ. The smile line as a guide to anterior esthetics. Dent Clin North Am 1989;33(2):157–164.

Moss JP, Linney AD, Lowey MN. The use of three-dimensional techniques in facial esthetics. Semin Orthod 1995;1(2):94–104.

Nanda RS, Ghosh J. Facial soft tissue harmony and growth in orthodontic treatment. Semin Orthod 1995;1(2):67–81.

Peck S, Peck L. Selected aspects of the art and science of facial esthetics. Semin Orthod 1995;1(2):105–126.

Peck S, Peck L, Kataja M. Some vertical lineaments of lip position. Am J Orthod Dentofacial Orthop 1992;101(6):519–524.

Peck S, Peck L, Kataja M. The gingival smile line. Angle Orthod 1992;62(2):91–100.

Philips E. The anatomy of a smile. Oral Health 1996;86(8):7–9, 11–13.

Philips E. The classification of smile patterns. J Can Dent Assoc 1999;65(5):252–254.

Sabri R. The eight components of a balanced smile. J Clin Orthod 2005;39(3):155–167.

Sarver DM. The importance of incisor positioning in the esthetic smile: The smile arc. Am J Orthod Dentofacial Orthop 2001;120(2):98–111.

Sarver DM. Principles of cosmetic dentistry in orthodontics. Part 1. Shape and proportionality of anterior teeth. Am J Orthod Dentofacial Orthop 2004;126(6):749–753.

Sarver DM, Ackerman MB. Dynamic smile visualization and quantification: Part 1: Evolution of the concept and dynamic records for smile capture. Am J Orthod Dentofacial Orthop 2003;124(1):4–12.

Sarver DM, Ackerman MB. Dynamic smile visualization and quantification: Part 2: Smile analysis and treatment strategies. Am J Orthod Dentofacial Orthop 2003;124(2):116–127.

Skinazi GLS. Intento de evaluacion de los labios y su mimica. Rev Esp Ortod 2005;35(3):179–187.

Skinazi GLS. Die bewertung des gesichts profils anhand impressionistischen porträts. I.O.K. 1995;4:407–419.

Skinazi GL, Lindauer SJ, Isaacson RJ. Chin, nose, and lips. Normal ratios in young men and women. Am J Orthod Dentofacial Orthop 1994;106(5):518–523.

Tjan AH, Miller GD, The JG. Some esthetic factors in a smile. J Prosthet Dent 1984;51(1):24–28.

Tarantili VV, Halazonetis DJ, Spyropoulos MN. The spontaneous smile in dynamic motion. Am J Orthod Dentofacial Orthop 2005;128(1):8–15.

Wong NK, Kassim AA, Foong KW. Analysis of esthetic smiles by using computer vision techniques. Am J Orthod Dentofacial Orthop 2005;128(3):404–411.

Zachrisson BU. Esthetic factors involved in anterior tooth display and the smile: Vertical dimension. J Clin Orthod 1998;32:432–445.

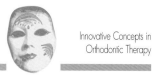

Innovative Concepts in
Orthodontic Therapy

Achieving Facial Balance and Harmony

IV

Section Editor:
Michael Scheflan

Val Lambros
Peter J. M. Fairbairn
Gilbert C. Aiach
Maurício de Maio
Michael Scheflan
Noam Hai

Facial Aging 16

Val Lambros, MD

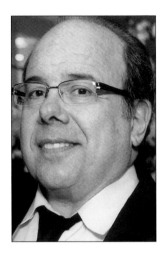

Val Lambros, MD, FACS

Val Lambros earned his MD degree at Rush Medical College (1974) and is a diplomate of the American Board of Plastic Surgery. He is a clinical instructor at the University of California, Irvine. He is a member of the American Society for Aesthetic Plastic Surgery, American Society of Plastic Surgery, California Society of Plastic Surgery, Lipoplasty Society of North America, Orange County Medical Association, and Orange County Society of Plastic Surgeons.

In practice in Orange County since 1984, Dr Lambros has been on the forefront of new thought and technique in plastic surgery on a national and international level.

He is a frequent speaker at local regional and national meetings and has challenged traditional plastic surgery assumptions about many aspects of facial aging and facial surgery. Dr Lambros is an authority on how the face actually ages, not how it is supposed to age.

Email: LAMBROSONE@aol.com

Fairly or not, superficially or not, human beings in most cultures inhabit a hierarchy of attractiveness and youth. When people look good, the rest of the world looks at them as being healthier and more vibrant than otherwise. When people perceive that they look good, they project that feeling into the world.

Why Cosmetic Surgery?

If people perceive their appearance as an obstacle to self-expression, relationships, or other goals, they may turn to cosmetic surgery as a solution. Cosmetic surgery of the aging face is an attempt to regain what has been lost, and this loss is accompanied by psychic pain. Some people have been carried through life by their looks, and a large part of their personality may be tied into their appearance. Many have lost spouses or have been divorced and are unwilling to give up on the potential for future relationships. Though these concerns may seem trivial or shallow, one of the duties of a physician is to alleviate suffering, a condition that brings many patients into the office. Many physicians do not appreciate issues about aging and appearance until they themselves grow older and feel those losses more poignantly.

In general, the craft of cosmetic surgery may be viewed as a process of making people look better and increasing the part of their self-confidence that is based on appearance. In fact, cosmetic surgery may be considered not so much an art form as a way to make people happy.

Most patients presenting for revitalizing surgery of the face are female; however, the issues of aging are very similar for both women and men, though their concerns might be expressed differently. Because faces age in generally similar ways, every plastic surgeon hears the same concerns and eventually becomes a minor expert in the psychology of aging and an observer of human self-perception. To help these patients, the plastic surgeon needs to be a sympathetic listener. Most patients coming for consultation will say that they look tired and older than they feel. Women in particular seem to have a horror of looking like their mothers, and both men and women express concerns about staying competitive in the workplace.

Plastic surgeons come to rely on instinct and the instant gestalt perception. That is, in the second or two after greeting a patient, they have formed an opinion of the patient's facial appearance and how it makes them feel, which gives them a reliable understanding of how it makes most other people feel.

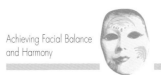

Physical Assessment

Expressive versus structural features

The face can be described as having an emotional foreground and a structural background. Glabellar frown lines express anger. Deep tear troughs and lower lid fat pads look tired. Marionette lines look unhappy or bitter. And hollow cheeks look haggard and unhealthy. The structural background of the face comprises the relationships between facial masses and landmarks and nonexpressive wrinkles and folds. The structural background does not have an expressive or emotional impact, but it gives impressions of weight, age, photogenicity, and other attributes.

In discussions with the patient, the relative importance of these areas to both of us becomes clear. Many patients—more than half—say they look tired all the time. When asked which feature makes them look so, they point to virtually every feature on the face, from the upper lids to the marionette lines to the jowls. Many others complain of looking angry when they are not. People tend to notice problems on their necks, mouths, and eyes more than those on their foreheads.

The skin

The covering of the face, the skin, is one of the most readily observed features of a person's appearance. The skin's quality, thickness, smoothness, and response to stretching and shortening are all noticeable. Likewise, the presence of shadows on the face, created by adjacent hollows and bulges such as fat pads in the upper and lower lids, are also noticeable, as are perioral and muscle-induced wrinkles.

What cannot be seen cannot be fixed. Therefore, patients considering cosmetic surgery are asked to animate their faces and necks to reveal the effects of muscle activity on the skin. The patients are asked to grimace, showing the activity of the plastysma, and in the neck, the submandibular glands are palpated. Young skin is, above all, smooth skin, and traction is placed on the face to see how it responds. These observations take only a minute or two yet provide a pretty clear notion of the materials of the face, how they behave, and how they will respond to cosmetic surgery.

Psychologic Assessment

The patient examination should not be limited to physical characteristics. Every careful plastic surgeon also performs a psychologic examination, though not a formal one. With experience, one learns which personality types one can operate on safely. Listening closely is a virtue that both the physician and the patient should cultivate. If the physician does not lis-

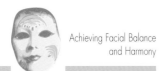

ten closely to the patient or vice versa, both will be unhappy. If there is easy communication between the two, progress will be made much more easily. Communication is a key ingredient for happy outcomes.

Some people are slaves to bizarre self-images and usually are not candidates for surgery, though they frequently seem to find it. They look at their own reflection and see themselves as if looking in a fun house mirror. The clinical experience of the physician can help patients to see themselves more realistically. It also enables physician and patient to work together in identifying those factors that most contribute to the appearance of aging and can be treated most successfully.

Surgical Model of Facial Aging

It was probably very soon after the invention of the mirror when people discovered that tugging on the cheeks made the older face look better. A whole medical industry has been based on this observation, though it is frustrating that what seems to be so easy to accomplish temporarily with fingers has been so difficult to accomplish surgically—an illustration of the fact that aging is not a surgical disease. Nevertheless, the "lift" procedures, face-lift, brow lift, and neck lift, are the current state of the surgical art.

Briefly, the surgical model of facial aging states that the face falls down and grows excesses, and it is the job of cosmetic surgery to lift and remove soft tissues. Surgery achieves just those things; it is very good at removing, tightening, and rearranging tissues. Thus, when cosmetic surgery is applied to the aging face, the components of facial aging that are amenable to these treatments are improved with predictable consequences. The eyes are more defined; the excesses of skin are removed and smoothed; and the neck and jawline are improved.

In a universe of youngish people with good skin desiring cosmetic surgery, this model would work fairly well. A full upper lid, which may have changed very little over time, would become more defined by a blepharoplasty, resulting in a crisper look that the patient may never have had. Small fat pads of the lower lid would be removed, leaving smoother lower lids. A little traction would make the youngish face look distinctly better. These are the patients who fit the surgical model and represent both the easiest subset of facial cosmetic surgery and its biggest triumphs.

However, the face does not age entirely by descent and the growing of excesses, and much can be learned by examining old photographs of patients. After even a short time of comparing patients with their old photographs, doubts as to the effectiveness of the surgical model develop. Many faces age by thinning. They seem to deflate, and as they do so, they become wrinkled in repose or with animation. Faces like this, when

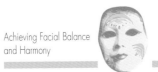

Achieving Facial Balance
and Harmony

subjected to standard cosmetic surgery, have fewer wrinkles, but they become overly defined. That is, the skin gets closer to the bone, and when the swelling of surgery subsides, the patient may look even older than before. Similarly, many upper eyelids and brows lose volume with age. A young photograph may show the presence of full brows and tight overlying skin. With age and deflation of subcutaneous tissues, that fullness is lost, leaving excesses of skin. Removing those excesses gives more definition but may make the eye more prominent in a now visible and hollow orbit. The eye looks more defined but older. If surgical alternatives exist, the physician can succeed in exercising judgment and making real choices about what will make the patient look better instead of making the same rote decisions. However, the final judgment about what looks better should probably be left to the patient.

One improvement in cosmetic surgery in the last 15 years has been an appreciation of the effects of volume in the face. By adding volume, hollow cheeks can look full instead of skull-like. Overly round orbits can appear fuller and more oval. Cheekbones can be elevated. Jawlines can be separated from the neck. Initially, the tools of volume alterations of the face were limited to implants and injected fat. Each has technical advantages and disadvantages. As more fillers become available, there is greater flexibility in addressing issues of volume in the aging face.

By examining photographs taken of people over a long span of time, cosmetic surgeons have learned that the process of aging is more complex than the surgical model describes. Creating an anatomically correct young face frequently looks quite odd in aging patients because of the temptation to correct problems intrinsic to the skin; for instance, filling the subcutaneous space often leads to an overfilled face. In any of the hubs of Western civilization, one can see people who have had cosmetic surgery and look obviously pulled, overly elevated, and overly defined. This realization has led to the liberating thought that the goal of cosmetic surgery is not to create an elevated and defined face but to create a better looking face, one that may be interpreted as younger. The cosmetic surgeon strives to create a complex illusion based on all available tools of surgery, skin smoothing, and filling.

Since the materials of the face are the key to its improvement and since the older one gets the more questionable the quality of the materials, there is an apparent paradox to facial cosmetic surgery: The more it is needed, the less it works. Compared with younger people with better skin, older people with thin, inelastic, and wrinkled skin do not get the same degree of improvement and are at a higher risk for distortions. Very overweight people do not see much improvement at all.

The face-lift is an imperfect operation and does not solve all problems on the face, which is why cosmetic surgeons have begun to conceptualize facial cosmetic surgery as component treatments. The jowls almost always need some reduction as well as some traction. The chin

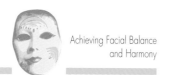

Achieving Facial Balance
and Harmony

hollows almost always need some fill, as do the cheek hollows. The tear troughs and deficiencies in the anterior malar area almost always need some volume fill as well. Before going to the operating room, the surgeon should have a fairly exact plan to encompass the various units of the face. Most of the surgery should follow the preoperative plan; clinical judgments based on a supine, anesthetized patient are not as good as those based on a vertical, mobile patient.

Conclusion

When the surgeon finally gets to the operating room, most of the analysis and conceptualization should have been completed, and the remainder is a technical effort to realize those changes. The fastest and flashiest technician never produces results as good as the thoughtful, careful surgeon.

Cosmetic surgeons operate on people with lives, friends, relatives—people who have to relate to other people on a daily basis. The surgery affects those patients' faces, their most exposed body part. Cosmetic surgeons are privileged to be allowed to intervene in their patients' lives, and it is imperative that such interventions be conducted in a thoughtful and careful way.

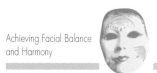

17

Lip Repositioning Surgery:
A Solution to the Extremely High Lip Line

Peter J. M. Fairbairn, BDS

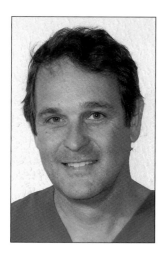

Peter J. M. Fairbairn, BDS

Peter Fairbairn is the principal dental surgeon at the Scarsdale Dental Aesthetic and Implant Clinic, London. He has had a special interest in esthetic dentistry and the perioral soft tissues since 1986 and consults with plastic surgeons to ensure optimal outcomes.

Dr Fairbairn spoke on dental and soft tissue esthetics at the British Academy of Cosmetic Dentistry (BACD) Forums in 2005 and 2006, at the International Academy of Advanced Facial Aesthetics (IAAFA) in 2007, and at the Association of Dental Implantology (ADI) Forum in 2006 and 2007. He has published numerous peer-reviewed articles on esthetics, implant placement, and synthetic bone grafting, and he is an active member of the BACD, the IAAFA, and the ADI.

Email: peterdent66@aol.com

The position of the inferior border of the upper lip during smiling determines the amount of gingiva displayed. A gingival display within a range of 1 to 2 mm at the central incisor position is deemed satisfactory. A high lip line that displays more than 2 mm of gingiva or, conversely, a low lip line that shows no gingiva is not esthetically desirable.

An extremely high lip line—that is, when more than 3 mm of gingiva is displayed during smiling (sometimes referred to as a "gummy" smile) (Fig 17-1)—often causes intense feelings of dissatisfaction in those affected. For these patients, treatment can be viewed as reconstructive and not merely cosmetic. Fortunately, this condition is relatively rare, though its prevalence varies in different cultural and racial groups, and it is more common in women (14%) than in men (7%).[1]

In working with more than 200 patients with an extremely high lip line over a 4-year period, the author has noted the following characteristics: lack of confidence; fear of being photographed, especially of being "caught" in an unrestrained smile; a tendency to smile with a hand in front of their mouth; and a desire to solve the problem. Most of these patients were referrals who often presented with the more extreme situations, and all the emotional hallmarks were immediately recognizable.

The extremely high lip line is generally less of a problem later in life because the lip becomes less active with age and gingival recession may occur. Furthermore, an extremely high lip line is not a problem for all patients; many become accustomed to this feature and live with it. Therefore, it is for patients to decide whether their lip line is unsatisfactory.

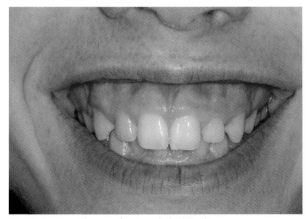

Fig 17-1a Frontal view of extremely high lip line.

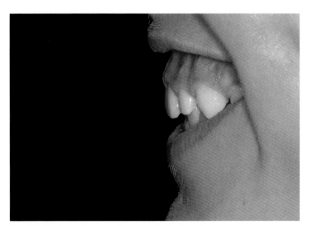

Fig 17-1b Lateral view of extremely high lip line.

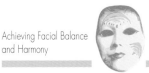

Achieving Facial Balance and Harmony

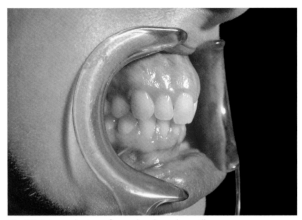

Fig 17-2 Lateral view of overdeveloped maxilla.

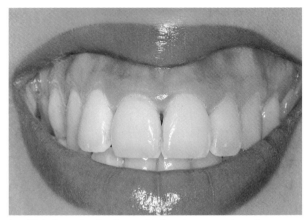

Fig 17-3 Example of a "bowed" effect due to muscle pull.

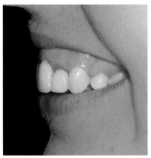

Fig 17-4 Example of extremely high lip line due to deficient upper lip length from nose to vermilion border.

Etiology

There are several causes of the extremely high lip line, including delayed eruption of the teeth, jaw deformities (eg, a protruding maxilla) (Fig 17-2), hypermobile musculature in the upper lip (Fig 17-3), and deficient upper lip length from the nose to the vermilion border (Fig 17-4). As with all aspects of dentistry, a preventive approach can be important, and in some cases, early monitoring and appropriate orthodontic treatment can prevent the situation. For patients who do have an extremely high lip line, however, the diagnosis is essential in the development of a treatment plan.

Assessment

The most important part of the assessment is a lengthy discussion with the patient so that the physician understands the patient's expectations. Is the patient happy with his/her profile? With the resting shape and position of the lips? How dramatic does he/she want the changes to be? (You can demonstrate by holding the lip.) Should asymmetries be corrected to prevent the lip from raising more on one side than the other (Figs 17-5 and 17-6)? How does he/she feel about extensive surgery (maxillary reduction) or dental surgery (crowns or veneers)? Generally, most patients are happy with a raised resting lip height, so it is not the resting position that needs to be altered but rather the excessive movement on smiling hard.

The assessment also should address the state of the patient's anterior teeth to determine whether complex dental work is needed. Frontal and profile photographs are needed of the "resting" and "maximum" smile positions, and a lateral cephalometric radiograph should be taken. This is used to take a series of measurements, as follows:

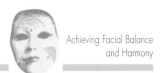

Achieving Facial Balance and Harmony

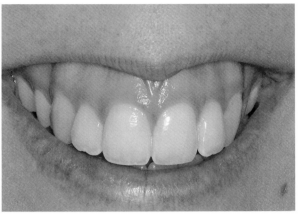

Fig 17-5 Frontal view of very active muscle pull.

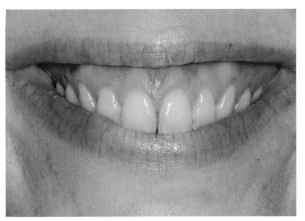

Fig 17-6 Frontal view of asymmetric smile.

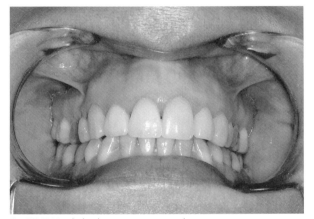

Fig 17-7 Vestibule showing gingiva and mucosa.

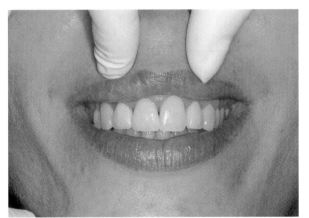

Fig 17-8 Holding the lip to visualize an outcome.

- Amount of attached gingiva: In a normal lip line, 10 to 12 mm of attached gingiva is typical. In an extremely high lip line, there can be as much as 20 to 30 mm of attached gingiva in the area of the lateral incisor (Fig 17-7).
- Depth of the vestibule: Because of the mobile nature of the soft mucosa, it is difficult and somewhat arbitrary to assess the vestibule depth. Experience helps, however. By holding the lip and asking the patient to smile (Fig 17-8), the experienced surgeon can visualize the outcome to decide how much mucosa to remove.
- Width of the upper lip from the vermilion border to the base of the nose (Fig 17-9): If this width is small, it is important that less mucosa be removed on the labial side of the vestibule.
- Strength and angles of pull of the elevating musculature: The muscles that need to be examined include the levator anguli oris, zygomaticus major and minor, levator labii superioris, levator superioris alaeque nasi, and depressor septi nasi (see Fig 17-5).

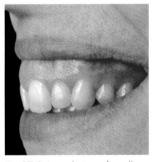

Fig 17-9 Lateral view of small upper lip.

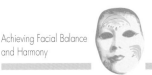

Achieving Facial Balance and Harmony

Once a diagnosis has been made, the patient should be presented with all the treatment options, including the long-term benefits and complications, in order to make an informed decision as to a treatment modality—surgical or nonsurgical.

Treatment Modalities

There are essentially five distinct approaches to treating the extremely high lip line, three surgical and two nonsurgical. Assessment of the individual case is critical in the choice of treatment plan. These different modalities emphasize the multidisciplinary nature of dealing with this situation, so it is often best to employ a team approach. The combined skills of dental surgeons, dental technicians, orthodontists, periodontists, and maxillofacial and cosmetic surgeons can help create a balanced dental and surrounding soft tissue end result.

Nonsurgical approaches

Orthodontic intrusion

Orthodontic intrusion can be an ideal treatment in younger patients, but the desired result may be difficult to achieve in severe cases of extremely high lip line.[2] This treatment option has been described and extensively performed by orthodontists. Therefore, case discussion with the orthodontic member of the team is essential in all treatment planning, as a combined approach is often the most successful.

Botulinum toxin

Botulinum toxin is a very new nonsurgical treatment option that is being pioneered by Dr Bob Khanna, president of the International Academy of Advanced Facial Aesthetics. It is primarily useful in patients with hypermobility of the upper lip. Administration of either Dysport (Ipsen; 30 U) or Botox (Allergan; 10 to 12 U) to the levator labii superioris, the levator labii superioris alaeque nasi, and, to a lesser extent, the depressor septi nasi muscles helps to stabilize the lip.[3] With this treatment, as with all botulinum toxin treatments, it takes 2 weeks to achieve the full result. Results last for about 4 to 6 months, after which the lip slowly returns to its original position on smiling hard. With repeated use, less toxin may be required because of muscle atrophy.

An advantage of botulinum toxin treatment is its noninvasiveness. However, its use is limited in more extreme cases involving the levator anguli oris and zygomaticus muscles. In addition, the use of botulinum toxin requires extensive knowledge about the number, location, and actions of the muscles in the upper lip area, making it a challenging treatment option. Finally, high doses (40 U) of botulinum toxin are required

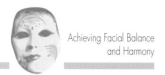
Achieving Facial Balance
and Harmony

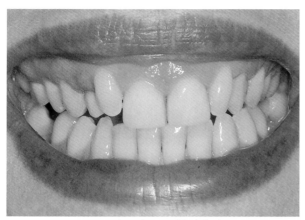

Fig 17-10a Preoperative frontal view of high lip line.

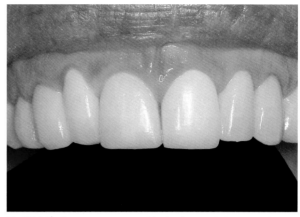

Fig 17-10b Postoperative view. Ideal soft tissue balance resulting from crown lengthening.

to achieve the desired effect, which may be uncomfortable for the patient (especially on a repeat basis).

Surgical approaches

Maxillary osteotomy

The maxillary osteotomy is well documented and regularly performed by oral and maxillofacial surgeons. This procedure is of great importance in the treatment of extreme skeletal deformities. It can be used to restore a normal occlusal relationship as well as to correct cosmetic issues. Orthognathic surgery can provide a viable solution in the treatment of patients with even the most severe cases of extremely high lip line.[4] However, it is associated with morbidity and possible paresthesia, which may deter the patient from choosing this option.

Crown lengthening

Crown lengthening is the most popular method of reducing the extremely high lip line. It is well documented[5,6] and used on a regular basis in general dental and periodontal surgery. Crown lengthening is an important treatment option for patients who need or want the associated dental work (crowns or veneers) when there is sufficient attached gingiva present. Its use is limited to the milder cases (Fig 17-10) in the 2- to 4-mm range (measured from the cervical margin to the lower border of the lip on hard smiling), and it involves the removal of both soft (gingiva) and hard (bone) tissue as needed to maintain the biologic width. Crown lengthening allows the creation of a balanced soft tissue (Fig 17-11), which is necessary in patients with an extremely high lip line.[7] A variety of instruments can be used for the soft tissue surgery, including lasers, electrosurgery, and scalpels.

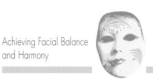

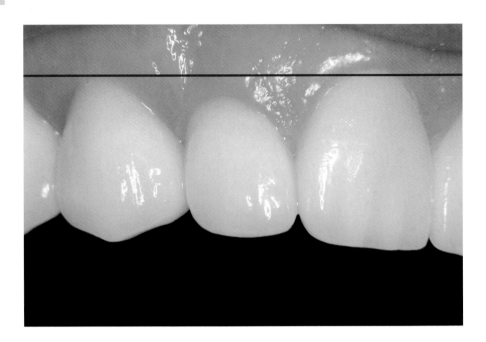

Fig 17-11 Ideal soft tissue balance.

Lip repositioning surgery

Lip repositioning surgery, a relatively simple procedure, involves the removal of a section of mucosa and (depending on the case) the attached gingiva. It results in a narrower vestibule and a more firmly attached mucogingival margin that restricts the muscular action of the upper lip, thereby reducing the visible gingiva on smiling. This procedure has its origins in the plastic surgery techniques of 30 years ago.[8] The author has treated patients with it for 4 years.[9] Once this treatment option has been chosen, the case must be reassessed to determine the shape and extent of the area of mucosa to be surgically removed. The patient must give informed consent, and the surgical procedure can then be performed, usually under sedation.

Surgical Procedure: Lip Repositioning Surgery

All parts of the assessment process must be completed before surgery is started. The patient should rinse with a chlorhexidine mouthwash, followed by the administration of a local anesthetic (lidocaine hydrochloride 2% with adrenalin 1:80,000) into the mucosa from the area of the first premolar to first premolar (Fig 17-12a). The inexperienced surgeon may choose to outline the incision lines with a marking pen prior to administration of the local anesthetic, which distorts the vestibule.

The incisions are made bilaterally using two no. 15 scalpel blades, one for each side.[10,11] Always start with the mucosal partial-thickness incision first, working from the centerline (Fig 17-12b) to the first pre-

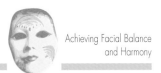

Achieving Facial Balance
and Harmony

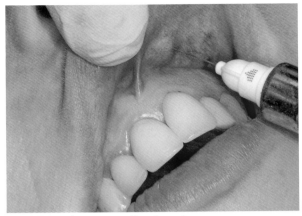

Fig 17-12a Administration of local anesthetic.

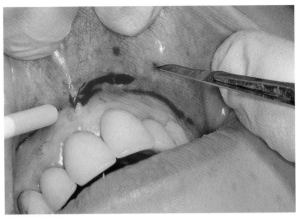

Fig 17-12b Initial incision of the mucosa.

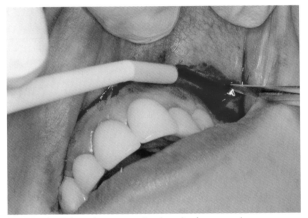

Fig 17-12c Taking the incision back to the first premolar area.

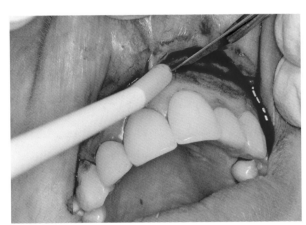

Fig 17-12d Making the gingival incision.

molar or even the second premolar area (Fig 17-12c) as this allows a certain stability from the attached gingiva. When making the incision, the tension of the mucosa-gingiva attachment will be released and can be felt; this tension will later be re-created on suturing. Next, proceed to the attached gingiva (Fig 17-12d), making the incision down to the periosteum, which is retained to provide the new attachment. The two incisions meet (Fig 17-12e) at the premolar area, and epithelial tissue is carefully removed (Fig 17-12f). The width of material to be removed varies based on case assessment and patient needs (more tissue for a more dramatic effect) (Fig 17-12g). Once the tissue is removed, use gauze to stem the blood flow (Fig 17-12h), and then proceed to the other side, being careful to avoid minor salivary glands and musculature. The result is an elliptical area where the epithelial layer has been removed, exposing the

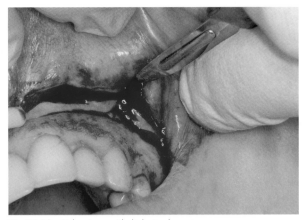

Fig 17-12e Releasing epithelial attachment.

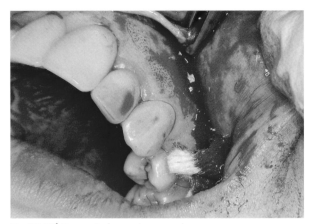

Fig 17-12f Removal of tissue between the incisions.

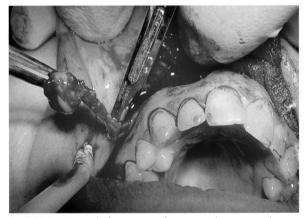

Fig 17-12g Removal of more tissue for a more dramatic result.

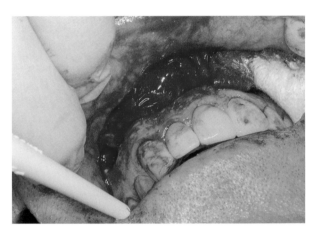

Fig 17-12h Use of gauze to stem blood flow.

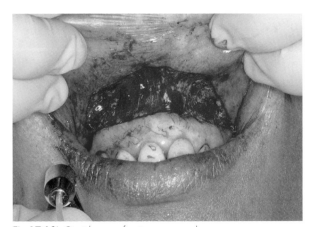

Fig 17-12i Ovoid area after tissue removal.

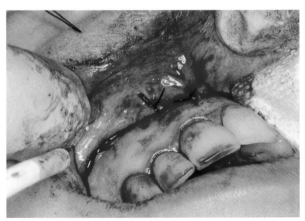

Fig 17-12j Centerline is sutured first.

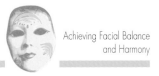

Achieving Facial Balance
and Harmony

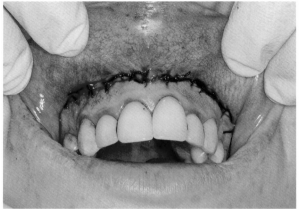

Fig 17-12k Completed suture line.

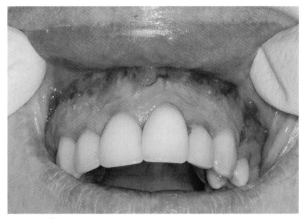

Fig 17-12l Resultant scar line at 2 weeks.

deeper connective tissue (Fig 17-12i). The two incisions can then be approximated and the possible outcome reassessed to determine whether more tissue needs to be removed on one or both sides (a decision that relies on experience), after which the suturing can commence.

Always begin the suturing at the centerline (frenum) to ensure that the position of the lip is retained in a lateral context (Fig 17-12j). Then, proceed to suture the remainder of the area, placing an interrupted suture (3-0 Mersilk [Ethicon] or vicryl [Ethicon], depending on the surgeon's preference) every 2 to 3 mm to ensure firm attachment of the mucosa to the periosteum and attached gingiva (Fig 17-12k). To resist the forces of facial expression and mastication for the next 2 weeks, the sutures must be well placed and firmly tied.

The patient is then instructed to use oral antibiotics, an anti-inflammatory medication, and an oral rinse (Corsodyl Mouthwash, GlaxoSmithKline). Most important, the patient is warned to avoid excessive use of lower facial expression for the following 2 weeks. Excessive smiling and other lip movement in this period can affect the strength of the new mucogingival bond or even rupture the sutures. This is a very important aspect of healing and must be stressed as such to the patient.

After 1 week, alternate sutures are removed to further aid the healing process, and then after 2 weeks the remaining sutures are removed, leaving a scar (Fig 17-12l) that is not visible because of the lip. The collagen fibers and even muscle fibers from orbicularis oris will now be firmly attached to the periosteum to form a strong bond that will resist actions of the musculature. When asked to smile hard during the postoperative assessment, patients generally report a tightness that is less marked than when the sutures were in place. The tightness eases over time, and patients become more used to the situation, as indicated by its

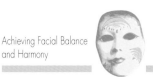

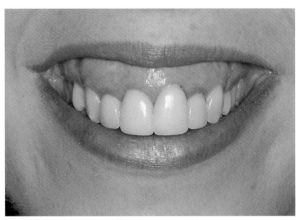

Fig 17-12m Preoperative frontal view on smiling.

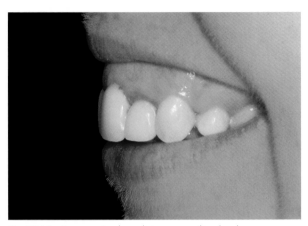

Fig 17-12n Preoperative lateral view on smiling hard.

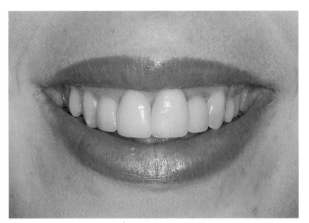

Fig 17-12o Postoperative frontal view on smiling.

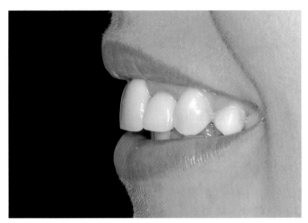

Fig 17-12p Postoperative lateral view on smiling hard.

not being an important issue at follow-up visits. Next, postoperative photographs are taken and shown to the patient (Figs 17-12m to 17-12p), allowing the physician to note patients' level of satisfaction.

As with all soft tissue surgical procedures, there can be some relapse, but the author has noted a low level of relapse over the 4 years of doing this procedure. Side effects of the procedure can be an increased fullness of the upper lip, especially on smiling (Fig 17-13), and reduced nasolabial folding, both of which appear to be desirable to most patients, especially to those with severe conditions.

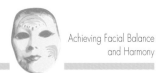

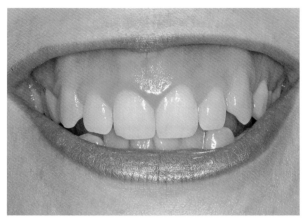

Fig 17-13a Preoperative frontal view of thin lips.

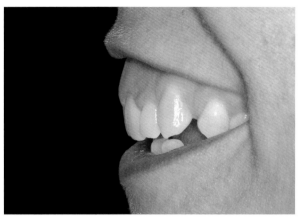

Fig 17-13b Preoperative lateral view of thin lips showing deep nasolabial lines.

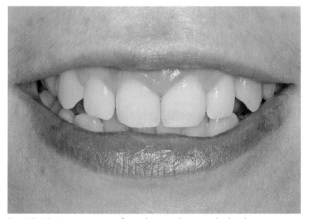

Fig 17-13c Postoperative frontal view showing thicker lips.

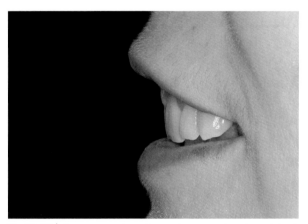

Fig 17-13d Postoperative lateral view showing reduced nasolabial lines.

Surgical variations

Minor surgical variations can be used in different cases to achieve the best solution for the patient. As with all esthetic procedures, there is often little fixed measurement and more "feel" to achieve the results that patients desire; thus dialogue in evaluation is necessary.

For the patient shown in Fig 17-14, the biggest issue is the width of the lip from the vermilion border to the base of the nose, which correlates to less labial mucosal tissue in the vestibule. In such cases, less mucosal tissue

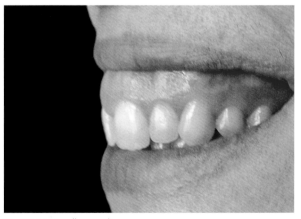

Fig 17-14 Small upper lip.

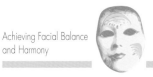

Achieving Facial Balance
and Harmony

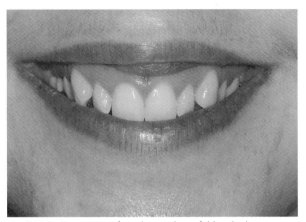

Fig 17-15a Preoperative frontal view shows fold in the lip on smiling.

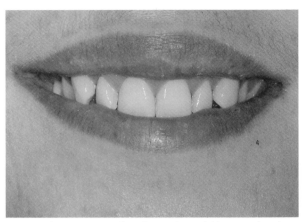

Fig 17-15b Postoperative frontal view shows fold removed and fuller lip.

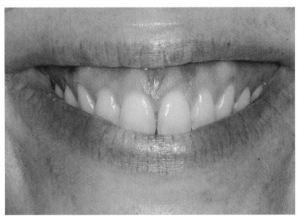

Fig 17-16a Preoperative frontal view of asymmetric smile.

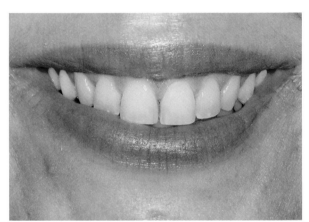

Fig 17-16b Postoperative frontal view shows smile line corrected by removal of more tissue on the higher side.

and more attached gingival tissue are removed, and at least 5 mm of attached gingiva is always left.[5] These modifications result in a surgical site that is less ovoid or elliptical than usual. In contrast, where there is a deep vestibule and wide upper lip, more labial mucosal tissue can be removed, resulting in a more ovoid site. Furthermore, the removal of more labial mucosal tissue prevents the eversion, or folding, that occurs on smiling in patients with thicker lips (Fig 17-15).

Lip repositioning surgery can correct an asymmetric smile by removing more mucosal tissue on one side (Fig 17-16). If the asymmetry is caused by a transverse cant in the dentition, however, orthodontic correction is needed.[2] Lateral corrections can also be made via lip repositioning surgery by resuturing in a corrected position (laterally), but this approach can be difficult and requires experience (Fig 17-17). Excessive muscular pull from the levator labii superioris and levator superioris

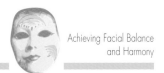

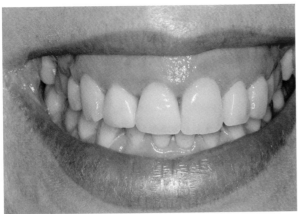

Fig 17-17a Preoperative frontal view of an off-center Cupid's bow.

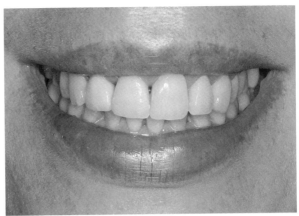

Fig 17-17b Postoperative frontal view shows Cupid's bow corrected by a lateral reposition.

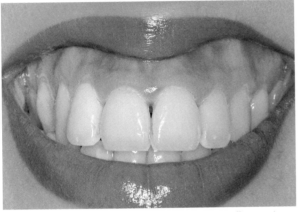

Fig 17-18a Preoperative frontal view of a "bowed" effect resulting from muscle pull.

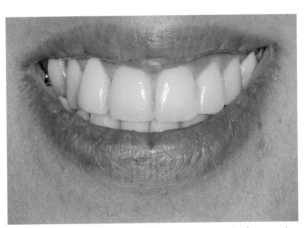

Fig 17-18b Postoperative view following correction by firm attachment in the lateral area.

alaeque nasi muscles can lead to a bowed effect on the lip, which is corrected by more tissue removal in the 2 and 3 areas (Fig 17-18). These cases though can be the most prone to relapse due to the strength of these muscles. Here botulinum toxin can be used 2 weeks prior to surgery to lessen the effect of the muscles during the healing phase.

Conclusion

An open-minded, multidisciplinary approach to the treatment of patients with an extremely high lip line is necessary for achieving the best possible results. Because of differing etiologies and patient preferences, some patients are treated with orthognathic surgery, some by orthodontic methods, and some via other modalities.

A combination of the modalities may be the preferred treatment plan for the patient. The most commonly used combination is crown lengthening with repositioning in severe cases where there is adequate attached gingiva, sufficient biologic width, and the need or desire for the associated dental treatment.

Although other surgical techniques (including myectomies) are used by plastic surgeons to treat extremely high lip lines, lip repositioning surgery is a relatively safe and uncomplicated procedure that yields satisfying results. The restriction in lip movement produced by the procedure is similar to that felt by people who have a low lip line (although here the aim is to achieve the ideal of 1 to 2 mm of gingiva showing) and does not affect the resting esthetics. Lip repositioning surgery has a future in the treatment of the extremely high lip line case, and combined with the other options, it gives the patient and physician more ways to achieve the most favorable esthetic result.

References

1. Saadoun A. All about the smile. In: Romano R, Bichacho N, Touati B (eds). The Art of the Smile: Integrating Prosthodontics, Orthodontics, Periodontics, Dental Technology, and Plastic Surgery in Esthetic Dental Treatment. Chicago: Quintessence, 2005:265–295.
2. Sarver DM, Ackerman MB. Dynamic smile visualization and quantification. In: Romano R, Bichacho N, Touati B (eds). The Art of the Smile: Integrating Prosthodontics, Orthodontics, Periodontics, Dental Technology, and Plastic Surgery in Esthetic Dental Treatment. Chicago: Quintessence, 2005:104–138.
3. Khanna B. Lip stabilisation with botulinum toxin. Aesthetic Dentistry Today 2007;1:54–59.
4. Bell WH, Guerrero CA (eds). Distraction Osteogenesis of the Facial Skeleton. Hamilton, ON: BC Decker, 2007.
5. Van Dooren E. Esthetics at the periodontal-restorative interface. In: Romano R, Bichacho N, Touati B (eds). The Art of the Smile: Integrating Prosthodontics, Orthodontics, Periodontics, Dental Technology, and Plastic Surgery in Esthetic Dental Treatment. Chicago: Quintessence, 2005:323–340.
6. Lee EA. Aesthetic crown lengthening: Classification, biologic rationale, and treatment planning considerations. Pract Proced Aesthet Dent 2004;16:769–778.
7. Blitz N, Steel C, Willhite C. Diagnosis and Treatment Evaluation in Cosmetic Dentistry. Madison, WI: American Academy of Cosmetic Dentistry, 2001.
8. Rubenstein AM, Kostainsky AS. Cirugia estetica. Pren Med Argent 1973;20:952.
9. Rosenblatt A, Simon Z. Lip repositioning for reduction of excessive gingival display: A clinical report. Int J Periodontics Restorative Dent 2006;26:433–437.
10. Fairbairn P. Lip repositioning surgery. Aesthetic and Implant Dent. 2006;9:33–37.
11. Fairbairn P. Lip repositioning surgery—A Photographic Guide. Aesthetic Dent Today 2007;1:66–73.

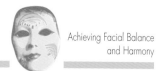

Achieving Facial Balance and Harmony

Secondary Rhinoplasty

18

Gilbert C. Aiach, MD

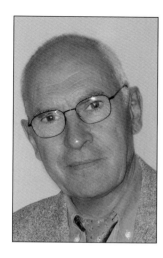

Gilbert C. Aiach, MD

Gilbert Aiach trained in Paris at the Fach Hospital with Dr Tessier and Dr Merville. He is a professor of the International Society of Plastic Aesthetic Surgery and past president of the Société Française de Chirurgie Esthétique et Plastique. Dr Aiach also holds membership in the Société Française de Chirurgie Plastique Recontructrice et Esthétique, the Société de Chirurgie Maxillo Faciale, the American Society for Aesthetic Plastic Surgeons, and the Rhinoplasty Society.

Dr Aiach has delivered numerous lectures, held courses, and performed several live surgery demonstrations around the world. He has also published many articles and two books on rhinoplasty, and he organizes a biennial rhinoplasty course in France.

Email: gaiach@club-internet.fr

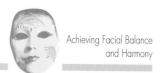

Rhinoplasty is the most difficult operation in the field of esthetic surgery because no two noses are alike and the extent of the defects does not parallel the difficulties encountered during surgery. The goal of this procedure is to obtain a nose that is harmonious with other components of the face and the overall appearance of the patient. Severe defects are caused by technical faults: Asymmetric or over-resections of the nasal pyramid affect not only the esthetics but also the function of the nose. However, errors in judgment can cause failures even when a rhinoplasty is performed with technical accuracy, sometimes resulting in a nose that does not suit the other facial components. The most frequently made mistakes that cause an unnatural, "operated on" appearance are *(1)* an overly shortened nose with an inadequately deepened nasofrontal angle, *(2)* an overly reduced dorsum that emphasizes a supratip deformity, and *(3)* a round nasal tip lacking definition.

To carry out a successful rhinoplasty, careful preoperative planning is essential. Not only unfavorable soft tissue and cartilage conditions but also narrow nostril orifices need to be identified. During the initial assessment, the following steps should be taken:

- Palpate the contour of the bony vault and the cartilages to check their condition (recoil, thickness, size).
- Press down the tip lobule to determine the resistance of the medial crura.
- Evaluate the condition (suppleness, thickness) of the soft tissues, which should adequately redrape the underlying skeleton reduced by resections or augmented by grafts. A thick, nonelastic soft tissue cannot redrape the underlying skeleton. A thin soft tissue is not forgiving of asymmetries or prominences of the underlying framework and may make these features more visible.
- As Aufricht used to say, the surgeon should have the nose "in his finger."
- Examine the endonasal region, including the endonasal mucosa and internal nasal valve area, to identify septal deformities and evaluate the potential for harvesting septal cartilage for grafting.

The most frequent approach to rhinoplasty is the open transcolumellar approach, which allows an accurate analysis of the deformities via a direct view of the cartilages. These deformities are usually corrected through a combination of the following techniques: *(1)* conservative resections of the cartilages; *(2)* cartilage grafts that augment deficient structures, improve the contour of tip and ala, and improve the function of the internal and external valve; and *(3)* suture techniques that permit the cartilages and grafts to be reshaped harmoniously.

Rhinoplasty is one of the most rewarding of all esthetic operations. The surgeon not only enhances the patient's appearance but

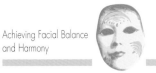

Achieving Facial Balance
and Harmony

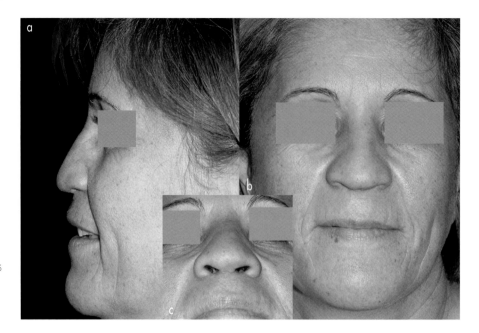

Figs 18-1a to 18-1c The patient underwent two previous rhinoplasties and a septoplasty. She presented with a flat nasal base, a short columella, and a severe loss of nasal tip supports. (a) Profile view. (b) Frontal view. (c) Basal view.

contributes to his/her self-confidence as well. In addition, the operation draws on a variety of skills, including artistic interpretation and technical finesse. The demanding surgeon can achieve excellent results, but not without significant effort.

Case Report

Preoperative planning

After two previous rhinoplasties and a septoplasty, this patient presented with a flat nasal base, a short columella, and a severe loss of nasal tip supports (Fig 18-1). A flat nose often results from a weak, short columella support and also from previous surgery in which the caudal septum and the lower lateral cartilages have been damaged or over-resected with significant loss of tip supports. Preoperative assessment of the patient revealed the following findings:

- Profile view (Fig 18-1a): Subsequent to the loss of the tip projection, there was a lack of balance between a retruded nasal tip and a false dorsal hump.
- Frontal view (Fig 18-1b): A wide dorsum, bony vault, and flat broad nasal tip without definition were present.
- Basal view (Fig 18-1c): The columella was very short, making the interalar distance appear wide in comparison. Pseudo alar flaring was caused by the severe loss of tip supports and projection, and the axis of the nostril orifices was horizontal.

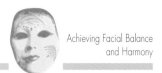

Achieving Facial Balance and Harmony

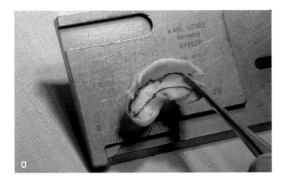
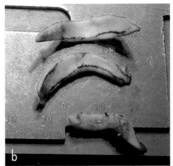

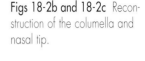

Fig 18-2a Ear cartilage harvested via a retroauricular approach.

Figs 18-2b and 18-2c Reconstruction of the columella and nasal tip.

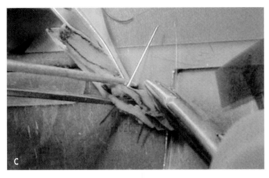
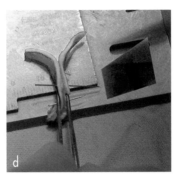

Fig 18-2d A rigid polydioxanone plate is used to enhance the stiffness of the two grafts.

- Endonasal examination: A large anterior septal perforation precluded any harvesting of septal material.
- Palpation: The nasal tip was easily depressed because of poor columella and septal support, and the alar cartilages appeared weak and soft on palpation.

From the assessment, it was determined that the main goal of surgery was to correct the flat nasal base by reconstructing the tip supports to provide more projection and definition and to narrow the bony vault with lateral osteotomies and dorsal augmentation. Usually, the best material for reconstructing such defects is a stiff, solid graft material, typically harvested from the septum. In this case, the large septal perforation precluded any harvesting at this level. Because the patient had refused a harvesting of costal cartilage, ear cartilage, which is often too soft, was harvested instead.

Procedure

The two conchae were harvested via a retroauricular approach (Fig 18-2a). Next, a transcolumellar incision was made at the base of the columella, where soft tissue elevation revealed the poor laxity of the alar cartilage, and a pocket was developed on the dorsum for placement of a dorsal graft. The columella and nasal tip were reconstructed with a fleur-de-lis–shaped graft using the two lateral edges of the harvested conchae (Figs 18-2b and 18-2c). The concavities of the two grafts were positioned back-to-back to provide more rigidity. To further improve the

Achieving Facial Balance and Harmony

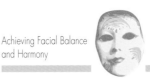

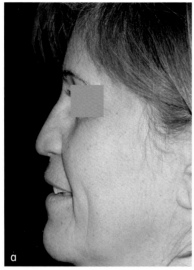 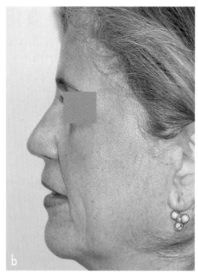 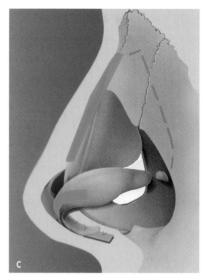

Figs 18-3a to 18-3c (a) A dorsal graft has been placed on the dorsum to balance the projection of the tip with that of the dorsum. (b and c) On profile view, there is a significant increase in tip projection.

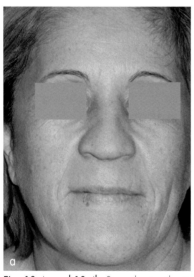 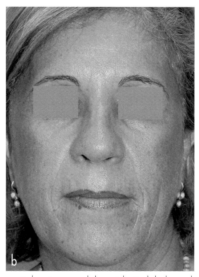

Figs 18-4a and 18-4b Strengthening the tip supports has improved the wide tip lobule and large interalar base distance. The wide dorsum has been corrected by lateral osteotomies and dorsal augmentation, as can be seen in the frontal view.

stiffness of these two grafts, a rigid 0.5-mm thick batten of a 15 × 5-mm polydioxanone (PDS) plate was placed between the two cartilages and sutured to them (Fig 18-2d).

PDS foil is produced in the form of violet sheet (plate) and various film strengths and thicknesses (0.25 and 0.50 mm). This material has already been used in reconstruction of the septum for stabilization of

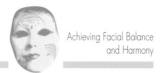

Achieving Facial Balance
and Harmony

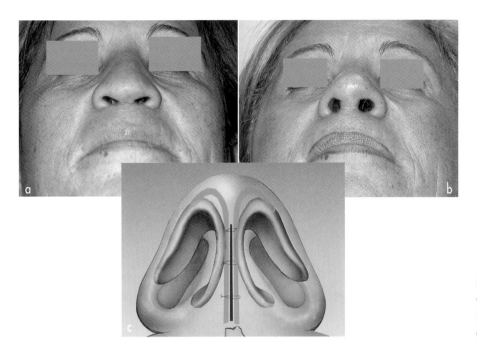

Figs 18-5a to 18-5c On basal view, the short columella has been lengthened, with subsequent correction of the alar flaring.

separate septal fragments and correction of fracture of the orbital floor. PDS is resorbable after 6 months but provides a temporary scaffold that enables the fibrous tissue to stabilize the involved structures. It was used in the columella with two objectives: *(1)* to provide stronger support to the columella by suturing PDS battens between two ear cartilage fragments, and *(2)* to stabilize a columellar strut to the nasal spine by suturing an extension of the PDS batten to the nasal spine.

The divergent anterior extensions of the grafts were positioned on top of the domes and sutured to the lateral crura (see Fig 18-3a). A single-layer graft was placed on the dorsum, and lateral and medial osteotomies were performed.

Results

Figures 18-3 to 18-6 show preoperative and 12-month postoperative photographs. On profile view, the nasal tip projection is in good balance with the projection of the dorsum. On frontal view, the nose is narrower, and the nasal tip is well defined. On basal view, augmentation of the nasal tip projection has produced a change in the shape of the nostril orifice. After 6 months, the PDS plate is totally resorbed and replaced by connective tissue.

 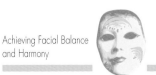

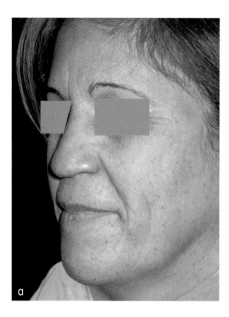 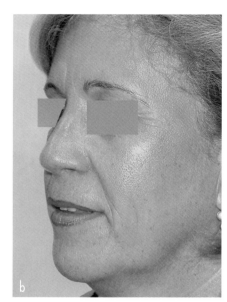

Figs 18-6a and 18-6b Oblique view displays the improved harmony and balance of the subunits of the nose.

Acknowledgment

All figures from Aiach GC, Kelly MH. Secondary rhinoplasty. In: Nahai F (ed). The Art of Aesthetic Surgery: Principles & Techniques. St Louis: Quality Medical Publishing, 2005:1634–1636. Reprinted with permission.

Facial Treatment with Botulinum Toxin

19

Maurício de Maio, MD, PhD

Achieving Facial Balance
and Harmony

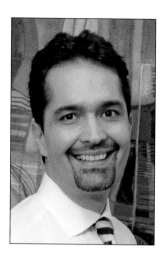

Maurício de Maio, MD, PhD

Maurício de Maio received his medical degree from the Medical School of the University of São Paulo in 1990. He specialized in plastic surgery in Brazil in 1996, obtaining his master of medicine in 1997 and doctor of philosophy degrees in 2006 from the University of São Paulo. He was a clinical assistant professor in the plastic surgery department of the University of São Paulo from 1996 to 2002.

Dr de Maio is a board-certified plastic surgeon in the Brazilian Society of Plastic Surgery and a member of the International Society of Aesthetic Plastic Surgery. He has authored scientific publications and articles as well as the following books: *Fillers in Aesthetic Medicine* (2006) and *Botulinum Toxin in Aesthetic Medicine* (2007), both by Springer-Verlag, Germany. He is actively involved in research and teaching in international training courses in North, Central, and South America, and in Europe and Asia.

Email: mauriciodemaio@uol.com.br

The aging process is a consequence of genetic and environmental influences. Genetic, or chronological, aging manifests mainly in saggy skin, gravitational folds, and loss of facial and neck definition. In contrast, environmental aging, or photo damage, is represented by wrinkles. Wrinkles are divided into five categories: static, dynamic, gravitational, sleeping lines, and combined.

Mimetic Muscles

Mimetic muscles are those used when a person expresses emotions. If muscular behavior falls outside normal patterns, communication between humans may be misinterpreted. If someone has vertical lines between the eyebrows that do not relax, an angry or sad expression may be what viewers perceive even if that person is completely happy. As a person ages, the muscular pattern undergoes modifications. Mimetic muscles are gradually used more for adaptation processes such as focusing the eyes and counteracting gravitational forces. As a result, undesirable wrinkling may appear.

Antagonist and Synergist Muscles

Antagonist and synergist mimetic muscles play an important role in facial esthetics. In an analysis of the face, a clinician may divide the mimetic muscles into two groups: elevators and depressors. The fibers of these muscles are not independent; they are interwoven, and they interact. When a muscle, or part of a muscle, is blocked, a reorganization occurs between the antagonist and synergist forces. In general, one specific muscle and its synergists only contract because the antagonists relax.

As an example, the muscles that influence the movements of the eyebrow include three depressors that are synergists and a single antagonist elevator, the m frontalis. The eyebrow lifts because the m frontalis contracts while the depressors relax. The eyebrow depressors include the m corrugator supercilii, the m procerus, and the m orbicularis oculi (pars orbitalis).

De Maio Grading of Muscle Activity

The correct treatment plan depends on the correct diagnosis. Categorizing the mimetic muscles into different types of behavior allows a better understanding of muscle reactions to proposed treatments. Dose selection, duration of muscle relaxation, and frequency of treatments throughout the year may be better identified when a patient can be placed correctly into one or more of the following six general groups:

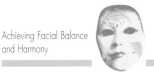

Achieving Facial Balance
and Harmony

- Group A (kinetic pattern): Patients in Group A have good control over facial expressions. They can move their muscles when they want. The contractions are in accordance with the type and level of emotion these people want to convey.
- Group B (hyperkinetic pattern): The facial muscles of patients in Group B contract in a faster rhythm although the patients may not be experiencing any particular emotion. These patients cannot control muscle contractions, and emotional expressions are disorganized.
- Group C (hypertonic pattern): The muscular pattern of patients in Group C is a result of years of hyperkinetic movement. The muscles cannot relax. These patients appear to be tense, unhappy, stressed, or angry, even when they are very happy.
- Group D (hypokinetic pattern): Patients in Group D display a reduction in the velocity of muscle cycling from slow to minimal or even a complete absence of visible movement. This is the pattern usually seen after treatment with botulinum toxin.
- Group E (hypotonic pattern): Patients in Group E lack muscle expression and may seem to be without any emotion. After botulinum toxin treatment, due to hypotonic muscle reaction, some patients may experience a feeling of heaviness, such as that found with the frontalis block.
- Group F (atonic pattern): Patients in Group F have lost even minimal muscle tone. This pattern occurs when excessive doses of botulinum toxin are given or injection sites are misjudged. This is the most feared result of treatment with botulinum toxin.

Clinical Cases

Please note that preferred injection sites may vary from clinician to clinician, and yet the same results may be obtained. The total dose range for each muscle may be found in Table 19-1.

Group A patients

Patient 1

Description

In this patient, two asymmetric vertical lines formed at the glabella during animation. The right line was smaller and more superficial (Fig 19-1a). There was no horizontal line at this level. The left medial eyebrow was slightly inferior to the right because of more intense muscle activity on that side.

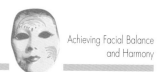

Achieving Facial Balance
and Harmony

Muscle	Botox (Allergan)	Dysport (Ipsen)
M frontalis	6–10 U	15–30 U
M corrugator supercilii	20–30 U	30–60 U
M procerus	3–6 U	7.5–15 U
M orbicularis oculi	12–30 U	30–60 U
M depressor septi nasi	2–4 U	8–12 U
M levator labii superioris alaeque nasi	2–6 U	4–8 U
M levator labii superioris	2–6 U	4–8 U
M zygomaticus minor	2–3 U	8–10 U
M zygomaticus major	2–6 U	6–18 U
M depressor labii inferioris	2–3 U	8–10 U
M depressor anguli oris	5–10 U	10–20 U
Platysma bands	10–40 U	30–100 U

Table 19-1 Range of suggested doses for each mimetic muscle*

*Doses include both sides, if applicable.

Anatomy

The muscle responsible for this feature is the m corrugator supercilii, the "frowning muscle." It originates in the medial end of the superciliary arch of the frontal bone and inserts into the eyebrow skin above the midpart of the orbital arch. This muscle draws the eyebrow medially and downward and forms the glabella vertical lines.

Technique

To allow an injection directly into the corrugator muscle, the injection site should be planned for the upper medial portion of the eyebrow (Fig 19-1b). Insert one half of the 30-gauge needle and direct it upward and laterally along the direction of the m corrugator fibers. It is advisable to protect the eye with the thumb. If bleeding occurs, a slight compression followed by upward movements with gauze is recommended.

Follow-up

When the patient returned for the next visit, a line remained on the left corrugator (Fig 19-1c).

Achieving Facial Balance and Harmony

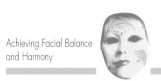

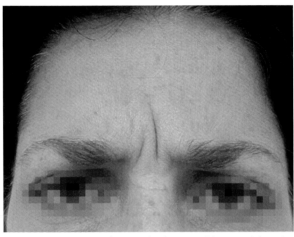

Fig 19-1a Pretreatment photograph. The vertical lines result from the contraction of the corrugator muscles. The left side is stronger.

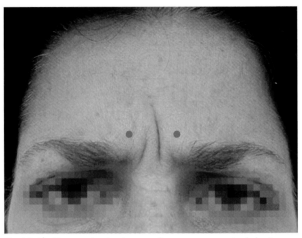

Fig 19-1b The standard selection of injection points (red dots). Note that the patient presents asymmetric strength.

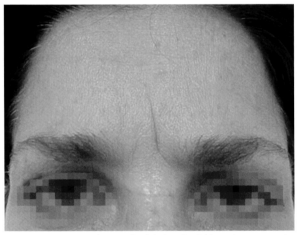

Fig 19-1c Remaining line on the left that should have been treated with higher dose compared to the right side.

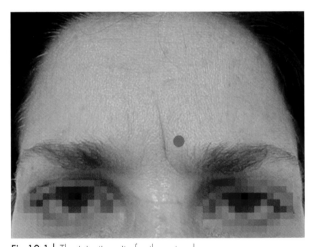

Fig 19-1d The injection site for the extra dose.

Explanation

An identical dose and symmetric injection sites led to this result. A higher dose on the left m corrugator should have been injected. To improve the situation, simply reinject the dose into the left m corrugator (Fig 19-1d).

Patient 2

Description

Along with the two small vertical lines in the glabella due to the contraction of the corrugator muscles, this patient presented with horizontal lines at the nose radix (Fig 19-2a). The muscle responsible for these lines is the m procerus. Here, the action of three depressors of the eyebrow can be noted.

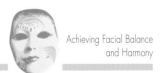

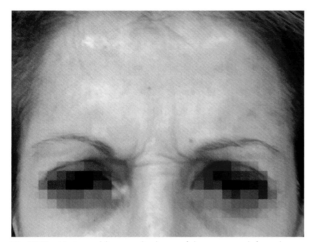

Fig 19-2a Horizontal lines at the base of the nose result from the contraction of the m procerus.

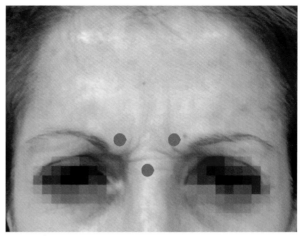

Fig 19-2b The three medial eyebrow depressors should be treated.

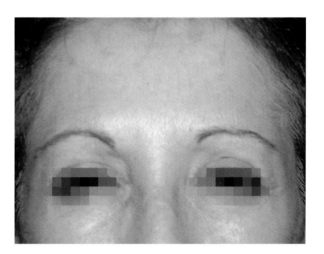

Fig 19-2c All the wrinkles at the glabella level are erased. Note that the medial aspect of the eyebrow is lifted.

Anatomy

The m procerus depresses the medial aspect of the eyebrow.

Technique

Selection of the injection sites should include all three depressors (Fig 19-2b). As the m procerus action is quite evident, it should receive the same dose as each m corrugator. The injection at this level should be superficial. In general, one-third of the 30-gauge needle should be injected.

Follow-up

The medial eyebrow is lifted by blocking the depressors (Fig 19-2c).

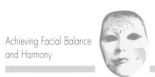

Achieving Facial Balance and Harmony

Group B patients

Patient 3

Description
The vertical lines in the glabella of this patient were nearly symmetric, although the contraction patterns of each side differed. On the right side, the m corrugator moved more medially and downward, while the left m corrugator appeared weaker (Fig 19-3a).

Observation
In contrast to Patient 1, the medial portion of the eyebrow moved only medially and not downward.

Explanation
The medial fibers of the m frontalis were partially contracted in opposition to the m corrugator, which lifts the medial eyebrow.

Technique
Because the corrugator muscles are asymmetric, the right m corrugator should be injected with a higher dose (Fig 19-3b).

Follow-up
Note that after blocking, the right eyebrow moved to a more outward position compared to the left (Fig 19-3c).

Patient 4

Description
When this patient contracted the m frontalis, the eyebrows were lifted, and horizontal lines were extremely evident on the forehead. The eyebrows were almost symmetric (Fig 19-4a).

Anatomy
The resultant eyebrow position is a balance between the forces of the antagonists that act upon it. The m frontalis fibers have to counteract the three eyebrow depressors described previously.

Technique
The injection sites may be distributed evenly (Fig 19-4b). The injections should be superficial and the doses should be balanced to avoid excessive weakness in the m frontalis lifting fibers.

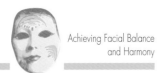

Achieving Facial Balance
and Harmony

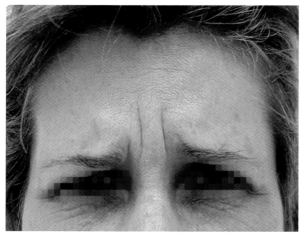

Fig 19-3a Although the corrugator muscles seem to be symmetric, there is a difference in the pattern of contraction.

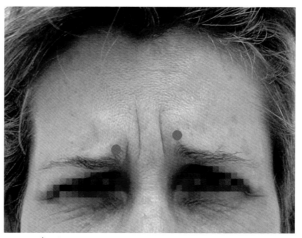

Fig 19-3b The injection sites should be adapted to avoid asymmetric results.

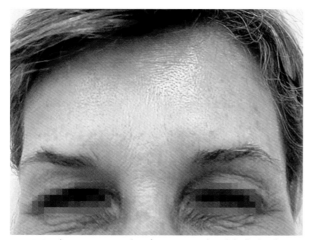

Fig 19-3c There is no more line formation at the glabella level.

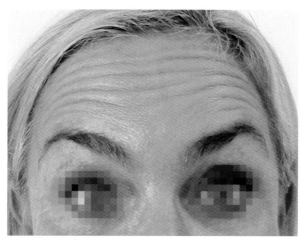

Fig 19-4a The forehead lines result from the contraction of the m frontalis, which is the sole eyebrow elevator.

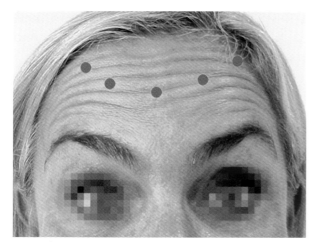

Fig 19-4b The injection sites should be evenly distributed. It is of utmost importance that the injection is superficial to avoid excessive weakening of the m frontalis and eyebrow droop.

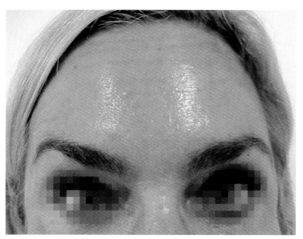

Fig 19-4c A superficial, low-dose injection allows maintenance of the lifted position of the eyebrows yet erases the wrinkles.

Achieving Facial Balance
and Harmony

Follow-up

Fifteen days posttreatment, the patient demonstrates the expected result from the treatment with botulinum toxin. On animation, the eyebrows lift, but the horizontal lines have been erased (Fig 19-4c).

Patient 5

Description

This patient had the same complaint as the previous one (Fig 19-5a). However, an excessive dose of botulinum toxin with multiple injection points distributed evenly into the whole forehead provoked a hypotonic response in the frontalis muscle. As a consequence, the patient experienced a sensation of heaviness in the forehead combined with excess skin in the upper eyelid (Fig 19-5b). The posttreatment musculature is an example of a Group F pattern.

Explanation

Excessive weakening of the m frontalis resulted in loss of its lifting effect. Care should be taken to balance the need to maintain a proper eyebrow position and muscle tone with the need for wrinkle removal.

What to do

There is nothing much to do at this point except wait. Muscular stimulation devices have been indicated but provide mild to no benefit.

Patient 6

Observation

Analysis of the diagram on this patient (Fig 19-6a) easily reveals some of the problems that may arise in the treatment of the m frontalis.

The forehead should be divided into three levels: The first level contains the m frontalis lower fibers and the eyebrow depressors; the second level consists of the m frontalis intermediate fibers; and the third level contains the m frontalis upper fibers.

Each side of the forehead should be divided into three columns: column A represents the medial aspect of the eyebrow; column B represents the intermediate portion of the eyebrow and where the mid-pupillary line lies; and column C represents the lateral aspect of the eyebrow. One should avoid deep injections in sites displayed in a single column, as this may excessively weaken the lower, intermediate, and upper elevating fibers of the frontalis and result in drooping of the medial eyebrow (Fig 19-6b).

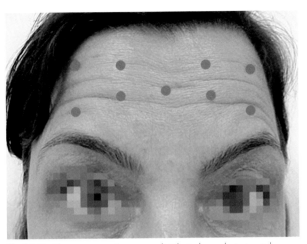

Fig 19-5a The injection sites were distributed evenly to treat the forehead lines.

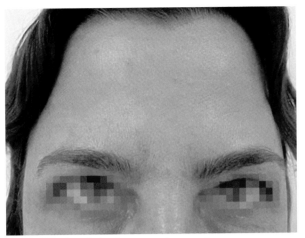

Fig 19-5b Although the dose was adequate, the injections were carried out too deeply, resulting in lowered eyebrows.

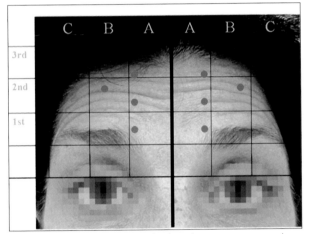

Fig 19-6a A helpful diagram to distribute the injection sites on the forehead.

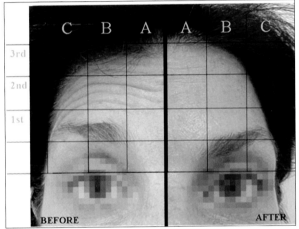

Fig 19-6b Pretreatment, the eyebrow is lifted, and the forehead lines are formed. Posttreatment, the lines disappear, and there is a tendency for the medial aspect of the eyebrow to be lower. Injection sites in column A at the first, second, and third level may excessively weaken the lifting fibers of the m frontalis.

Patient 7

Description and technique

The orbital wrinkling in this patient expanded to the cheekbone lateral aspect (Fig 19-7a). When treating cheek-lines or their lateral extensions to the cheekbones, the clinician should be careful. A slightly deeper injection or diffusion may affect the m zygomatic major, and ptosis of the upper lip may result. To treat these lines, only very superficial injections in a very low dose are advisable. Only the bevel of the needle should penetrate the skin in the three lower injection points (green dots).

The injection sites in red should be penetrated with only one third of a 30-gauge needle (Fig 19-7b).

Follow-up
After the m orbicularis oculi (orbital part) was weakened, the crow's feet disappeared (Fig 19-7c). If patients complain about dry eyes posttreatment, inadvertent diffusion to the m orbicularis (palpebral part) or excessive dosage may have affected the blinking or the lacrimal gland pumping mechanism.

What to do
Prescribe eye drops for lubrication. Many patients report complete recovery within 30 days after the injection.

Patient 8

Description
Wrinkles at the nasal dorsum are seen during animation. At this level, four muscles may have their fibers interwoven: m procerus, m nasalis, m levator labii superioris alaeque nasi, and m orbicularis oculi (Fig 19-8a). By injecting at this level, the clinician would interfere with all four muscles.

Technique
Two planned injection sites in each lateral wall of the nasal dorsum are usually sufficient because the m procerus is usually injected at a higher point (Fig 19-8b). However, a third injection site in the middle of the dorsum may be beneficial. At this level, the injection is superficial. Only one third of the 30-gauge needle should penetrate the skin. Bruising in the lateral walls may occur.

Follow-up
To evaluate the result, the clinician should check the botulinum toxin's effect on each treated muscle: elevation of the medial portion of the eyebrow and reduction of some of the horizontal lines (m procerus); reduction of the wrinkles at the lateral nasal dorsum (m nasalis); relaxation of the wrinkles at the inner palpebral canthus (m orbicularis oculi); and finally, the reduction in nasal flare (m levator labii superioris alaeque nasi) (Fig 19-8c). This case elucidates how an injection into a single point can affect surrounding muscles.

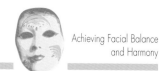
Achieving Facial Balance and Harmony

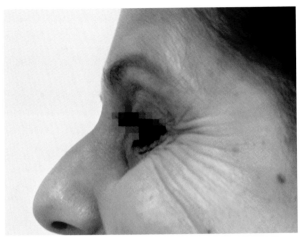

Fig 19-7a The crow's feet may expand down to the malar area.

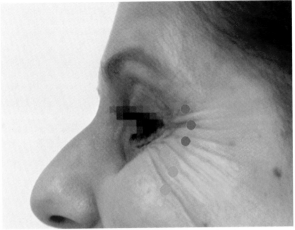

Fig 19-7b All the injection points should be superficial. However, for the intradermal injections (green dots), only the needle bevel should penetrate the skin.

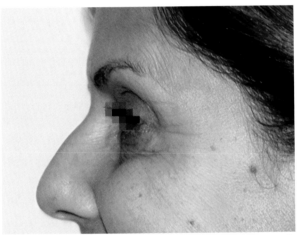

Fig 19-7c Respecting the depth of injection, the clinician may easily treat the cheek lines with a low dose to avoid a droop of the upper lip due to impairment of the m zygomatic major.

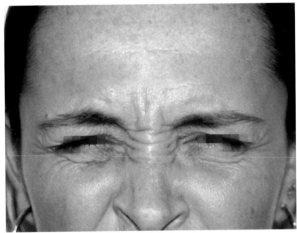

Fig 19-8a Four muscles interact at the nose level to cause this wrinkling: the m procerus, m nasalis, m levator alaeque nasi labii superioris, and m orbicularis oculi.

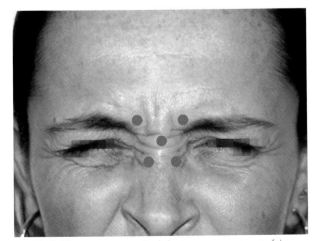

Fig 19-8b The injection sites (red dots) promote treatment of the glabella and nasal lines.

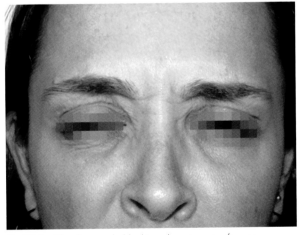

Fig 19-8c After the muscle blocking, there is a significant improvement of the lines at this level.

Achieving Facial Balance and Harmony

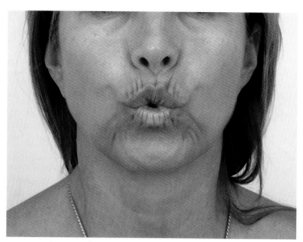

Fig 19-9 The superficial fibers of the orbicularis oris cause the dynamic wrinkling of the perioral region when the lips are pursed.

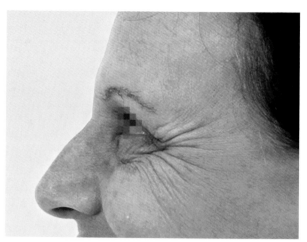

Fig 19-10a Due to the contraction of the m orbicularis oculi (orbital part), crow's feet appear, and there is a droop in the tail of the eyebrow. The dynamic lines are present in the upper, middle, and lower parts of the lateral orbit. (Used with permission from De Maio M, Rzany B. Botulinum Toxin in Aesthetic Medicine. New York: Springer Science and Business Media, 2007.)

Patient 9

Description

Perioral wrinkles may be only dynamic or also be present at rest. When present at rest, the botulinum toxin treatment combined with fillers may promote better longevity. Generally, fillers are the first option for the treatment of vertical lip lines. The treatment of these wrinkles is a challenge with botulinum toxin.

Anatomy

The m orbicularis oris is a complex muscle that contains superficial and deep fibers. The deep fibers bring the lips together and promote direct lip closure; the superficial fibers, which are principally the decussating fibers, protrude the lips (Fig 19-9). The superficial fibers should be targeted in treatment with botulinum toxin.

Technique

Because there is practically no subcutaneous fat in the upper lip and the dermis is quite thin, any injection may be too deep at this level. Inadvertent needle penetration and diffusion may compromise the deep fibers and impair lip function. It is advisable to penetrate only the bevel into the skin and inject low volume at low doses.

The transition line between the mucosa and the skin is considered the best injection site. One or two injection sites close to the philtrum suffice for the upper lip. Excessive treatment in the upper and especially in the lower lip may result in oral incontinence.

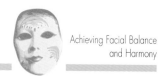

Achieving Facial Balance and Harmony

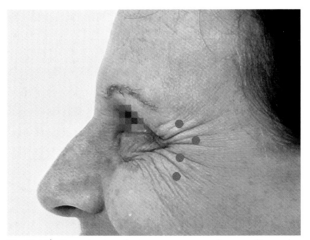

Fig 19-10b The selection of injection sites is made according to the extension of wrinkles. Usually, three to four sites are located in a row in the lateral orbit. (Used with permission from De Maio M, Rzany B. Botulinum Toxin in Aesthetic Medicine. New York: Springer Science and Business Media, 2007.)

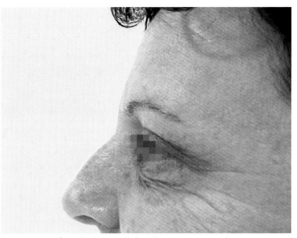

Fig 19-10c After blocking with botulinum toxin, mainly in patients with skin excess, unwanted wrinkling in the lower eyelid may result. (Used with permission from De Maio M, Rzany B. Botulinum Toxin in Aesthetic Medicine. New York: Springer Science and Business Media, 2007.)

Observation

It is not necessarily true that because the clinician blocks the action of the m orbicularis oris and removes the lines, the patient has a positive experience. On the contrary, it is not uncommon for the patient to refuse further treatments with botulinum toxin in this area because of unnatural results or even the presence of eyebags after muscle relaxation.

What to do

For successful treatment, select a patient with few initial wrinkles. Place the injections as superficially as possible.

Group C patients

Patient 10

Description

Due to the contraction of the m orbicularis oculi (orbital area), crow's feet appear, and the tail of the eyebrow droops. The dynamic lines are present in the upper, middle, and lower parts of the lateral orbit (Fig 19-10a).

Anatomy

The m orbicularis oculi is composed of three smaller muscles: the orbital, the palpebral, and the lacrimal. The orbital muscle action protrudes the eyebrows, closes the eyelids (voluntary action), and forms the

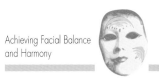

Achieving Facial Balance and Harmony

crow's feet. The palpebral muscle closes lids during blinking, and the lacrimal muscle draws the lids and lacrimal papillae medially and compresses the lacrimal sac.

Technique
The selection of injection sites is made according to the extension of wrinkles. Usually, three or four sites are located in a row in the lateral orbit (Fig 19-10b). The injection should be very superficial to avoid deep vessels and consequent bruising.

Follow-up
After blocking with botulinum toxin, mainly in patients with excess skin, undesirable wrinkles in the lower eyelid may result (Fig 19-10c).

Patient 11

Description
The tip of the nose may droop due to the contraction of the m depressor septi nasi during smile. This short muscle may remain in a hypertonic state and droop the tip of the nose even in static position (Fig 19-11a). Botulinum toxin may relax it, and as a result, the tip of the nose may be maintained in an elevated or neutral position at rest and during animation.

Anatomy
The m depressor septi nasi draws the tip of the nose downward. Some of its fibers are interwoven with those of the m orbicularis oris. During smile, the medial and lateral upper lip elevators contract, and their antagonist, the m orbicularis oris, relaxes.

Technique
Insert one third of the 30-gauge needle into the nasolabial angle, at the collumella base. Usually, one injection site is enough. There may be two injection sites at this level if necessary, though.

Observation
Not all candidates present the same reaction to treatment. Botulinum toxin may lift the tip of the nose but not sustain it in position (Fig 19-11b). A prominent anterior nasal spine may provide enough support for the tip, for example. The nasolabial angle is another important landmark to be observed. If in a static position this angle is greater than 90 degrees, it will enable an adequate response. In patients with an angle less than 90 degrees and without support at the nasal base, the addition of fillers is essential.

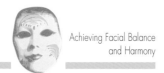

Achieving Facial Balance
and Harmony

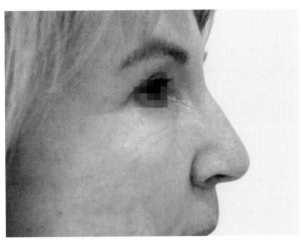

Fig 19-11a The m depressor septi nasi may droop the tip of the nose at rest and mainly during animation. (Used with permission from De Maio M, Rzany B. Botulinum Toxin in Aesthetic Medicine. New York: Springer Science and Business Media, 2007.)

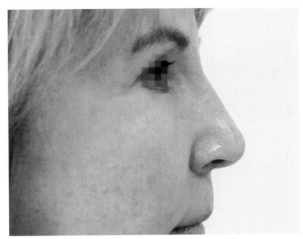

Fig 19-11b The muscle blocking may lift the tip of the nose yet be unable to maintain it in position. So, fillers should be associated. (Used with permission from De Maio M, Rzany B. Botulinum Toxin in Aesthetic Medicine. New York: Springer Science and Business Media, 2007.)

Patient 12

Description

The dynamic, gummy smile results from the overcontraction of the two upper lip medial elevators (Fig 19-12a). The ideal smile results when the upper lip hides the upper third of the central incisors, and that was the goal of this patient's treatment with botulinum toxin.

Anatomy

The two upper lip medial elevators are the m levator labii superioris alaeque nasi (previously described) and the m levator labii superioris. The latter muscle is located between the lateral slip of the m levator labii superioris alaeque nasi and the m zygomatic minor. Its action is to elevate and evert the upper lip.

Technique

The injection site can vary from patient to patient (Figs 19-12b and 19-12c). At this level, the m orbicularis oris fibers are more superficial than those of the m levator labii superioris. To avoid the m orbicularis fibers, a deeper injection is necessary. Usually, penetration of one-half of the 30-gauge needle will suffice.

Observation

One complication of the treatment of the nasolabial fold and the gummy smile with botulinum toxin would be the excessive weakening of

Achieving Facial Balance and Harmony

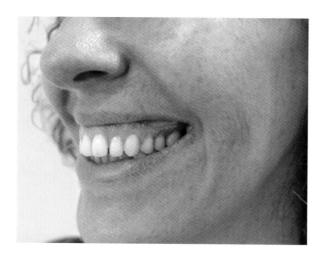

Fig 19-12a The dynamic gummy smile results from the overcontraction of the two upper lip medial elevators. (Used with permission from De Maio M, Rzany B. Botulinum Toxin in Aesthetic Medicine. New York: Springer Science and Business Media, 2007.)

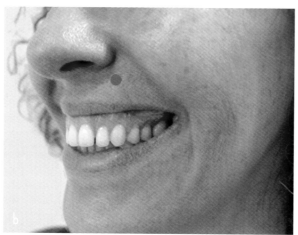

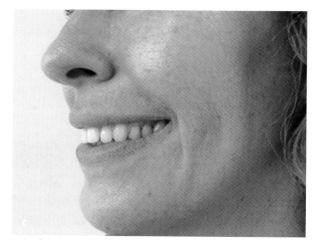

Figs 19-12b and 19-12c The injection site may vary according to the needs of the patient. (Used with permission from De Maio M, Rzany B. Botulinum Toxin in Aesthetic Medicine. New York: Springer Science and Business Media, 2007.)

the medial elevators, which could result in upper lip ptosis or elongation. With weaker medial elevators, the lateral upper lip elevators get stronger and give the appearance of a "joker" smile.

What to do
To reduce the risk of this undesirable feature, the m zygomatic major should be weakened.

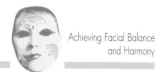

Patient 13

Description

Marionette lines may result from lack of mechanical support, from muscle hyperactivity, or both. When both components are present, a combination of fillers and botulinum toxin is preferred.

Anatomy

The muscle responsible for the marionette lines is the m depressor anguli oris. It depresses the modiolus and the angle of the mouth (Fig 19-13a). At this level, fibers from the m levator anguli oris, m zygomatic major, and m orbicularis oris are also found. At the oblique line of the mandible, the fibers of the m depressor anguli oris are lateral and more superficial to those of the m depressor labii inferioris. These are interwoven with the fibers of the platysma. That is why both muscles may be seen contracting together during animation.

Technique

The better and safer injection site to block the m depressor anguli oris is at the mandibular level (Fig 19-13b). The injection site should be lateral to an imaginary line that starts at the oral commissure and extends inferiorly to the mandible. The needle should penetrate to one-third or one-half of its length depending on the fat content at this level.

Observation

As faces are normally asymmetric, care should be taken during injection into the m depressor anguli oris because it may cause asymmetries or worsen any that were previously there.

Follow-up

The elevation of the corner of the mouth is obtained by the counteraction of the weakened m depressor anguli oris by its antagonists, the m zygomatic major and m levator anguli oris. The blocking should not be excessive because it may lead to an unpleasant sensation of heaviness perceived by the patient. The lifting of the corner of the mouth should be evident in static analysis (Fig 19-13c). On animation, it would be preferable to maintain partial action of the m depressor anguli oris so that the patient still retains a natural range of expressions (Figs 19-13d and 19-13e).

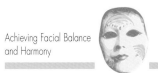

Achieving Facial Balance
and Harmony

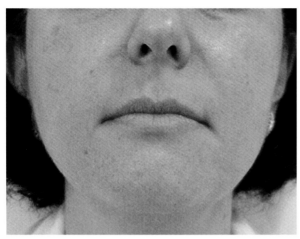

Fig 19-13a The overcontraction of the depressor anguli oris may depress the oral commissure.

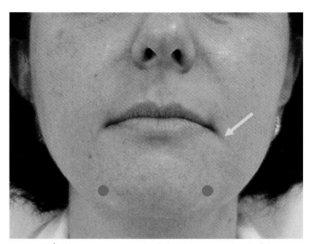

Fig 19-13b The injection sites *(red dots)* are at the level of the depressor anguli oris origin.

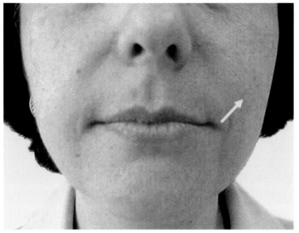

Fig 19-13c After the blocking, the corner of the mouth is elevated.

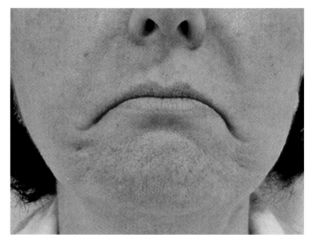

Fig 19-13d On animation, the muscle depresses the corner of the mouth.

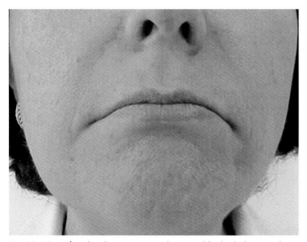

Fig 19-13e After the depressor anguli oris is blocked, the muscle is weakened but still keeps its function.

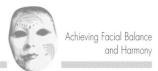

Achieving Facial Balance
and Harmony

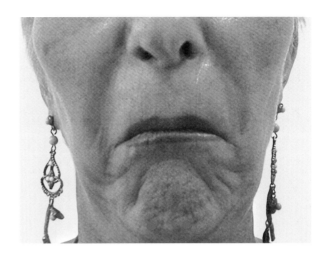

Fig 19-14 The injection sites *(red dots)* for the treatment of the cobblestone chin. The m mentalis should be injected deeply at one or two sites. Lower injections are preferred to upper injections. (Used with permission from De Maio M, Rzany B. Botulinum Toxin in Aesthetic Medicine. New York: Springer Science and Business Media, 2007.)

Patient 14

Description

This patient presented with the cobblestone chin on animation. Some patients present skin wrinkling and a deep line at the mentolabial sulcus even at rest. Botulinum toxin promotes an astonishing result through relaxation of the overcontracting muscle.

Anatomy

The m mentalis raises the mental tissues, mentolabial sulcus, and base of the lower lip. As it inserts into the skin of the chin, it produces wrinkles.

Technique

The m mentalis should be injected deeply at one or two injection sites. More inferiorly positioned injections are preferred (Fig 19-14). Full needle penetration is usually required for this treatment.

Follow-up

Not only do the wrinkles and mentolabial sulcus improve, but a reduction in the muscle bulk may also occur. A less prominent and more delicate chin may result.

Patient 15

Description

The platysmal bands are an undesirable sign of aging in the neck. They may become very visible and form the so-called turkey neck. Platysmal bands are divided into medial and lateral portions. Contraction of the lateral platysmal bands deforms the mandible shape and renders a saggy appearance in the face (Fig 19-15a).

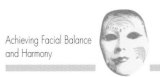

Achieving Facial Balance
and Harmony

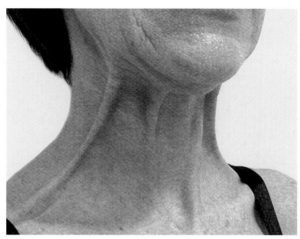

Fig 19-15a Contraction of the lateral platysmal bands deforms the mandible shape, rendering a saggy appearance in the face. (Used with permission from De Maio M, Rzany B. Botulinum Toxin in Aesthetic Medicine. New York: Springer Science and Business Media, 2007.)

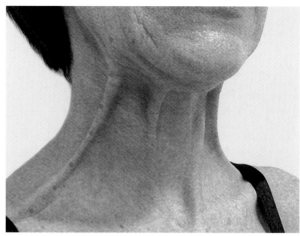

Fig 19-15b An even distribution of injection sites into the medial and/or lateral bands will provide information about the final quantity of points. The distance between them should be around 1.5 to 2 cm. (Used with permission from De Maio M, Rzany B. Botulinum Toxin in Aesthetic Medicine. New York: Springer Science and Business Media, 2007.)

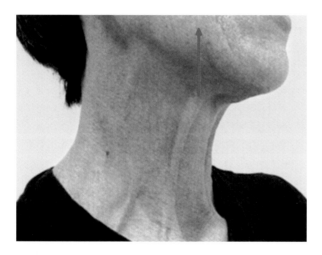

Fig 19-15c The platysma is the strongest depressor of the face and by blocking it, a lifting effect at the mandible level may result. (Used with permission from De Maio M, Rzany B. Botulinum Toxin in Aesthetic Medicine. New York: Springer Science and Business Media, 2007.)

Anatomy

The platysma is divided into three groups of fibers. The anterior fibers assist mandible depression; the intermediate fibers (pars labialis) depress the lower lip; and the posterior fibers (pars modiolaris) depress the buccal angle.

Technique

The patient is asked to contract the platysma. An even distribution of injections into the medial and/or lateral bands provides information about the final quantity of injection points. The distance between them should be approximately 1.5 to 2 cm (Fig 19-15b).

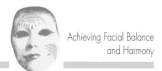

Achieving Facial Balance and Harmony

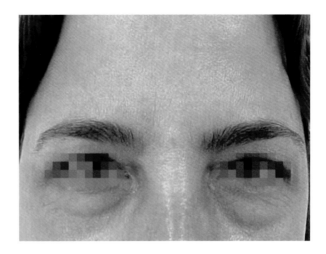

Fig 19-16 Be careful with patients who present with a combination of crow's feet and eye bags. The use of botulinum toxin at this level may provoke or worsen the eyebags.

Follow-up
The platysma is the strongest depressor of the face. After it is blocked, a lifting effect at the mandible level may result (Fig 19-15c).

Observation
Patients with hypertonic medial and lateral bands may complain of a sensation of heaviness on the neck and difficulties while swallowing and getting out of bed. They use the platysma as a compensatory muscle for daily activities, instead of using other muscle groups such as the abdominal musculature.

Group E

Patient 16

Description
This patient presented with eye bags in the lower eyelid and wrinkles (Fig 19-16). The fat bags are a result of the weakened m orbicularis oculi. One of the relative contraindications of treatment of crow's feet with botulinum toxin is the presence of eye bags.

Observation
When the orbicularis oculi are weakened in treatment, eye bags may get worse. Some patients may complain that these have appeared after the injection.

Explanation
Botulinum toxin is an agent that weakens muscles. By injecting this into the crow's feet, the clinician also reduces the power of the muscle contractions in that area. When eye bags appear at rest, this indicates that the

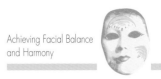

Achieving Facial Balance and Harmony

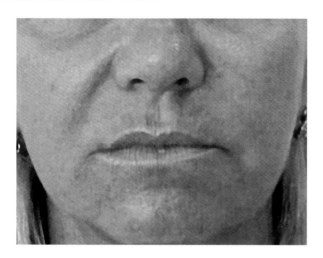

Fig 19-17 The nasolabial fold on the patient's right side is best treated with injection of botulinum toxin, and the left side should be treated with fillers. The use of fillers on the right side could result in a sausage-like appearance of the fold.

muscle tone was affected and reduced, causing protrusion of the fat bags. Reduction of the muscle contraction power affects the local lymphatic drainage and leads to swollen eyes.

What to do

Manual lymphatic drainage may be helpful, but the result is limited. Reversal of this feature may take up to 4 months. Therefore, concomitant treatment of crow's feet in patients with eye bags should be avoided or handled only by experienced injectors. With this patient, the formal indication is surgery.

Mixed Groups

Patient 17

Description

This patient presented with a Group C pattern on the right and a Group B pattern on the left. The prominent nasolabial fold may have resulted from (1) redundant skin drooping over the sulcus; (2) excessive fat deposits positioned laterally to the sulcus; (3) ptosis and/or laxity of the malar fat pad; or (4) muscular hyperactivity. The correct diagnosis enables the appropriate treatment plan. If at rest there is a prominent nasolabial fold and a bulge at the nasal flare level that worsens during animation, the feature may induce muscle hyperactivity. This patient allows a comparison of the indication for botulinum toxin versus fillers for treatment of the nasolabial fold (Fig 19-17). The right nasolabial fold is a perfect indication for blocking, while the left would benefit from volume replacement. On the right, there is a sausage-like shape of the nasolabial fold. If fillers are injected into this fold, this "sausage" will go

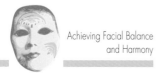
Achieving Facial Balance and Harmony

upward and result in a fat appearance. On the left, although botulinum toxin is also indicated, the use of fillers is more effective.

Anatomy

The m levator labii superioris alaeque nasi comprises the medial and the lateral slips. The medial slip dilates the nostril and displaces laterally the curvature of the inferolateral convex malar furrow. The lateral slip raises and everts the upper lip. It also raises the curvature of the nasolabial furrows' superior part.

Technique

The injection site is at the lateral upper part of the nasal flare, where the two slips separate. The 30-gauge needle should penetrate to only one-third its length into the skin.

Observation

Before treatment with botulinum toxin is begun in the perioral area, the clinician should be aware of the potential complications of treatment. Blocking one of the medial upper lip elevators may result in upper lip elongation or lip ptosis. It is advisable to have a two-step treatment for beginners, with half of the suggested dose given at each step.

Bibliography

Carruthers A, Carruthers J. Eyebrow height after botulinum toxin type A to the glabella. Dermatol Surg 2007;33(special issue 1):26–31.

Carruthers J, Carruthers A. The use of botulinum toxin type A in the upper face. Facial Plast Surg Clin North Am 2006;14(3):253–260.

Carruthers J, Carruthers A. Complications of botulinum toxin type A. Facial Plast Surg Clin North Am 2007;15(1):51–54.

De Boulle KL. Botulinum neurotoxin type A in facial aesthetics. Expert Opin Pharmacother 2007;8(8):1059–1072.

De Maio M, Bento RF. Botulinum toxin in facial palsy: An effective treatment for contralateral hyperkinesis. Plast Reconstr Surg 2007;120(4):917–927.

De Maio M. Challenges in the mid and the lower face. J Cosmet Laser Ther 2003;5(3–4):213–215.

De Maio M. Botulinum toxin in association with other rejuvenation methods. J Cosmet Laser Ther 2003;5(3–4):210–212.

De Maio M. Use of botulinum toxin in facial paralysis. J Cosmet Laser Ther 2003;5(3–4):216–217.

De Maio M. The minimal approach: An innovation in facial cosmetic procedures. Aesthetic Plast Surg 2004;28(5):295–300.

De Maio M, Wahl G (eds). Expert Approaches to Using Botulinum Toxins. Cirugiá Plástica Ibero-Latinoamericana 2(5):2–12, 2006.

De Maio M, Rzany B (eds). Botulinum Toxin in Aesthetic Medicine. New York: Springer-Verlag, 2007.

De Maio M, Rzany B (eds). Injectable Fillers in Aesthetic Medicine. New York: Springer-Verlag, 2006.

Flynn TC. Update on botulinum toxin. Semin Cutan Med Surg 2006;25(3):115–121.

Frankel AS, Markarian A. Cosmetic treatments and strategies for the upper face. Facial Plast Surg Clin North Am 2007;15(1):31–39.

Kim NH, Chung JH, Park RH, Park JB. The use of botulinum toxin type A in aesthetic mandibular contouring. Plast Reconstr Surg 2005;115(3):919–930.

Lee CJ, Kim SG, Han JY. The results of periorbital rejuvenation with botulinum toxin A using two different protocols. Aesthetic Plast Surg 2006;30(1):65–70.

Maas CS. Botulinum neurotoxins and injectable fillers: Minimally invasive management of the aging upper face. Otolaryngol Clin North Am 2007;40(2):283–290.

Pena MA, Alam M, Yoo SS. Complications with the use of botulinum toxin type A for cosmetic applications and hyperhidrosis. Semin Cutan Med Surg 2007;26(1):29–33.

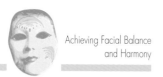

Rebalancing the Aging Face Through Lipomodeling

20

Michael Scheflan, MD

Noam Hai, MD

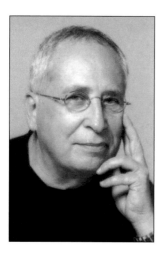

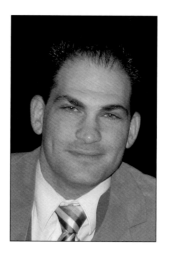

Michael Scheflan, MD

Michael Scheflan is an ISAPS (International Society of Aesthetic Plastic Surgery) professor, a past president of the Israel Society of Plastic Surgeons and the Mediterranean Society of Plastic Surgeons. He currently serves as the medical director of Atidim Medical Center in Tel Aviv, Israel, and teaches at the Tel Aviv University Sackler School of Medicine. In addition, he practices esthetic and reconstructive plastic surgery in a private setting.

Dr Scheflan has written and edited 4 books and numerous scientific publications.

Email: scheflan@medigroup.co.il

Noam Hai, MD

Noam Hai is a board-certified plastic and reconstructive surgeon and an associate esthetic plastic surgeon at the Atidim Medical Center in Tel Aviv, Israel. A cum laude graduate of the Faculty of Medicine of the Technion, Israel, he fulfilled most of his training at the Sha'are Zedek Medical Center in Jerusalem and continued his more advanced surgical training as a fellow while working with some leading plastic surgeons around the world. He received many awards during his training, including the Elkin Award for the best surgical MD thesis, the AFIPE award for the outstanding Israeli resident in plastic surgery, and the Kaplan Prize for the best basic science research presentation.

Dr Hai is currently involved in some research programs on the use of adipose-derived stem cells in various fields of medicine.

Email: noamhai@walla.com

Facial aging is more than just a result of gravitational laxity and descent. Rather, it is a complex of degenerative processes that leads to loss of volume and tissue atrophy that affects all of the supportive structures of the face. These processes include *(1)* resorption of the bony skeleton; *(2)* gradual muscular weakening and flaccidity in some areas, or hypertonicity and hyperactivity in others; *(3)* fat absorption in some areas, or accumulation of fat in others; *(4)* skin wrinkling; *(5)* pigmentation; and *(6)* loss of elasticity and thickness. All of these elements act together on the facial contours and proportions to create an aged and tired appearance.

The understanding that aging is affected by volume loss and wasting is the foundation of the contemporary approach to facial rejuvenation surgery. The reversal of facial aging is not a single-mode surgical intervention. Rather, it is a balanced, carefully planned, and skillfully executed multitude of surgical and nonsurgical procedures that attempt to create a long-lasting, younger appearance while maximizing safety and minimizing patient downtime, risks, and complications. Methods to restore volume vary widely among surgeons. During face-lift procedures, the surgeon generally redistributes sagging tissues such as jowls and cheeks to a higher, more youthful location by redraping excess loose tissues in the lower parts of the face and replenishing lost volume in the upper parts of the face.

Aging is a gradual process that affects different people in different ways; usually the cheeks sag medially and centrally over the nose and the mouth and accentuate the nasolabial folds and marionette lines. Further inward sagging over the jaw line creates the infamous jowls, and neck skin redundancy results in the undesirable turkey neck appearance. In general, a young face appears short, full, convex, and round; an old face is long, narrow, concave, and rectangular.

In the past, most patients seeking rejuvenation were in their late 50s. Now more women seek facial rejuvenation in their early and mid-40s. This younger age group shows early signs of facial aging that mostly involve facial volume depletion. The forms of facial aging that specifically involve volume depletion are referred to as *gaunting* patterns of aging. Patients with these patterns typically present with soft tissue atrophy that is advanced for their chronological age, accompanied by facial laxity and sagging. Common features of volumetric facial aging include the following:

- *Temporal and periorbital fat atrophy* results in sunken eyes; a distinct lower eyelid–cheek junction, often with dark circles and a prominent tear trough; a malar-facial groove; and possible prominent lower eyelid fat bags.
- *Mid-cheek atrophy* with prominent cheekbones results in a skull-like appearance. Flat malar bones and submalar depressions also result in a sunken and old appearance.

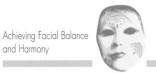

Achieving Facial Balance and Harmony

- *Perioral fat atrophy* leads to a longer upper lip, thin lips, prune-like lip furrows, and mandibular marginal notching that creates a pointy chin appearance.

Extreme examples of such facial atrophy are HIV-related facial lipoatrophy and Parry-Romberg syndrome (hemifacial atrophy). These two conditions are treated with lipomodeling or other resorbable or semipermanent fillers.

Lipomodeling Philosophy

Fat grafting is a commonly practiced surgical tool used to enhance facial esthetics and reverse the aging process. In the past, fat grafting was considered an unreliable and inconsistent surgical tool, ranging from only 30% to 80% retention, and to some extent, it still is considered too risky by some surgeons. Past procedures depended solely on technique and experience of the surgeon, and proponents of fat grafting claim that strict surgical technique is of paramount importance to maximize graft retention.

The authors' experience with the LipoStructure technique over the last 12 years has been extremely positive. This surgical technique of micro–fat grafting was described and popularized by Dr Sydney Coleman as a way to harvest, process, and place the patient's own fat. If strictly followed, the technique may prove to be a rewarding and effective surgical method that should be a part of every plastic surgeon's armamentarium.[1]

In recent years, as tissue engineering technology has continued to evolve, fat has been targeted as one of the most researched donor tissues for adult stem cells. Fat is the richest source of adult stem cells; compared to bone marrow, it contains 100 times the concentration of stem cells per milliliter of tissue. In 2002, the breakthrough research of a group of scientists from UCLA headed by Dr Zuk opened new horizons in tissue engineering research by showing that lipoaspirate can be processed to produce adult stem cells.[2] These adipose-derived stem and regenerative cells (ADRCs) were shown to be the body's native repair cells, with the ability to repair and replace tissues lost to daily wear and tear, injury, or disease.

ADRCs can proliferate and differentiate into tissues including fat, skeletal and smooth muscle, tendon, cartilage, bone, and even neural elements. They are used to enhance fat graft retention through stimulation of vessel growth and revascularization of the fat graft. Enrichment of fat grafts with ADRCs has been shown to improve fat graft retention by 20% to 50% (unpublished data).

Lipomodeling should be viewed as a sculpting procedure. Sculpting is all about volumes and proportions. The sculptor's experience and tech-

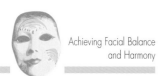

Achieving Facial Balance
and Harmony

nical skills enable him or her to analyze the face and then structurally add volume to some areas while subtracting volume from others.

A scheme, a frame, a model, or a blueprint should be set as an initial guide and a planning tool. The starting point is the patient's face. It is essential that the clinician study the entire face and neck first, and then ask the patient what it is that would make him or her look better, refreshed, younger, and prettier. The patient's answer should be combined with the clinician's experience and knowledge to formulate a feasible treatment plan. Some areas of the face may need volume restoration and enhancement, while other areas necessitate fat removal through liposuction, and still others require tightening and redraping. Hence the phrase *facial rebalancing* is used to encompass all of these procedures.

Although attempts at fat grafting for recontouring started much earlier, liposuction was established as an effective surgical technique by Dr Illouz in the early 1980s and is now considered a standard surgical tool. When sculpting living tissues, volumes may be added and retained (or "engrafted") only if basic concepts of tissue engrafting are strictly respected. Small pearls of intact fat can be introduced into areas of healthy tissue so that each "fat parcel" is surrounded by the recipient tissue, which supports and nourishes the graft by diffusion and imbibition until a new blood supply integrates the transplanted fat.

Fat grafting allows the clinician to restore volume not only to the face but also to many other areas of the human body (eg, breasts, neck, dorsum of hands, chest wall, torso, and extremities) for esthetic and reconstructive purposes. Depressions and irregularities caused by disease, injury, or irradiation that include radionecrotic ulcers, ischemic venous and arterial ulcers, tracheal fistulas, and inflammatory bowel disease fistulas have all been treated successfully with the grafting of fat.

Since 2008, the authors have used the Celution System platform (Cytori Therapeutics), a fully automated system that extracts autologous ADRCs from lipoaspirate. We believe that our work as plastic surgeons today has the potential to change the face of medicine tomorrow.

Surgical Technique

Fat grafting is governed by the same physiologic principles that govern a successful simple skin graft. Harvested tissue should suffer minimal trauma during harvesting and must be kept in a physiologic environment for the least possible amount of time until grafted. Graft mass should be small and thin enough to be supported and embraced by the recipient's normal tissue, and it should be placed in intimate contact with recipient tissue. The recipient "bed" must nurture the graft by means of plasmatic imbibition (diffusion) and inosculation (blood vessel alignment) until normal blood flow is restored.

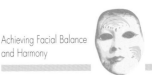

Achieving Facial Balance and Harmony

Minimal trauma to aspirated fat cells is possible if the surgeon uses low-pressure, handheld aspiration syringes. These should be equipped with harvesting cannulae specifically designed to retrieve small parcels of intact adipose tissues in an atraumatic fashion so as to minimize tissue breakdown.

The graft is processed to separate the intact fat from the unwanted debris of fragmented tissue, ruptured fat cells, blood cells, oil, and tumescent fluids. This is traditionally achieved by centrifugation of the lipoaspirate at 1,500 rpm for 3 minutes. Harvested, spin-dried intact fat is then loaded into small Luer Lock syringes (Becton Dickinson) capped with fine injecting cannulae. After the preparatory steps have been accomplished, the most important variable determining fat graft survival is the injection technique. The surgeon's expertise is especially challenged at this stage of the procedure.

A surgeon involved in facial rejuvenation and lipomodeling should be able to meticulously follow all of these steps to achieve an ideal esthetic result. This procedure is not a panacea for every patient, nor is it something that can be performed by every surgeon or physician. In summary, the following suggestions should be applied:

1. Study a patient's aging face to determine whether lipomodeling and volume restoration are able to achieve the desired esthetic goal as a stand-alone procedure, or if lipomodeling should be used as an ancillary procedure to augment other surgical maneuvers (eg, face-lift, browpexy, blepharoplasty, and chemical or laser peeling).
2. Analyze the face and plot areas to be augmented versus areas to be reduced, transitioned, or feathered. Create a surgical plan that includes estimates of how much volume needs to be added or subtracted in each subunit. This latter ability is the most demanding of the clinician's skills and necessitates an understanding of facial balance and esthetics in addition to a talent for three-dimensional visualization and extrapolation.
3. Minimal-access surgery requires complete familiarity with and knowledge of the facial anatomy, similar to that needed for standard face-lift procedures. Lipomodeling is a three-dimensional volumetric transformation and restoration that uses meticulous surgical principles and techniques.

Case Analysis

The patient shown in Figs 20-1 to 20-5 represents a commonly encountered scenario of early signs of facial aging that are mainly related to volume depletion. This 40-year-old healthy woman sought a surgical solution to her tired appearance.

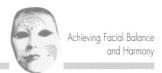

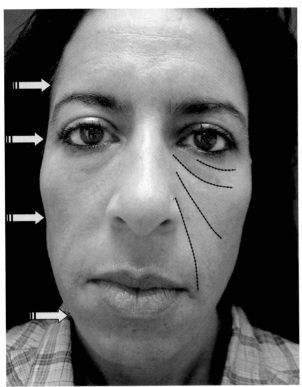

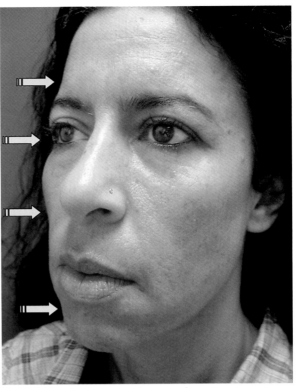

Fig 20-1 Anterior photograph of patient demonstrates facial aging with volume depletion. Right: Contour depressions *(arrows)*, from top to bottom: temple, lateral orbital, submalar (lower cheek), and mandibular. Left: Linear depressions *(dotted lines)* that accentuate and demarcate areas of lost volume, from top to bottom: lower eyelid crease, tear trough (nasojugal crease), malar-facial groove, and nasolabial fold.

Fig 20-2 Three-quarter view with contour depressions *(arrows)*.

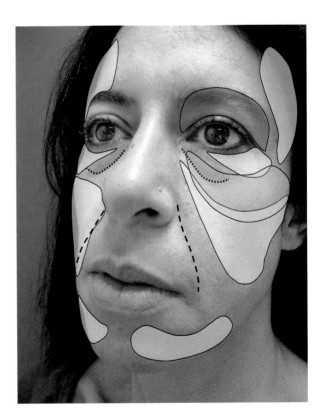

Fig 20-3 Surgical treatment plan: areas of volume depletion marked for micro–fat grafting.

Achieving Facial Balance
and Harmony

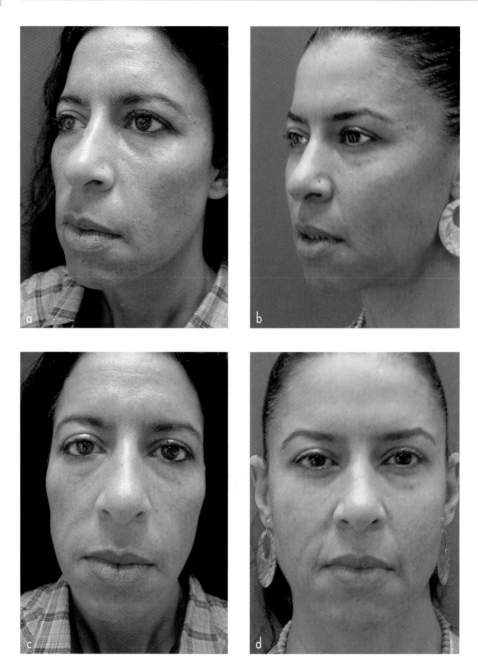

Figs 20-4a to 20-4d Comparisons of preoperative (a, c) and 1-year postoperative (b, d) views.

The pretreatment anterior facial photograph shows good overall skin color and tone and a smooth forehead with some degree of gravitational descent of the eyebrow and the upper eyelid (see Fig 20-1). In noting issues with volume, the clinician should consider the cascade of depressions that hollow the face and are most visible in the three-quarter view (see Fig 20-2). These depressions can be seen in the temple area, the lateral lower eyelid, the tear trough, the malar area, the submalar zone, and the nasolabial fold.

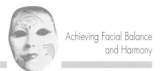

Achieving Facial Balance and Harmony

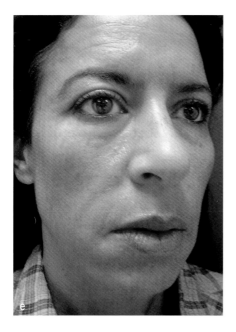
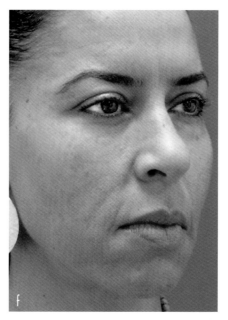

Figs 20-4e and 20-4f Comparisons of preoperative (e) and 1-year postoperative (f) views.

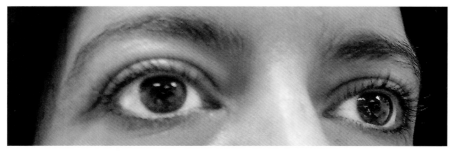

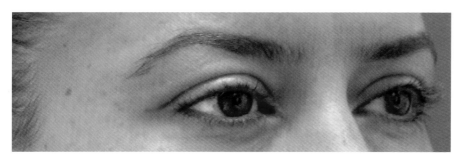

Fig 20-5 Periorbital rejuvenation through lipomodeling.

Since most of the aging stigmata in her case consisted of midface volume depletions, surgical planning included lipomodeling of the described areas (see Fig 20-3). Lipomodeling was done using fat grafts enriched with ADRCs. These were extracted from the lipoaspirate using the Celution System platform. This fully automated closed system washes the lipoaspirate, digests the fat cells using collagenase, and concentrates stem and regenerative cells using differential centrifugation. The procedure was done with the patient under local anesthesia and deep sedation.

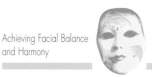

Achieving Facial Balance and Harmony

Table 20-1   Summary of fat grafting volumes in the face

	Left hemiface (mL)	Right hemiface (mL)
Temporal area	9.9	10.3
Upper eyelid area	4.2	4.1
Lower eyelid and tear trough	3.6	3.5
Malar area	20.3	23.3
Submalar area	12.3	13.0
Total volume	50.3	54.2

A total volume of 104.5 mL of fat enriched with ADRCs was grafted to the face (Table 20-1) using Coleman's LipoStructure technique. Microdroplets of fat parcels were placed in the subcutaneous, suprafascial, and supraperiosteal planes (see Figs 20-4 and 20-5).

Conclusion

Lipomodeling is a powerful surgical technique that in selected patients may be the sole modality required to provide facial rejuvenation.

More advanced facial aging requires more drastic measures, which in the authors' opinion should always be integrated with volume replacement through lipomodeling. When combined with face-lift procedures, fat grafting as an adjunct treatment creates a more youthful, more harmonious, and natural appearance than can face-lift procedures alone. Lipomodeling techniques are the next level of expertise that should be taught to and learned by clinicians who wish to create a beautiful and natural rejuvenation. ADRCs and other products aimed at enhancing fat graft retention may further revolutionize our surgical skills and may offer some level of delay or modification in facial aging by influencing the activation and initiation of repair mechanisms within the body itself.

References

1. Coleman SR. Facial recontouring with lipostructure. Clin Plast Surg 1997;24:347–367.
2. Zuk PA, Zhu M, Ashjian P, et al. Human adipose tissue is a source of multipotent stem cells. Mol Biol Cell 2002;13:4279–4295.

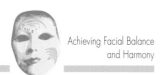

Achieving Facial Balance and Harmony

Patient Communication and Motivation

V

Roger P. Levin

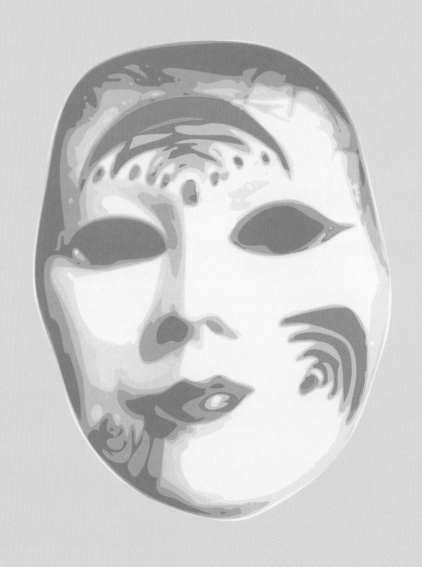

How to Increase Case Acceptance

21

Roger P. Levin, DDS

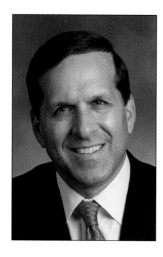

Roger P. Levin, DDS

Roger P. Levin is chairman and chief executive officer of Levin Group, the leading dental practice management firm. Levin Group provides Total Practice Success, the premier comprehensive consulting solution for lifetime success to dentists in the United States and around the world. A third-generation dentist, Dr Levin is one of the profession's most sought-after speakers, bringing his Total Practice Success seminars to dentists and dental professionals throughout the country.

For more than two decades, Dr Levin and Levin Group have been dedicated to improving the lives of dentists.

Email:customerservice@levingroup.com.

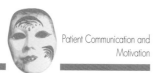

Case presentation is a science and an art. It involves more than simply educating patients about their dental condition and laying out the different treatment options. Clinicians must also achieve a very delicate balance between influencing or persuading patients to make choices that are in their best interests and benefiting practice productivity. Achieving this balance can make a difference between a practice that "just gets by" and one that excels.

Case presentation can be challenging because of factors such as the following:

- Many practitioners have not received adequate training in case presentation. Dental schools provide students with clinical training to become dental professionals. Communication and leadership training are not priorities at most dental schools, although some are beginning to change this situation.
- Clinicians tend to focus on the technical and clinical features of cases rather than the benefits, which are of more interest to most patients.
- Successful case presentation takes time and training. Given the pace of most practices today, it is becoming increasingly difficult for many doctors to allow adequate time to describe all aspects of individual cases to the patient, answer questions, address objections, and work through other issues to help the patient make a decision.

Making Case Presentation Work

To achieve greater case acceptance, practitioners need to think differently about case presentation. The first step is to understand that most patients are not motivated to accept comprehensive treatment. Their motivation is to get only what is absolutely necessary (sometimes not even that). Consumers do not mind spending money, but they want to spend it at places that give them enjoyment or satisfaction. Rarely is this the dental practice. In addition, patients are often unaware of a practice's available services. The following steps can help create greater patient interest and motivation.

Comprehensive patient education

Educate every patient about every service provided. One of the most effective opportunities to educate patients occurs during the hygiene visit. The hygienist usually spends more time than the dentist with the patient. Provide standard scripts for hygiene visits to educate patients about all the potential services in the practice, especially cosmetic and elective dentistry. Most patients do not know what cosmetic services are available, and therefore they do not ask questions to determine whether

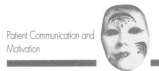

Patient Communication and
Motivation

they have an interest in cosmetic enhancement. The same is true for implants. The first time a patient hears about a dental implant should not be after the loss of a tooth. It should be a service that the patient is familiar with and automatically assumes is the next step when teeth are lost.

Collateral materials

Use supporting educational materials, such as brochures, videos, and posters, to educate patients about your services. These materials alone do not sufficiently motivate or influence patients, but they are tools that act as effective "conversation starters" or "treatment reinforcers." The right collateral materials get patients to ask questions about possible treatment or reinforce what has already been discussed.

No-cost consultation

If the doctor does not have time to fully discuss a potential case during a hygiene exam, then the patient should be rescheduled at no charge for a consultation. Most practices do not handle follow-up consultations very well. Instead, the doctor spends 2 minutes with a hygiene patient talking about a potential service that rarely leads to case acceptance for larger cases. The patient should be rescheduled for a 20- or 30-minute uninterrupted appointment to meet with the doctor and treatment coordinator to discuss the potential case and all treatment options. Successful dentists realize that a no-cost consultation is often necessary to help a patient make a decision about going forward with treatment, especially for larger and more complex cases. If these appointments are handled well, the vast majority of patients will accept treatment, and practice production will increase.

Follow-up call

Finally, any patient who receives a case presentation and does not schedule for treatment should receive a follow-up phone call within 48 hours. Many patients are extremely interested in having treatment and just need a slight additional prompt to schedule. Many cases are lost every year because patients are not able to find time to fit in the dentistry. You simply have to make it easy for the patient. By having a front desk staff follow up to schedule the patient, you have a much greater opportunity of the patient following through on a decision to have treatment.

The scripting can be easy. If a patient says, *"I will call you tomorrow because I don't have my book,"* you simply respond by saying, *"Mrs Jones, as a service to you, where can I conveniently call you tomorrow morning?"* The best way to reach patients is usually via their cell phones.

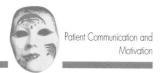

Patient Communication and Motivation

Five Key Questions to Address in the Case Presentation

Every case presentation should answer these five questions:

- What is it?
- What will it do for me?
- How long will it take?
- Will it hurt?
- How much will it cost?

These are the questions that patients want answered, and when they are answered properly, case acceptance often follows. The clinician's response to these five questions during treatment presentation determines how likely the patient will accept the treatment plan.

What is it?

Every case presentation should begin by informing the patient of the various treatment options. Most conditions have a number of treatment options. When presenting possible treatments, you need to provide a quick clinical overview.

The operative word in the previous sentence is *quick*. Most clinicians give far too much technical information, which results in a loss of patient interest. A rule of thumb is that the clinical explanation of a presented case should never exceed 3 minutes. In the dental profession, very few subjects require more than a 3-minute clinical explanation. After 3 minutes, the patient quickly loses interest in the clinical parameters. Specific subjects such as biochemistry, biomedical issues, biocompatibility, bond strengths, etc, do not normally interest patients. They are mostly interested in the treatment benefits (Question 2).

To maintain patient interest, technical information must be presented in a manner that is easily understood by the patient. One way to do this is to follow each clinical statement with a reference to the procedure's benefits: "Mrs Jones, you definitely need a crown. It will match your other teeth beautifully and should last many, many years."

The more benefit references made while addressing patients' needs and desires, the better the chances that the patient will accept treatment. Patients are definitely interested in the technical aspects of their cases, to a point. However, most are equally interested in the skill, compassion, and concern of the clinician treating them. Dental cases are rarely sold by extensive clinical details but rather by the trust and motivation engendered by the doctor.

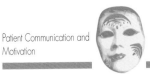

What will it do for me?

This is the key question that patients want answered. They want to hear about the benefits of treatment rather than in-depth clinical details. If a patient wants to know more about clinical details, it is certainly possible to take the time to answer those questions. By spending the majority of the presentation time focusing on benefits, the practitioner motivates patients much more to accept treatment.

Practitioners should identify the three main benefits of every service, and then mention these to the patient and review them at least three times in a case presentation. The only exception would be if a patient were to identify one specific reason why he or she is interested in treatment; in this situation, the clinician should focus mainly on that particular benefit.

Patients do not get excited about clinical aspects of care, but they do have a tremendous interest in how that treatment will enhance their quality of life. Whether the main issue is prevention, health, attractiveness, or something else, all people are interested in how treatment allows them to enhance some aspect of their daily lives. A failure to emphasize benefits likely results in a low case acceptance.

Although each patient's primary reason for treatment should be systematically identified and referenced, be sure to address *all* the advantages of the procedure. Keep stating the benefits as the presentation progresses. Careful explanation of each life-enhancing benefit motivates patients to undergo care. If, after treatment presentations, patients habitually say, "I need to think about it," their questions have not been sufficiently answered, or they have not been properly motivated.

How long will it take?

The answer to this question is somewhat obvious to the clinician. However, merely telling patients that the case will take 2 weeks or 6 months does nothing to help sell the treatment. Today, everyone worries about time. To patients, time for dental procedures equals inconvenience, work absences, and lengthy discomfort.

Therefore, time must be presented as a benefit. Explain to patients that 2 weeks or 6 months is necessary to complete their cases thoroughly and effectively. Let patients know that the treatment will progress as quickly as possible and that the office will attempt to schedule convenient appointments. However, emphasis continually should be placed on quality as the most important factor.

When longer cases are presented, the treatment duration should be divided into segments of time. For example, the patient can be told that Phase I will last 2 months, Phase II will last 3 months, etc. Patients should always be told the length of time necessary to complete the

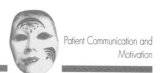

procedure, how many visits will be involved, and that convenient appointments will be scheduled whenever possible. Every year, more procedures are turned down because patients believe they do not have time in their lives to proceed with treatment. More and more people are delaying dental treatment until they find time in their schedules, which often never occurs. Making appointments as convenient as possible is an effective way to combat the time crunch patients face in their lives.

Will it hurt?

This is an area that many doctors want to avoid during treatment planning and discussion. Unfortunately, it is also an area of major concern for most patients. If the issue of pain is not addressed, people assume the worst and often reject treatment with the thought that the discomfort will be far worse than expected.

Most procedures today can be performed without excessive discomfort. Postoperative discomfort is relatively short-term and can be controlled through medication. Patients can be assured that the clinician and staff will do everything possible to keep them comfortable. All steps and expectations of postoperative care should be explained. Patients should feel informed about the level of care and should know that their comfort is a top priority.

How much will it cost?

Ultimately, this is the question that most often derails case presentations. Generally, however, the intent of this question is not "How much does it cost?" but rather "How am I going to pay for it?"

Patients have to weigh the expense of dental treatment against other expenses in their lives. Some of those expenses are essential (e.g., mortgages and car payments) while others are elective (eg, vacations and jewelry). Either way, these expenses are real for the patient, who has to decide where to allocate money. The clinician's job is to minimize the role that cost plays in the decision-making process. Most people find the money to pay for what they want. Therefore, it is essential to motivate patients to *want* treatment.

Flexible payment options are critical. Let patients know that the practice has created financial arrangements that enable almost every patient to take advantage of treatment. Emphasize, too, that a financial coordinator (not the clinician) is available to work with each patient regarding all financial considerations.

While not an easy or pleasant experience for most clinicians, fee presentation is critical. However, if the treatment plan presentation has been properly handled by building a sense of value and motivation, the fee discussion should go smoothly. If at any point the patient appears unwilling to pay the fee in question, then sufficient value has not been created to justify the treatment cost. Remember, it is not how much the treatment costs that concerns patients, but how they are going to pay for it.

Dental Insurance

Dental insurance, or the lack of it, is a factor in many case presentations. Every clinician should take the time to educate all current patients about their insurance plans and all new patients about the key factors of insurance. Because patients are concerned with out-of-pocket expenses, information can be included such as maximum allowable benefits, percentage of coverage for various services, predetermination factors, filing of insurance, co-payments, and covered and noncovered services.

The next step that may benefit many practices is to ensure that patients not only understand the basics of their insurance plans but also how these factors link to treatment options that may be presented. Many treatment plans are rejected in the later stages of discussion when the patient realizes dental insurance will not cover certain procedures such as cosmetic or implant dentistry.

When patients suddenly discover that there will be a significant co-payment or no insurance coverage at all, they may be unable to make a decision, and the process of treatment acceptance is brought to a grinding halt. At this point, patients need to decide whether they have sufficient funds and if the suggested procedures are worth the amount of the co-payments.

The author suggests that explanations about dental insurance (especially co-payments, noncovered, and covered services) take place either before or very early in the treatment presentation process. This allows the clinician to overcome the obstacle of dental insurance issues and still recommend excellent need-based treatment or potential elective treatment to a patient. Any discussion of insurance should occur in the context of other financial options offered by the practice.

Financial Options

The following four financial options should be offered to every patient during case presentation. They can be offered together to give the patient four choices and to create a strong awareness that financing is available:

- A 5% discount for full cash payment on any amount over $300.
- Acceptance of major credit cards.

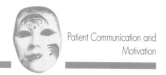

- A payment of 50% at the start of treatment and the balance paid before the end of treatment. The patient should be reminded about the balance at least three times prior to the final appointment so that there is no question about the amount owed to the practice.
- Outside patient financing. A number of companies provide this service. With this option, the office can be paid in full in less than 48 hours.

These four financial options create the framework of the entire financial system for the practice. Proper review of the four financial options and discussing them with patients leads to higher case acceptance and higher patient satisfaction. Best of all, patients receive treatment that otherwise may have been unaffordable.

The Case Is Not Closed

Even after a financial option has been accepted, the real definition of a closed case is when a patient has scheduled an appointment (keep in mind that the patient can always cancel it later, and it would need to be rescheduled). All too often, patients are very excited and motivated by the presentation and agree to a financial arrangement, only to arrive at the front desk and realize that they do not have their schedule with them. It is recommended that all large cases be started within 7 to 10 days. If not, many patients who have agreed to treatment will not follow through. Other life factors, combined with the loss of motivation, often cause patients to cancel appointments. This lack of follow-through is even more frequent with patients who never even schedule the appointment.

Follow-Up

Following up with any patient is simple. When patients announce that they don't know their schedule or that they "will call tomorrow," the standard response from the office should be to tell patients to expect a call the next morning. One sample script would be to respond, "Mrs Jones, as a service to you, when can I conveniently call you tomorrow morning to schedule the appointment?" This will not push a patient into scheduling who really does not want treatment. Instead, it allows the office to follow up with the majority of patients who actually want treatment. A phone call the next morning allows the office to reach the patient, take control of the situation, and provide a high level of customer service. Be certain to acquire the patient's cell phone number, as this is a much easier way to reach patients, and most individuals check their cell phone messages on a daily basis. Telling patients to expect a call the next morning creates an artificial deadline for them to check their schedules and identify potential treatment times.

Conclusion

Effectively addressing the above five questions usually results in the acceptance of treatment. Conversely, spending a great deal of time on the clinical aspects of a case, which many clinicians focus on due to their own natural instincts and education, often results in patients rejecting treatment. Patients may decide to wait and think about whether or not they want to have treatment performed. Ultimately, though, they are likely to lose their motivation and not follow through with treatment unless the clinician and office staff follow up with scheduling and payment options.

Practice success depends on case presentation. If the doctor and team members excel at presenting a variety of need-based and esthetic cases, the practice will achieve a significant increase in productivity and position itself for long-term profitable growth. However, many practices do not maximize opportunities to increase case acceptance due to a variety of factors that include poor verbal skills, office inefficiencies, and a lack of documentation.

Good case presentation skills require that the clinician be completely committed to understanding the patient's point of view. Without a willingness to take this empathetic view and clarify treatment philosophy accordingly, it is nearly impossible to positively influence patient behavior and the choice to pursue treatment. A clinician who understands the viewpoint of the person in the chair has a far better chance of relating to each patient. Strong relationships with patients is often a prerequisite for achieving a high case acceptance ratio.

Patients interpret each new experience through past experiences, beliefs, and values. The best communicators understand this phenomenon and break down resistance by using education, compelling stories, and testimonials to help patients understand the benefits of treatment within each individual's unique frame of reference. Customized information that addresses each patient's priorities and concerns is the foundation of the finest case presentations.

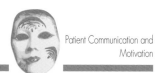